Public Health in Europe

Springer
Berlin
Heidelberg
New York
Hong Kong
London
Milan
Paris
Tokyo

W. Kirch (Ed.)

Public Health in Europe

– 10 Years European Public Health Association –

Selected Manuscripts from the 10th Annual Congress of the European
Public Health Association, 28–30 November 2002, Dresden, Germany

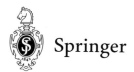 Springer

Editor:
Prof. Dr. med. Dr. med. dent. WILHELM KIRCH
President European Public Health Association
Chairman Public Health Research Association Saxony
Medical Faculty, Technical University Dresden
Fiedlerstr. 27
D-01307 Dresden
Germany

I am sincerely thankful to my co-workers Dr. rer. medic. PEGGY GÖPFERT, M.A. Päd. NICOLE WAGNER, Dipl.-Soz. DIRK MEUSEL, Dipl.-Oec. INES KUBE, Mrs. BEATRIX HÖRGER from the BMBF Research Association Saxony, Mrs. SIMONE ARRAS and Dipl.-Päd. CHRISTIANE HAGEDORN for their important help in editing the underlying book "Public Health in Europe".

ISBN 3-540-40240-3 Springer-Verlag Berlin Heidelberg New York

Library of Congress Cataloging-in-Publication Data
Public health in Europe: 10 years EUPHA / Wilhelm Kirch, (Ed.).
p. cm.
Based on contributions to the 10th annual congress held by EUPHA in Dresden, Germany, from 28 to 30 November 2002.
Includes bibliographical references.
   ISBN 3-540-40240-3 (alk. paper)
1. Public health – Europe – Congresses. 2. Medical policy – Europe – Congresses. 3. Health planning – Europe Congresses. I. Kirch, Wilhelm.
RA483.P826 2003
362.1′094–dc21   2003053932

Springer-Verlag Berlin Heidelberg New York
a member of BertelsmannSpringer Science+Business Media GmbH

http://www.springer.de

© Springer-Verlag Berlin · Heidelberg 2004
Printed in Germany

Hardcover-Design: Erich Kirchner, Heidelberg

Production Editor: Frank Krabbes, Heidelberg

SPIN 10910924   14/3109-5 4 3 2 1 0 – Printed on acid-free paper

During the 10th Annual Congress of EUPHA from 28–30 November 2002 in Dresden **Honour Medals** of the German Society of Public Health (DGPH) were presented to:

- **Prof. Dr. Jouke van der Zee**, Utrecht, The Netherlands, one of the founders of EUPHA and member of its Executive Council, for this attainments concerning in the development of Health Services Research in Europe and the European Public Health Association.
- **Prof. Dr. Dr. Dres. h. c. Heinz Häfner**, Director emeritus of the Central Institute of Mental Health in Mannheim, Germany for his merits for Public Health in Germany. Professor Häfner was Chairman of the Scientific Council of the German Government from 1976-1983 and Chairman of the Evaluation Board of the German Research Ministry (BMBF) for the 5 Public Health Research Associations (Bavaria [Munich], Berlin, Northern Germany [Hanover], North Rhine-Westphalia [Bielefeld/Duesseldorf] and Saxony [Dresden]) from 1990–2002.

Preface

"La patience et l'amour peuvent seuls nous conduire au coeur battant du monde."
'Le vent à Djémila'
ALBERT CAMUS

After foundation of the European Public Health Association (EUPHA) 1992 in Paris, yearly conferences took place in Maastricht, Copenhagen, Budapest, London, Pamplona, Gothenburg, Prague, Paris, and Brussels. From 28 to 30 November 2002 the 10th Annual Congress was held in Dresden, Germany. Thus, on the occasion of EUPHA's anniversary the idea came up to publish a book with the most important contributions of this conference. In particular some retrospectives and perspectives of the development and achievements of EUPHA should be reflected. This demand was fulfilled for the present book publication. Therefore, scientists like Professor Louise Gunning-Schepers, who was the first president of EUPHA, or Professor Jouke van der Zee, who has been EUPHA's secretary for many years, had to be recruited as authors. Of course, further manuscripts with interesting themes were included.

In conclusion, we very much appreciate that we were able to edit a book on the occasion of a EUPHA conference, namely its 10th annual meeting.

The main sponsors of our congress and the present book publication were the European Commission in Luxembourg, Directorate – General Health & Consumer Protection SPC.2002270, the Open Society Institute (OSJ) of the Soros Foundation, New York 20008644, the German Ministries of Research (BMBF) 01EG0201 and of Health (BMG) Z21-4005, the German Research Federation (DFG) 4851/36/02 and the State Ministry of Research Saxony (SMWK) 4-7531.50-05-02/1. This book publication was produced in kind cooperation and with the support of the WHO/Euro Copenhagen, Denmark.

Concerning the future of EUPHA, let me close with two sentences from Franklin D. Roosevelt's Jefferson Day Speech in 1945: *"The only limit of our realization of tomorrow will be our doubts of today. Let us move forward with a strong and active faith."*

Dresden, May 2003   WILHELM KIRCH

Contents

Editorial XIII
Prof. Dr. Dr. W. KIRCH
Faculty of Medicine, Dresden University of Technology, Germany

List of Contributors XVII

I.   10 years European Public Health Association (EUPHA)

1.   Public health at the turn of the 20th century, Europe coming of age   3
     Prof. Dr. LOUISE J. GUNNING-SCHEPERS
     University of Amsterdam, The Netherlands

2.   The future of EUPHA   9
     Dr. VIVIANE VAN CASTEREN
     Belgian Association of Public Health, Dept. of Epidemiology, Brussels, Belgium

3.   EUPHA 10 Years: the annual conference 15
     Prof. Dr. J. VAN DER ZEE, Dr. MADELON KRONEMAN, Dr. TINA DORN,
     NIVEL, Utrecht, The Netherlands

4.   European Journal of Public Health and EUPHA – 10 years on 33
     Prof. Dr. M. MCKEE
     London School of Hygiene and Tropical Medicine, UK

II.   Public Health Research and Practice

5.   Public Health and the way forward 41
     Prof. Dr. G. TELLNES
     Dept. of General Practice and Community Medicine, University of Oslo,
     Norway

6.   Public Health Research Strategies in Europe and the WHO 47
     Dr. G. THIERS
     Scientific Institute of Public Health, Brussels, Belgium

7.   Public Health and Public Health Research in the European Union.
     The need for a new alliance 51
     Dr. H. STEIN
     German Federal Ministry of Health, Bonn, Germany

8. **Public Health in the Netherlands** 59
    Dr. ELS BORST-EILERS
    Ministry of Health Welfare and Sports, The Hague, The Netherlands

9. **Public Health in France** 63
    Prof. Dr. M. BRODIN
    Dept. de Sante Publique, Faculte Xavier Bichat, Paris, France

10. **Public Health in Germany** 71
    Prof. Dr. F. W. SCHWARTZ, Dr. WISMAR, PD Dr. ULLA WALTER,
    PD Dr. MARIE-LUISE DIERKS
    Medical School of Hanover, Germany

11. **Ageing and Health Policy** 81
    Dr. MARGOT FÄLKER
    Federal Ministry of Health, Bonn, Germany

12. **Ferenc Bojan Memorial Lecture – The Meaning of life expectancy**
    for the individual, for Public Health and for Social Security Systems 89
    Prof. Dr. C. VON FERBER
    University of Cologne, Germany

13. **The significance of drug utilization for Public Health** 99
    PD Dr. LISELOTTE VON FERBER, Dr. H. MCGAVOCK,
    Dr. I. SCHUBERT, Dr. R.H. VANDER STICHELE, Dr. E.J. SANZ
    University of Cologne, Germany

14. **Gender bias – research in Public Health** 119
    Prof. Dr. ULRIKE MASCHEWSKY-SCHNEIDER, Dr. JUDITH FUCHS
    TU-Berlin, Germany

III. Health Care Services

15. **From patient-centred medicine to citizen-oriented health policy-making** . . . 131
    Prof. Dr. B. BADURA
    University of Bielefeld, Germany

16. **Influenza surveillance** 135
    Prof. Dr. P. CROVARI, Prof. Dr. R. GASPARINI
    Department of Health Sciences, University of Genoa, Italy

17. **The mental health care system on its way to integration**
    in general health care 145
    Prof. Dr. Dr. H. HÄFNER
    Zentralinstitut für Seelische Gesundheit, Mannheim, Germany

18. **The role of acute day hospital treatment for mental health care:**
    research context and practical problems of carrying out the
    international multi-centre EDEN-study 153
    PD Dr. T. KALLERT, Dr. S. PRIEBE, Dr. M. SCHÜTZWOHL,
    Dr. J. BRISCOE, Dr. M. GLÖCKNER and the EDEN-study group
    Dresden University of Technology, Germany

19. Evidence-based mental health services research: the contribution
    of some recent EU-funded projects 173
    Prof. Dr. T. Becker, Dr. Lorenza Magliano, Dr. Stefan Priebe,
    Dr. Hans-Joachim Salize, Dr. Matthias Schützwohl,
    PD Dr. Thomas Kallert
    University of Ulm, Germany

20. Cost-effectiveness of mental health service systems in the European
    comparison 189
    Prof. Dr. M. C. Angermeyer, Dr. Christiane Roick, Prof. Dr. T. Becker,
    Dr. Reinhold Kilian
    University of Leipzig, Germany

21. Hypertension and diabetes care among primary care doctors in Germany:
    results from an epidemiological cross-sectional study 203
    Dr. D. Pittrow, Prof. Dr. U. Wittchen, Prof. Dr. Dr. W. Kirch for the
    HYDRA-study group, Faculty of Medicine, Dresden University
    of Technology, Germany

22. Cardiac rehabilitation 219
    Prof. Dr. P. Dylewicz, Dr. Ślawomira Borowicz-Bieńkowska,
    Dr. Ewa Deskur-Smielecka, Dr. Izabela Przywarska
    Clinical Centre of Rehabilitation, University School of Physical Education,
    Poznan, Poland

23. Spatial patterns of cancer mortality in Europe 227
    Dr. Carolyn Davies, Dr. A. H. Leyland
    Medical Research Council, Social and Public Health Sciences Unit,
    Glasgow, UK

24. Evidence-based dentistry and dental Public Health:
    a German perspective 245
    Prof. Dr. K. W. Böning, Dr. B. H. Wolf, Prof. Dr. M. H. Walter
    Dresden University of Technology, Germany

IV. Information and Promotion

25. Public Use Files – the dissemination of empirical research data
    of the German Research Associations Public Health via the internet 259
    Dipl.-Soz. D. Meusel, Dr. Peggy Göpfert, Prof. Dr. Dr. W. Kirch
    Faculty of Medicine, University of Technology, Dresden, Germany

26. The span in information from researching new tools to accessible
    presentation – experience from child and adolescent health 275
    Prof. Dr. M. Rigby, Dr. S. Denyer, Dr. A. MacFarlane,
    Dr. Ann McPherson, Dr. A. Quinlan, Dr. U. Ravens-Sieberer
    Keele University, Staffordshire, UK

27. **Hospital patient migration: analysis using an utility index** 293
Prof. Dr. N. NANTE, Dr. O. AL FARRAJ, Dr. S. MORGAGNI, Dr. G. MESSINA,
Dr. ROBERTA SILIQUINI, Prof. Dr. G. RICCIARDI, Dr. R. SASSI
University of Siena, Italy

28. **The impact of disasters: long term effects on health** 317
Prof. Dr. C.J. YZERMANS, KDr. G.A. DONKER, Dr. P. VASTERMAN
NIVEL, Utrecht, The Netherlands

29. **Impact of medicines on Public Health: EURO-MED-STAT** 343
Prof. Dr. P. FOLINO-GALLO, Dr. T. WALLEY, Dr. K. DEJONCHEERE,
Dr. R. VAN DER STICHELE
Italian National Research Council, Rome, Italy

30. **Health risks of psychosocial stress at work: Evidence and implications
for occupational health services** 355
Prof. Dr. J. SIEGRIST
Department of Medical Sociology, University of Duesseldorf, Germany

31. **Accreditation and professionalisation in (Public) Health related
education – consequences of Bologna** 365
Prof. Dr. J. VON TROSCHKE, Dr. DANIELA MAUTHE,
Dr. GEORG RESCHAUER, Dr. KARL KÄLBLE
German Coordinating Agency for Public Health, University of Freiburg,
Germany

Subject Index 373

Editorial

As outlined in the preface, on the occasion of the 10th anniversary of EUPHA a book publication with some of the main contributions of the conference is here published for the first time in EUPHA history. This is particularly important as the 10th annual EUPHA meeting gave the opportunity for a plenary on 10 years EUPHA with reflections on EUPHA's history and future. Therefore, in the present book publication four lectures on *Ten Years EUPHA* are contained ("Public Health at the turn of the 20th century, Europe coming of age", "The future of EUPHA", "EUPHA 10 years: the annual conference", "European Journal of Public Health and EUPHA – 10 years on").

Furthermore, contributions are presented on the topics *Public Health Research and Practice* and on *Health Care Services*. Finally, as a fourth major theme of the underlying book, articles on *Information and Promotion in Public Health* are given. Thus, the contributions cover in general the main headlines of the Dresden conference.

In the section *10 Years European Public Health Association (EUPHA)*, **Louise Gunning-Schepers** provides an overview on aspects of Public Health at the turn of the century. This contribution gives an outline of Public Health history and new aspects and developments in the last decades of the 20th century in Europe. In detail under the head "The future of EUPHA", **Viviane van Casteren** presents an outlook of EUPHA perspectives. She particularly emphasizes the mission that EUPHA will pursue during the next 10 years: being a platform of exchange between health professionals in research and practice and taking over a bridging function between these professionals and policymakers. **Jouke van der Zee et al.** give a review on past and present conferences of EUPHA, since the organisation and coordination of those is one of EUPHA's main tasks. In his contribution he outlines the history of EUPHA meetings from the beginning in Paris (1992) and Maastricht (1993) via Copenhagen (1994), Budapest (1995), London (1996), Pamplona (1997), Gothenburg (1998), Prague (1999), Paris (2000), Brussels (2001) to 2002 in Dresden. The fourth lecture under the head *Ten Years EUPHA* was presented by **Martin McKee** on the topic "European Journal of Public Health and EUPHA – 10 years on". His article portrays the development of the European Journal of Public Health describing the beginning as well as the original conditions that led to the birth of this journal, up to its current position.

The article "Public Health and the Way Forward" by **Gunnar Tellnes** gives an overview of the development of research in public health and epidemiology up to the 21th century. He presents a new approach to health promotion with the Nature-Culture-Health concept. The contribution "Public Health and Public Health research in the European Union. The need for a new alliance" by **Hans Stein** gives an insight into the current situation of Public Health and Public Health research in the European Union. He addresses problems and needs, and draws conclusions for future actions. **Godfried Thiers** considers "Public Health Research Strategies in Europe and the WHO". He describes the meaning of public health research for the European and international health policy. **Els Borst-Eilers** presents the development of Public Health in the Netherlands. She describes current issues and dilemmas of Public Health. A view on "Public Health in France" is presented by **Marc Brodin** in his article. This contribution describes structures and processes in the French health care system. **Friedrich Wilhelm Schwartz et al.** show in "Public Health in Germany" the context of Public Health aspects, prevention and the health care system in Germany. An important concern of Public Health research and practice is the ageing population and its impact on the health care system. **Margot Fälker** describes in "Ageing and Health Policy" the demographic changes that we are facing and their influence on financing the health care system including propositions how solidarity can be saved. **Christian von Ferber** gave the Ferenc Bojan-Memorial lecture. He presents data on the "Meaning of life expectancy for the individual, for Public Health, and for social security systems" and points out that research in life expectancy is still neglected and describes perspectives for future activities. Dealing with another important topic is the contribution of **Liselotte von Ferber et al.** "The Significance of Drug utilization for Public Health". They discuss issues of inadequate drug prescribing by physicians and inadequate drug use by the patient that may result in illnesses and even death. Finally they point out methodologies of drug utilization research and Public Health research that helps to improve the prescribing of drugs and utilisation techniques. Another aspect of Public Health research and practice is presented by **Ulrike Maschewsky-Schneider & Judith Fuchs**. In their manuscript "Gender bias – gender research in Public Health" they introduce results of a project that evaluated public health aspects of sex and the sensitivity of scientists for this topic as well as the frankness of scientific journals for gender based analysis.

The first contribution in the area *Health Care Services* is the article by **Bernhard Badura** "From patient-centred medicine to citizen-oriented health policy-making" discussing patient participation and cooperation of representatives of the health care system and patients up to an involvement of the citizens in health policy-making. **Pietro Crovari** and **Roberto Gasparini** provide an insight to "Influenza surveillance". Characteristics, objectives, methods of surveillance and other indicators of influenza activity are presented. The authors conclude that it is necessary to combine several methods to have a sufficient picture of the virus. **Heinz Häfner** focuses another important aspect that needs to be considered. His contribution deals with "The mental health care system on its way to integration in general health care". This issue is particularly important when we look at the great number of people suffering from mental illnesses. Another paper discussing issues from the field Public Mental Health is written by **Thomas Kallert et al.** "The role of acute day hospital treatment for mental health care: research context and practical problems of carrying out the international multi-centre EDEN-study" supported by the EU. The authors introduce results of the European Day Hospital Evaluation (EDEN) study that analyses the effectiveness of acute psychiatric day hospitals in different European countries. **Thomas Becker et al.** also present a contribution to the field of Public Mental Health. They discuss current research outcomes of some EU-funded projects for the development of evidence-based mental health services. The importance of cost-effectiveness-analyses increases against the background of permanently arising costs in health care systems. **Matthias Angermeyer et al.** introduced a European project, comparing the cost-effectiveness of mental health services in several European countries. He points out that the empirical basis of this topic is small in European context and further adequate investigations are necessary. **David Pittrow et al.** present "Hypertension and diabetes care among primary care doctors in Germany: results from an epidemiological cross-sectional study". This contribution gives an overview of the HYDRA-study, its aims, methodology and selected results. The study aims to describe representatively the prevalence, duration and severity of both illnesses. The authors also describe the current health practise for these indications. Finally, differences in East- and West-Germany in diagnosis and treatment are characterised. The contribution of **Piotr Dylewicz et al.** deals with aspects of "Cardiac Rehabilitation". They describe the usefulness of cardiac rehabilitation in the Public Health system that was proven during the past four decades and finally they outline goals of cardiac rehabilitation and secondary prevention for the 21st century. An analysis of geographical variations in cancer mortality and their relationships with population characteristics is given in the paper by **Carolyn A. Davies & Alastair H. Leyland** "Spatial patterns of cancer mortality in Europe". They are able to show that a high variability in cancer mortality between and within countries in EU is evident. Another important Public Health issue is covered by the article of **Klaus Boening et al.** In their contribution "Evidence-based dentistry and Dental Public Health: a German perspective" they state that evidence-based dentistry is a field that belongs to the Public Health discipline but that is still undervalued in current practice.

The section *Information and Promotion* starts with an article by **Dirk Meusel et al.** "Public use files – the dissemination of empirical research data of the German Public Health research associations via the internet" describing an opportunity to distribute research data gained and make them accessible for further research and analysis, and thus to open a way to share information among researchers. **Michael Rigby et al.** state in their manuscript "The span in information from researching new tools to accessible presentation – experience from child and adolescent health" that it is highly important to focus the particularities of certain population groups such as children when developing health information systems. A study aiming on determination of a statistical model capable of explaining the choices of patients and their doctors regarding hospital admission is introduced by **Nicola Nante et al.** in the paper "Hospital patient migration: analysis using a utility index". They list several determinants for the choice of a place for treatment. The contribution of **Joris Yzermans et al.** "The impact of disasters: long term effects on health" describes the influences of catastrophes on the health of involved persons. The effect of expenditures and utilisation of medicinal products in the European Union is illustrated by **Pietro Folino-Gallo et al.** in the paper "Impact of medicines on Public Health: EURO-MED-STAT". The authors present some results of this European project. In his paper "Health risks of psychosocial stress at work: evidence and implications for occupational health services" **Johannes Siegrist** provides a selective overview of recent progress in research of psychosocial stress at work and its impact on the workers' health. The meaning of Public Health education as postgraduate programs at universities has increased. **Jürgen von Troschke et al.** give an insight into new accreditation systems for Public Health studies following the so called Sorbonne declaration and discusses it in the context of the Bologna process.

In conclusion, the present book contains a number of highly interesting and topical contributions in the field of Public Health and it is pleasing for us that we were able to edit it in a reasonably short period after our congress.

Dresden, May 2003   WILHELM KIRCH

List of Contributors

Dr. Oussama Al Farraj
Laboratory for the Planning and Organisation
of the Health Services
Institute of Hygiene
Siena University
Via Aldo Moro
I-53100 Siena, Italy

Prof. Dr. Matthias C. Angermeyer
Clinic and Policlinic for Psychiatry
University of Leipzig
Johannisallee 20
D-04317 Leipzig, Germany

Prof. Dr. Bernhard Badura
Faculty of Health Sciences, Bielefeld School
of Public Health
University of Bielefeld
Post Box No. 10 01 31
D-33501 Bielefeld, Germany

Prof. Dr. Thomas Becker
Department of Psychiatry II
University of Ulm
Ludwig-Heilmeyer-Str. 2
D-89312 Günzburg, Germany

Dr. Slawomira Borowicz-Bieńkowska
Clinical Center of Rehabilitation
University School of Physical Education
ul. Uzdrowiskowa 2
PL-60-488 Poznań, Poland

Dr. Jane Briscoe
Unit for Social and Community Psychiatry
Newham Centre for Mental Health
Queen Mary and Westfield College
Gled Road
UK-E13 85P London, England

Prof. Dr. Klaus W. Böning
Department of Prosthetic Dentistry
Faculty of Medicine
University of Technology
Fetscherstr. 74
D-01307 Dresden, Germany

Prof. Dr. Marc Brodin
Faculté Xavier Bichat, Santé Publique
16, rue Henri Huchard
F-75018 Paris, France

Dr. Carolyn A. Davies
MRC Social and Public Health Sciences Unit
University of Glasgow
4 Lilybank Gardens
UK-912 8RZ Glasgow, Scotland

Dr. Kees DeJoncheere
Regional Adviser for Pharmaceuticals
and Technology
WHO-Regional Office for Europe
8, Scherfigsvej
DK-2100 Copenhagen, Denmark

Dr. Ewa Deskur-Śmielecka
Clinical Center of Rehabilitation
University School of Physical Education
ul. Uzdrowiskowa 2
PL-60-488 Poznań, Poland

Prof. Dr. Sean Denyer
North Western Health Board
Best Health for Children
Park Road, Manorhamilton
Co. Leitrim, Ireland

PD Dr. Marie-Luise Dierks
Department of Epidemiology,
Social Medicine and
Health System Research
Hanover Medical School
OE 5410
D- 30623 Hannover, Germany

Dr. Gé Donker
NIVEL (Netherlands Institute
for health services research)
PO Box 1568
NL-3500 BN Utrecht, The Netherlands

Prof. Dr. PIOTR DYLEWICZ
Clinical Center of Rehabilitation
University School of Physical Education
ul. Uzdrowiskowa 2
PL-60-488 Poznań, Poland

Dr. MARGOT FÄLKER
Federal Ministry of Health
Am Probsthof 78
D-53121 Bonn, Germany

Prof. Dr. PIETRO FOLINO-GALLO
Institute for Research on Population
and Social Policies
National Research Council of Italy
Via Nizza, 198
I-00198 Rome, Italy

Dr. JUDITH FUCHS
Department of Health Sciences
University of Technology
Ernst-Reuter-Platz 7
D-10587 Berlin, Germany

Dr. MATTHIAS GLÖCKNER
Clinic and Policlinic for Psychiatry
and Psychotherapy
Faculty of Medicine
University of Technology
Fetscherstr. 74
D-01307 Dresden, Germany

Dr. PEGGY GÖPFERT
Research Association Public Health Saxony
Faculty of Medicine
University of Technology
Fiedlerstr. 33
D-01307 Dresden, Germany

Prof. Dr. LOUISE J. GUNNING-SCHEPERS
Academic Medical Center
Meibergdreef 9
NL-1105 Amsterdam, The Netherlands

Prof. Dr. Dr. Dres. h.c. HEINZ HÄFNER
Schizophrenia Research Unit
Central Institute of Mental Health J5
D-68159 Mannheim, Germany

PD Dr. THOMAS KALLERT
Clinic and Policlinic for Psychiatry
and Psychotherapy
Faculty of Medicine
University of Technology
Fetscherstr. 74
D-01307 Dresden, Germany

KARL KÄLBLE
German Coordinating Agency for Public Health
Albert-Ludwigs-Universität Freiburg
Hebelstr. 29
D-79104 Freiburg, Germany

Dr. REINHOLD KILIAN
Clinic and Policlinic for Psychiatry
University of Leipzig
Johannisallee 20
D-04317 Leipzig, Germany

Prof. Dr. Dr. W. KIRCH
Research Association Public Health Saxony
Institute of Clinical Pharmacology
& Therapeutics
Faculty of Medicine
University of Technology
Fiedlerstr. 27
D-01307 Dresden, Germany

Dr. ALASTAIR H. LEYLAND
Medical Research Council
Social and Public Health Sciences Unit
University of Glasgow
4 Lilybank Gardens
UK-G12 8RZ Glasgow, Scotland

Dr. AIDAN MACFARLANE
Independent Consultant in Planning
of Health Services
6 Cobden Crescent
UK-OX14LJ Oxford-England

Dr. LORENZA MAGLIANO
Department of Psychiatry, University of Naples
Largo Madonna delle Grazie
I-80138 Naples, Italy

Prof. Dr. ULRIKE MASCHEWSKY-SCHNEIDER
Department of Health Sciences
University of Technology
Ernst-Reuter-Platz 7
D-10587 Berlin, Germany

MANUELA MAUTHE
German Coordinating Agency for Public Health
Albert-Ludwigs-Universität Freiburg
Hebelstr. 29
D-79104 Freiburg, Germany

Prof. Dr. HUGH MC GAVOCK
Northern Ireland Council for Postgraduate
Medical and Dental Education
University of Ulster
55 Culcum Road, Cloughmills
UK-BT44 9NJ Co Antrim, Northern Ireland

Prof. Dr. MARTIN MCKEE
European Centre on Health of Societies
in Transition
London School of Hygiene
and Tropical Medicine
Keppel Street
UK-WC1E 7HT London, England

Prof. Dr. ANN MCPHERSON
Department of Primary Care
University of Oxford
Old Road, Headington
UK-OX3 7LFOxford, England

Prof. Dr. GABRIELE MESSINA
Institute of Hygiene
Laboratory for the Planning and Organisation
of the Health Services
Siena University
Via Aldo Moro
I-53100 Siena, Italy

Dipl.-Soz. DIRK MEUSEL
Research Association Public Health Saxony
Faculty of Medicine
University of Technology
Fiedlerstr. 33
D-01307 Dresden, Germany

Dr. SERGIO MORGAGNI
Institute of Hygiene
Laboratory for the Planning and Organisation
of the Health Services
Siena University
Via Aldo Moro
I-53100 Siena, Italy

Prof. Dr. NICOLA NANTE
Institute of Hygiene
Laboratory for the Planning and Organisation
of the Health Services
Siena University
Via Aldo Moro
I-53100 Siena, Italy

Dr. DAVID PITTROW
Research Association Public Health Saxony
Institute of Clinical Pharmacology
& Therapeutics
Faculty of Medicine
University of Technology
Fiedlerstr. 27
D-01307 Dresden, Germany

Dr. STEFAN PRIEBE
Unit for Social and Community Psychiatry
Newham Centre for Mental Health
Queen Mary and Westfield College
Gled Road
UK-E13 85P London, England

Dr. IZABELA PRZYWARSKA
Clinical Center of Rehabilitation
University School of Physical Education
ul. Uzdrowiskowa 2
PL-60-488 Poznań, Poland

Dr. AILIS QUINLAN
Best Health for Children
Conygham Road
I-Dublin 8, Ireland

Prof. Dr. ULRIKE RAVENS-SIEBERER
Research Unit in Child and Adolescent Health
Robert-Koch-Institute
KIDSCREEN Project
Nordufer 20
D-13353 Berlin, Germany

GEORG RESCHAUER
German Coordinating Agency for Public Health
Albert-Ludwigs-Universität Freiburg
Hebelstr. 29
D-79104 Freiburg, Germany

Prof. Dr. GUALTIERO RICCIARDI
Institute of Hygiene
Catholic University of "Sacro Cuore"
Largo F. Vito 1
I-00168 Rome, Italy

Dr. MICHAEL RIGBY
Centre of Health Planning and Management
Keele University
Darwin Builing
UK-ST5 5BG Keele-Staffordshire, England

Dr. CHRISTIANE ROICK
Clinic and Policlinic for Psychiatry
University of Leipzig
Johannisallee 20
D-04317 Leipzig, GErmany

Dr. HANS-JOACHIM SALIZE
Central Institute of Mental Health, J 5
D-68159 Mannheim, Germany

Dr. EMILIO J. SANZ
Department of Clinical Pharmacology
School of Medicine
University of La Laguna
E-38071 La Laguna, Tenerife, Spain

Dr. FRANCO SASSI
Institute of Hygiene
Laboratory for the Planning and Organisation
of the Health Services
Siena University
Via Aldo Moro
I-53100 Siena, Italy

Dr. INGRID SCHUBERT
Primary Health Care Research Unit
Clinic for Child and Adolescent Psychiatry
and Psychotherapy
University of Cologne
Herderstr. 52
D-50931 Köln, Germany

Dr. Matthias Schützwohl
Clinic and Policlinic for Psychiatry
and Psychotherapy
Faculty of Medicine
University of Technology
Fetscherstr. 74
D-01307 Dresden, Germany

Prof. Dr. F. W. Schwartz
Department of Epidemiology,
Social Medicine and Health System Research
Hanover Medical School
OE 5410
D-30623 Hanover, Germany

Prof. Dr. Johannes Siegrist
Department of Medical Sociology
University of Düsseldorf
P.B. 10 10 07
D-40001 Düsseldorf, Germany

Dr. Roberta Siliquini
Institute of Hygiene
Laboratory for the Planning and Organisation
of the Health Services
Siena University
Via Aldo Moro
I-53100 Siena, Italy

Dr. Hans Stein
Rudolf-Stöcker-Weg 23
D-53115 Bonn, Germany

Prof. Dr. Gunnar Tellnes
Department of General Practice
and Community Medicine,
Section of Occupational Health
and Social Insurance Medicine
University of Oslo
PO Box 1130 Blindern
NO-0318 Oslo, Norway

Prof. Dr. Godfried Thiers
Scientific Institute of Public Health
Louis Pasteur Bureau of Quality Assurance
J. Wytsmanstraat 14
B-1050 Brussels, Belgium

Dr. Viviane Van Casteren
Scientific Institute of Public Health,
Louis Pasteur Bureau of Quality Assurance
J. Wytsmanstraat 14
B-1050 Brussels, Belgium

Dr. Robert van der Stichele
Heymans Institute of Pharmacology
University of Ghent
De Printelaan 185
B-9000 Ghent, Belgium

Prof. Dr. Jouke van der Zee
NIVEL (Netherlands Institute
for health services research)
PO Box 1568
NL-3500 BN Utrecht, The Netherlands

Dr. P. Vasterman
Faculty of Communication and Journalism,
School for Journalism
PO Box 8611
NL-3503 RP Utrecht, The Netherlands

Prof. Dr. Christian von Ferber
Auf dem Ufer 7
D-40593 Düsseldorf, Germany

PD Dr. Liselotte von Ferber
Primary Health Care Research Unit
Clinic for Child and Adolescent Psychiatry
and Psychotherapy
University of Cologne
Herderstr. 52
D-50931 Köln, Germany

Prof. Dr. Jürgen von Troschke
German Coordinating Agency
for Public Health Studies
Albert-Ludwigs-Universität Freiburg
Hebelstr. 29
D-79104 Freiburg, Germany

Dr. Tom Walley
Department of Pharmacology and Therapeutics
University of Liverpool
70 Pembrooke Place
UK-Liverpool L69 3GF, England

Prof. Dr. Michael H. Walter
Department of Prosthetic Dentistry
Faculty of Medicine
University of Technology
Fetscherstraße 74
D-01307 Dresden, Germany

PD Dr. Ulla Walter
Department of Epidemiology,
Social Medicine and Health System Research
Hanover Medical School
OE 5410
D-30623 Hannover, Germany

Dr. Matthias Wismar
Department of Epidemiology,
Social Medicine and
Health System Research
Hanover Medical School
OE 5410
D-30623 Hannover, Germany

Prof. Dr. HANS-ULRICH WITTCHEN
Department of Clinical Psychology
and Psychotherapy
University of Technology
Chemnitzer Str. 46
D-01187 Dresden, Germany

Dr. BURKHARD H. WOLF
Department of Prosthetic Dentistry
Faculty of Medicine
University of Technology
Fetscherstr. 74
D-01307 Dresden, Germany

Prof. Dr. JORIS YZERMANS
NIVEL (Netherlands Institute
for Health Services Research)
PO Box 1568
NL-3500 BN Utrecht, The Netherlands

Part I 10 Years of European Public Health Association (EUPHA)

Public health at the turn of the 20th century, Europe coming of age

Louise J. Gunning-Schepers

Introduction

The twentieth century is often denoted as the era in which health care became effective. Both preventive programmes such as vaccination and curative interventions such as antibiotic treatment, surgical interventions and drugs vastly changed the population's health landscape in both developed and developing countries. Especially after the second world war, in the second half of that century, with social health insurance achieving universal access to health services in most European countries and health research generating ever more clinically relevant results, the sense of a new era full of promise was pervasive.

Public health by many associated more with the 19th century of social reform and the hygienist movement, provided the infrastructure necessary to achieve the promised results. Maternal and child health services already reached almost all pregnant women before the childhood vaccinations and birth control pills provided the effective tools to greatly reduce both maternal and early childhood mortality. In the 20th century public health departments switched their attention from environmental control to infectious disease monitoring and screening, case finding and treatment for tuberculosis and sexually transmitted diseases. However as the visible threat of infectious diseases diminished, so did the interest and attention for public health. In the 1960's public health seemed to have been outlived by health care services.

That changed abruptly when in the 1970's important epidemiological studies such as Framingham and the British physicians study yielded results on the risk factors associated with non-communicable diseases such as cardiovascular disease and cancers which in the wake of the decline of infectious disease mortality had become the major causes of premature mortality. The life style factors identified, such as smoking and diet, as well as the availability of new drugs against hypertension and later high cholesterol suggested that these causes of death might be avoidable, given good preventive programmes. Evidence of the effectiveness of early detection and treatment in both cervical and breast cancer started the interest in population screening programmes. Motor vehicle accidents which had become more important as car ownership increased dramatically were also amenable to prevention, be it that these required more structural interventions such as construction of double motorways and legislation requiring the use of seat belts. The Canadian health policy model of Lalonde, which showed the determinants of health from a public health perspective, is often quoted as the starting point of the WHO Targets for Health for All strategy in which prevention was very prominent. Public health was back in business.

Public health in the last quarter of the 20th century, promise of a renaissance

This was the period in which epidemiology was again reinstated as the backbone of public health. Large population studies identified numerous risk factors and health promotion used both health education and more structural measures to help the population adopt a healthier life style. In the beginning these were remarkably successful. Sex education together with widely available birth control clinics helped to reduce the number of unwanted pregnancies, especially teenage pregnancies. Early health education programmes on smoking cessation halved the prevalence of smoking in men in many countries, and halted the very rapid increase of smoking in women. Many adults knew their "number" (cholesterol) and jogging was a common feature of every large city in the world. Hypertension was detected and treated more often, although there was an increasing debate between GP's and cardiologists about the medicalisation of hypertensive patients. Many occupational and environmental risk factors were eliminated through legislation and health education.

Public health also became prominent again in health policy in many countries. Partly this was the result of the WHO Health for All strategy that asked member states to make national target documents. At that time however many countries were worried about the increase in health care costs and primary prevention appeared to promise a health gain at a decreased cost. One could speculate about the political gain to be achieved through giving much policy emphasis and media coverage to public health and preventive programmes, while at the same time trying to cut hospital beds and institute cost control measures through health care reforms. The public health message also echoed the general feeling about the power of medicine and its institutions and represented a change in policy making an appeal to the responsible individual to take care of his or her own health.

European public health research

As epidemiological studies looked for the variation necessary to identify risk factors, one sees three distinct types of studies emerge: comparative studies between countries, studies on socio-economic differences in health and studies on differences between ethnic groups. All have yielded important scientific knowledge. Think for instance of the much quoted inter country comparison on cancer incidence by Doll and Peto, the comparison on cardiovascular mortality in the Seven country study, the work on social inequalities by Diederichsen, Whitehead and Mackenbach, the studies on thalassaemia amongst immigrants from Mediterranean countries and diabetes amongst immigrants from Asian decent.

All served to bring researchers from European countries together since the European Union provided a unique opportunity to study the effect of variation in life style and in health services delivery, in relatively homogenous populations, but it also provided funding specifically for such comparative studies in research programmes such as Biomed. The European Public Health association (EUPHA) was to a certain extent but the formalisation of this reality.

European public health practice

These comparative studies also served to identify sub populations for which the gains in health had not been as spectacular as for the average population. This led to a whole range of innovative public health programmes to reach out to these populations and a large body of health services research to evaluate projects. Healthy cities, healthy schools, healthy regions, healthy factories, community intervention projects, large-scale prevention programmes involving large areas such as Heart Beat Wales, all slowly shifted the emphasis from health education geared towards the individual (blaming the victim) to holistic movements trying to empower communities. In doing so it changed the professional emphasis away from doctors and the health services towards change agents and social work.

Rude awakenings at the end of the century

In retrospect the first cracks appeared when HIV/AIDS signalled that the public health threat of infectious diseases might be controlled but not eliminated. On the one hand the new epidemic showed the potential of health education in many Western countries, but it also made clear that the globalisation no longer allowed us to limit our public health policies to our national territory. With the political changes in Eastern and Central Europe, the optimism of post communist regimes proved insufficient to maintain proper preventive programs like childhood vaccination and provide universal access to basic health services. Despite the support of WHO the health status of population in those countries deteriorated.

In the Western countries impressive gains had been obtained in cardiovascular disease and for some cancer types. However contrary to the expectations that did not result in lower health care costs. On the contrary. As more people lived to older age, more chronic, degenerative diseases replaced the "killers of middle age". Although life expectancy increased, healthy life expectancy and disability adjusted life expectancy showed that survival was associated with increasing disabilities and need for health services. Demographic analyses showed that the large post-war baby boom would greatly increase the need for services in the coming decades in many countries, while the generations who would need to provide both the professionals and the funding for those services were much smaller as a result of effective family planning.

Finally contrary to what might have been expected, the economic growth and social welfare programmes which all but eliminated poverty, the effective preventive services with a near 100% coverage, adequate nutrition in childhood, universal access to effective medical care, did not prevent the continuous existence of socio-economic inequalities in health. To many this may have been the most disappointing evidence that the optimism of conquering disease and providing an environment in which good health would be the capital with which each individual could shape his or her life, may not be justified.

2001 A new millennium, back to basics

Infectious diseases are here to stay

In later years the full realisation of this rude awakening may well be pinpointed on the September 11th tragedy in New York. For the first time the threat of bio terrorism became a real possibility. The response of the public health system both in the US and in Europe showed painfully the loss of expertise in infectious disease management and the need for a government supported network with authority to mobilise and direct the available health care potential in case of emergency. In the Netherlands this echoed earlier unease about the response to a large legionella outbreak and the publics reaction to "man made disasters" such as the fire work explosions in Enschede and the El Al plane crash in the Bijlmer.

The public health service had difficulty in convincing both the public and the politicians about the balancing of risks and benefits in the prevention of new such disasters. The rules and regulations concerning the prevention of legionella infection are so costly that one may well question the expected health benefits of such policy decisions in the context of alternative preventive programmes or the need for extra funding in curative services, for instance in the treatment of cancer patients. With the Enschede and especially with the Bijlmer disaster, it proved very difficult for public health workers to convince the public that there had been no identifiable exposure that could epidemiologically explain the symptoms and health complaints that were reported. The political support for further research at great expense, did not alleviate the fears as could be expected, but did undermine the ability of government to use good public health research as evidence to base policy decisions on. Both these examples illustrate the need for an authority on public health for politicians to refer to and to use in making difficult decisions.

Equitable health benefits

The interest in socio economic differences in health, led to a renewed interest in looking at the reach of public health programmes. As the global migration and the mobility of (illegal) immigrant groups within the European Union became more of a political issue, public health services had to admit that there were yet again sub populations who lagged behind in health status and that to a certain extent this was theoretically avoidable. Just as in the early years of the twentieth century some groups needed outreach programmes to achieve the same level of effectiveness of preventive measures as in the general populations. Whether this concerned childhood vaccinations, the prevention of HIV infection at birth, access to family planning for young girls, or good nutritional or psychological advise to new parents, just having a good network of services designed for the original population proved insufficient. To maintain the high average both in the uptake of services and in the health outcome necessitates more effort and a different approach.

Sustainable financing of health services

During that same period some European countries started to acknowledge that the policy of cost containment for health services, be it through a National health service or a social insurance system, had resulted in under funding of health care services to the extent that the benefits individuals had a right to expect, could not be delivered. The result was long waiting lists and sometimes longer waiting times than might be considered acceptable from a medical perspective. Here the European context proved both beneficial and detrimental. Beneficial in the sense that some of the more long-term policy decisions were not taken identically in the different member states of the European Union. Some counties limited the number of doctors and nurses trained, some countries tried to greatly reduce the number of hospital beds. Others did not. This provided an over capacity in some member states which is now gladly used to treat patients on waiting lists elsewhere. At the same time it is the European free market for goods and individuals, which may well threaten the national systems. Policies of social insurance with professional guidelines to limit unnecessary interventions and health services with a limited supply to maintain an incentive for efficient use of services, now find themselves in a system dictated by the European court of Justice that allows individuals to seek care across national borders and maintains that guidelines for evidence based health care are to be determined at a European rather than national level. All of these are likely to increase health care costs, and the political challenge will be to make a system that will continue to guarantee universal access to a benefit package of basic health services for all Europeans.

A public health response, three priorities

To some the disappointing results of the "new public health" with its health promotion approach may seem to herald the end of the renaissance of public health. I think on the contrary that the needs assessment made above warrants a renewed investment and strong positioning of public health. Provided public health goes back to basics.

I see three priorities that the public health community could and should contribute to, both with good public health research and with effective policies.

Reinforce basic public health programmes

Let us aim at a good coverage of public health services that concentrate on the important public health issues. That means using available resources to first achieve the following results for most of the population, before considering investing in additional programmes:

- ▶ *Maternal and child health services*, including a rational childhood vaccination programme. This may well mean additional investments to make sure that on the one hand immigrant populations are well served with possibly additional programmes (hepatitis B, BCG, good anti malarial prophylaxis) to assure a limited risk when visiting home countries. On the other hand some of the well-educated parents may have to be convinced again of the health benefits of traditional vaccinations and prevention programmes, which have become so much less visible as the diseases concerned have become invisible.
- ▶ *Infectious disease control.* Although infectious diseases are no longer very visible in the statistics on the health of the population in most Western European countries, globalisation, bio terrorism but may be even more important the resurgence of resistant strains of infectious agents such as tuberculosis and HIV in countries such as the former Soviet Union, will make infectious diseases and threats of epidemic a major concern for public health services anywhere. The fact that research in public health and in microbiology are no longer automatically intertwined needs addressing, both in our public health practice and in public health training.
- ▶ Maintaining the expertise and the *infrastructure to address large disasters.* The ability to respond rapidly to outbreaks and epidemics, but also to environmental disasters with the knowledge of the public health risks involved and the ability to organise large scale emergency services when needed, requires an infrastructure that is costly to maintain and often difficult to explain to the politicians. The events after September 11th have provided a great boost for that type of public health investment. It should be well used.
- ▶ The credibility and the effectiveness of *health education* is probably helped if it is limited to a number of important issues. After all changing peoples behaviour is difficult at the best of times, and here especially it pays to concentrate on the big issues. Epidemiology has generated a large body of knowledge on potential risk factors, many of which if controlled will have limited benefits on the populations health. Let us save our efforts to continue to change behaviour on a limited number of potentially important risk factors such as for instance smoking and safe sex including effective birth control.

▶ Knowing where to find and how to *reach high-risk populations*. With the larger immigrant populations and more fluid European migrant groups, it becomes easy to miss groups in any prevention programme. Since these are often groups at high risk through exposure of many kinds, it pays to have the knowledge and the infrastructure to reach such groups with tailor made preventive interventions.

Universal access to basic health services

▶ As European countries acknowledge the fact that they will not be able to pay all services to all individuals, it will be necessary to devise an *equitable system of social insurance* to delimitate both the societal responsibility for access for all citizens to health services and the necessary solidarity between young and old, healthy and sick, poor and rich. This will not be an easy task at a time when other elements of the welfare state are being questioned and market forces drive in a different direction. Public health is the only discipline that has the tradition to defend the populations health in political debate and as such has a major role to play.

▶ However universal access with an aging population will necessitate the definition of *a basic benefits package*. Limits to funds and solidarity will no longer allow us to provide everything to everybody. Here again it should be the rational weighing of the potential health benefits in a population in return for the necessary funding of those services that ought to determine what is more and what is less urgent. Public health science (epidemiology, cost effectiveness analysis and modelling) provides the tools to do so.

▶ If European policy will continue to force a common health services market, we need to invest more than we have done in producing *evidence based guidelines* for care that are acceptable in all of Europe. This will not be easy. Although the evidence may be universal, culture, traditions and health care systems have led to amazingly varying interpretation of those scientific data in different styles of evidence based medicine.

▶ *Health services research* can help in identifying the reasons for these traditional differences in health care practice between European members states. They can and should however also contribute to a more uniform and transparent system of quality assurance in Europe. This will help assess the cost benefit ratio of treating patients in different settings and may well lead to supra national specialisation of services.

A common European public health policy

Public health has never been limited by national borders. As the globalisation of our world continues and the borders within the European union become less and less important, it will be crucially important to develop a common European public health policy. However I am convinced that this should be initiated and supported by the public health community instead of EU directorate. The European Public Health Association has a crucial role to play in that. After a successful coming of age, it now needs to be a powerful advocate of the public health community, as it exists in the European Union, consisting both of public health researchers and practitioners. A good evidence based approach of public health policy will determine the future health of the European populations.

The future of EUPHA

Viviane van Casteren

10th Annual EUPHA Meeting, Dresden, 28–30 November 2002

This paper outlines the new mission for EUPHA (European Public Health Association) to be pursued in the coming 10 years. The new mission is to become the proactive platform for public health professionals in research and practice and to become the bridge between these professionals and policymakers. This mission can be achieved by intensifying the spreading of existing information, by intensifying the exchange of information between researchers, policymakers and practitioners, by developing a facilitating role and by responding proactively to all aspects of public health in Europe.

Introduction

In the course of its ten years existence, EUPHA has become the umbrella organisation for 31 public health associations from 27 different European countries, covering more than 9000 public health experts. Historically, EUPHA can be seen as an organisation mainly based on research with two tools of spreading and exchanging information: the EJPH and the annual EUPHA conferences.

The EJPH has grown from a European publication to an international well-known, indexed scientific journal, with innovative plans for the future, as already outlined by Prof. Martin McKee. The EUPHA annual conferences have become more professional, with a steady increase in participation and a wider focus on public health. These are without any doubt great successes and we have to express our thanks to all those who have contributed to these important achievements.

However, during our ten years of existence, we have observed one recurrent problem: how can research results be adequately translated into action (policy and practice) and how can policy and practice experiences be used to formulate new research questions. EUPHA has tried to address this problem, but rather in a reactive and passive way. The 10th anniversary of EUPHA, is an ideal occasion to present you with a new mission for EUPHA to be pursued in the coming 10 years.

New strategy for EUPHA

This new strategy was elaborated by the working group, which was installed by our Executive Council to propose a plan of action for EUPHA's second decade. The working group consisted of nine public health experts from 5 different countries. The strategy they have developed was approved by the Executive and Governing Council.

The new mission of EUPHA is to become the proactive platform for public health professionals in research and practice and to become the bridge between these professionals and policymakers. EUPHA will expand its tools to achieve this new mission and has the intention to become a more visible partner for public health in Europe. How can this new mission be achieved?

By intensifying the spreading of existing information

For this purpose, EUPHA already disposes of important and well developed tools. Research results should continue to be published in the EJPH, whereas practice and evidence-based experiences should be published either in a newsletter (to be developed) or on the new EUPHA website. The latter is also an ideal tool to highlight the policies and practices in the different member states as well as the activities of the European Commission, WHO/EURO, etc. The EJPH could offer in every issue e.g. half a page for a WHO/EURO and half a page for a EU column. The annual conference will remain an important moment to spread information.

By intensifying the exchange of information between researchers, policymakers and practitioners

The EUPHA annual conferences should continue to be the meeting place of researchers, policymakers and practitioners. The two sorts of abstracts (research-based and practice-based) should become standard. Parallel sessions should mix research and practice on a same subject to favour exchange of information between different disciplines.

The EJPH is already distributed to all EUPHA members, including policymakers and practitioners. To make the published research more accessible for all members, translations of abstracts should be offered.

Besides the annual EUPHA conference, EUPHA should organise workshops on specific subjects throughout the year and should set up clear and concise reports on specific health subjects or practices (e.g. country overview, different practices) and distribute them through the website, the EJPH (summaries), distribution lists etc.

By developing a facilitating role

A recurrent problem is that public health experts lack tools to bridge between research and policy/practice. To overcome this problem, at each EUPHA conference, skills-building workshops can be organised to provide tools to bridge between research and policy/practice (e.g. how to implement research results). EUPHA should offer, together with ASPHER, different training courses throughout the year and should actively pursue projects that facilitate the bridge between research and policy/practice.

By responding proactively to all aspects of public health in Europe

With the large database of public health experts EUPHA has set up, we should be able to provide statements on urgent or new public health subjects within a limited time frame, combining the current state of research/research needs with examples from practice and policy. The EJPH should continue with proactive editorials. EUPHA should be more proactive and steering at its annual conferences. We should actively invite key persons to set up specific workshops/sessions. EUPHA should actively pursue projects in this area.

EUPHA's future and the 10th EUPHA conference

This is a very ambitious plan, which needs a thorough analysis regarding its financial needs, personnel resources etc. However, several of the innovative ideas and activities formulated by the working group are in the meantime initiated and could already be discovered, experienced during the 10th EUPHA conference.

First of all, we are very proud to announce you our new website www.eupha.org, which is more complete than ever before and which will greatly improve our visibility. It includes not only information on EUPHA, but also gives detailed country-specific public health information with a link to WHO and the European Observatory on Health Care Systems. The new website offers possibilities to interact with both our national and their individual members. Online registration is now possible. Links with other European and international organisations, such as ASPHER (Association of Schools of Public Health in the European Region) and WFPHA (World Federation of Public Health Association) are present. We noted in September 31 000 hits, in October so far 25 000, illustrating the general interest in our website.

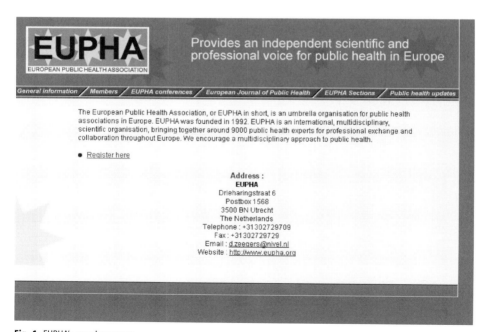

Fig. 1. EUPHA's new homepage

For the first time, there were two sorts of abstracts submitted for the conference: research abstracts and abstracts on practice, health information systems and health reform, thereby stimulating more practice-related presentations.

258 research abstracts were submitted, 210 were presented (82% acceptance rate), 57 practice abstracts were submitted, 51 were accepted (88% acceptance rate).

All accepted abstracts were published as a supplement to the EJPH, in this way strengthening the relation between EUPHA and the EJPH, which is not always obvious to our members, as well as wide spreading the research and practice presented at the conference.

The training side of EUPHA was further developed by a first skills-building workshop on how to write a scientific article. Staffan Janson and Anita Kallin from the EJPH editorial office and Martin McKee, EJPH editor-in-chief will participated in this workshop.

The working group on EUPHA's future stated that by giving more priority to specific projects, EUPHA can both increase its visibility as well as its financial situation. Presently, EUPHA is working on three projects, two of which were "visible" at the conference. The kick-off workshop of the project on the future of public health in Europe took place at this conference. This project is set up as five consecutive workshops, the first being held in Dresden, the last in Rome to gather researchers, policymakers and practitioners to talk about future public health problems and strategies to tackle these in Europe. The aim is to set up a concise report summarising the outcome of the workshops.

Together with the Open Society Institute of the SOROS foundation, EUPHA started a project for the support of public health associations as key links between government, the scientific community and the population in Central and Eastern Europe (CEE). The project invited key public health experts in selected countries (Albania, Armenia, Azerbaijan, Bulgaria, Estonia, Georgia, Kazakhstan, Kyrgyzstan, Latvia, Lithuania, Macedonia, Moldova, Mongolia, Romania, Tajikistan, Ukraine, Uzbekistan) to define the possible roles of a multidisciplinary public health association in their country that would meet national public health needs. On the basis of an application, a limited number of public health experts from up to twelve countries were sponsored to attend the Dresden conference. During this conference a "market place" was organised, where existing national public health associations in Europe will presented themselves. The goal is to prepare potential twinning partnerships between existing public health associations and the country representatives. This partnership will then be a central development tool for those applicants that receive grants in the following phase of the project. After the Dresden conference, country representatives will be invited to submit applications for 1-year funding up to 20 000 $ to either strengthen or create a public health association. This funding will include a multi-year membership of EUPHA, as well as membership in EPHA (the European Public Health Alliance), both of which include subscriptions to their periodic publications. Grant allocation will be made in mid 2003. The selected projects in 4 countries will begin shortly thereafter. EUPHA and its national members will actively offer support to the country teams.

Besides these two projects visible at the conference, EUPHA is also working with the Association of Schools of Public Health in the European Region (ASPHER) to set up an independent accreditation agency for public health training programmes (at master level) in Europe. An official cooperation agreement between ASPHER and EUPHA was established.

Continuous expansion of EUPHA's networking

2002 was characterised by an intensifying of EUPHA's international networking. ASPHER (Association of Schools of Public Health in the European Region) and EUPHA are, as already stated above, developing the accreditation project together.

EUPHA attended the annual meeting of the WFPHA (World Federation of Public Health Associations) and is actively collaborating in the international organising committee of their tri-annual congress to be held in April 2004 in Brighton UK.

IUHPE (International Union of Health Promotion and Education) and EUPHA had several contacts and both associations favour a closer collaboration. EUPHA is invited to participate in their VIth European conference in 2003.

EUPHA has extensive contacts with the Directorate General of Public Health of the European Commission. This DG has already attended and sponsored a number of EUPHA conferences and we are happy that they are interested in using the EUPHA tools (both conference and journal) to present their work in the field of public health. A delegation of EUPHA also attended the conference of DG research to launch the 6th framework on research in the European Union.

In October 2002, a delegation of EUPHA met with WHO/EURO regional director, Marc Danzon. WHO/EURO is very interested in using EUPHA as a channel to distribute information to a large network of public health experts. WHO/EURO also offered the use of their national offices in the EUPHA/Open Society Institute project to develop and encourage public health associations in Central and Eastern European countries.

Conclusion

Several of the activities proposed within the new strategy for EUPHA have already been initiated this year. We made great efforts to become more visible, to increase our networking, to become more proactive. This means, of course, only the start of EUPHA's future. Additional financial support and human resources will be needed to achieve the new goals. If the efforts already made are not only recognised by EUPHA's members and partners, but also noticed by possible sponsors, EUPHA's future is guaranteed.

EUPHA 10 years: the annual conference

Jouke van der Zee · Madelon Kronemann · Tina Dorn

Introduction

The annual conference forms one of EUPHA's main activities. It is one of the two 'pillars' of EUPHA, so to say. The second pillar is the European Journal of Public Health. The annual conference has in common with the Journal that the conferences already existed before EUPHA was officially founded. In 1989 NIVEL, the Netherlands Institute of Health Services Research, organised the first European Health Services Research meeting near Utrecht in the Netherlands in order to create an international platform for Health Services researchers and also for Public Health research. These Health Services Research conferences continued in 1990 (Cologne), 1991 (London) and 1992 (Paris) while the preparation for the foundation of EUPHA progressed. Even the 1993 conference (in Maastricht) was not yet a full EUPHA conference. The first genuine EUPHA conference was the conference in Copenhagen in 1994. So the Dresden conference is actually the ninth EUPHA conference and not the tenth.

Health Services Research and Public Health Research

The EUPHA conferences started as Health Services Research conferences; after EUPHA's foundation the focus gradually shifted to Public Health Research. The similarities and differences between the two types of research can be shown in a simple Venn-diagram (see graph 1).

In category I elements of the health services are studied without taking health (effects) into account (a study about remuneration of General Practitioners, for example). In category II (public) health is the research subject without taking health services into account (prevent adolescents to start smoking in schools). Category III forms the overlapping category: here the influence of 'health services' on 'health' forms the topic. EUPHA deals with the whole range of research subjects; Health services research forms an integrated part of EUPHA.

EUPHA conferences circulate through Europe with the rotating EUPHA-presidency according to a NEWS (North, East, West, South) scheme. Until the year 2000 the EUPHA-president acted as organiser and host to the conference; after 2000 it is the president-elect (next year's EUPHA president) who is charge of the conference. The aim of the conference is to provide a platform for researchers to present their work to research-colleagues and other interested conference-participants like policy-makers or public health practitioners. The most common way to participate as a researcher is by submitting an abstract for a poster or an oral presentation; since 1999 abstract submission for workshops is possible, too.

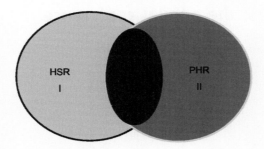

I.   HSR without health outcomes

II.   Public Health without health services

III.   a) HSR with health outcomes

        b) PHR with health services included

Fig. 1. Venn-diagram of similarities and differences between Health Services Research and Public Health Research

Abstracts are being judged by an international Scientific Committee, whose members score at least 100 to 150 abstracts and in some cases the total number of the abstracts on a 5 point scale (the score 5 represents excellent quality, the score 1 very low quality). These scores form the base of the decisions about acceptance and rejection of the abstracts[1]. Each abstract is rated by an average of 5–10 judges, which produces rather robust rates. The scientific committee consists of approximately 25 'permanent' members (one per EU-PHA member country), who, in principle, serve two three-year terms, completed each year by a group of approximately 5 local members, who participate one year only. The chair of the committee is appointed by the local organizer; he/she starts one year in advance and remains another year in the committee in order to communicate local experiences.

A jubilee is mostly a moment of reflection on the past and glances into the future. EU-PHA's 10th anniversary forms a good occasion to show how both the abstract submission and the evaluation developed over this 9-year period. As a reflection on the past, we would like to know what was achieved in the past conferences. We were curious who did submit papers and about what subjects and whether there could be demonstrated a development in subjects over the years. We also would like to gain insight in what the judges apparently find important features of the abstracts. In other words: what should an abstract look like to obtain a high score. As a glance in the future, we could give tips to improve future abstracts.

The EUPHA-office kept both the abstracts and the ratings of the judges as an electronic data-file for all the nine conferences since 1994. These files provided the basis to answer the following questions:

---

[1] The decision rules about acceptance or rejection of the abstracts are basically that the highest ranking 25% are accepted for oral presentation without discussion and the lowest ranking 25% are rejected. If, after this selection, there still is room left for oral presentations the second highest quartile serves as a source for further selection. This additional selection is also based on the ranking order but some adaptations may take place in order to correct an unbalanced distribution of the selected abstracts over the countries of origin of the (first) authors.

Research Questions

1. How did the number and origin of the submitted abstracts develop over the period 1994–2002 and what is the relationship between the conference location and the origin of the submitted abstracts?
2. What is the development in space (that is over the countries) and over time of the evaluation of the abstracts?
3. Can we identify determinants of the abstract evaluation? Can we answer the question what distinguishes a 'good' from a 'bad' abstract?

Method

The first two research questions will be answered by analysing the total database (that is the database with all the abstracts) with all submitted abstracts[2] and all judgements.

This database contains the following elements:

A conference year, location and conferencetheme (identical for all abstracts of a given conference)
B country of origin of the first author
C score of the judges
D outcome: acceptance for oral presentation, poster presentation or rejection

For answering the third research question (determinants of the average rating) abstracts of several years (the first two years (1994, 1995) and the last three years (2000, 2001, 2002[3])) were coded by the authors of this paper[4].

A scoring form (see Table 2) was developed to code the following characteristics:

A formal qualities of the abstract
   ▶ does it follow the guidelines for a structured abstract
   ▶ is it in English or in another language
   ▶ is it legible or generally comprehensible

B Study Design
   ▶ quantitative/qualitative
   ▶ descriptive/(systematically) comparative
   ▶ local/national/international scope

C Topic/subject of the study
   ▶ Fits this year's conference motto yes/no
   ▶ Fits last year's conference motto yes/no
   ▶ Topic classification into 5 main categories: Health services research/Epidemiology/ Health promotion/Health information or Methodology
   ▶ Disease related study or not disease related

---

[2] Only abstracts submitted for single presentations were selected for analysis; workshops were excluded (these were introduced in 1999).
[3] Originally when this study started the years 2000 and 2001 were the last two years. Later, the abstracts of 2002 have been added in order to provide an up-to-date overview at the Dresden conference.
[4] The data for 1994/1995 and 2000/2001 have been described in Tina Dorn's MPH thesis at Maastricht University: Dorn, Tina, Developments in European Public Health Research: towards more "new" Public Health? Maastricht University, MPH thesis, 2001.

Scoring procedure and inter judge reliability

The three authors of this paper all scored one third of the abstracts by means of the scoring form. The scoring on this form does not say anything about the quality of the abstract, but deals with structural parameters and the subject of the study (see above). In order to establish the inter-rater reliability among the authors, a set of 20 abstracts was scored by all three authors (Dorn, 2001, p 25). Cohen's Kappas were calculated as an indicator of the reliability. In total 18 categories have been scored (overall total of agreements: $3 \times 18 = 54$). Of these 54 possible agreements 18 (33%) were above 0.75 (very good agreement) and 6 (11 %) below 0.40 (low agreement); the other 30 had kappa's between 0.40 and 0.75. Agreement was especially low around classifying an abstract under the topic 'health promotion' and its subcategories (health education and policy). One of the three judges systematically deviated from the other two in this respect. A more comprehensive set of instructions and discussion among the raters was undertaken to improve the agreement on this point. For the rest the inter rater reliability was considered as sufficient.

Analysis

A multiple regression analysis (OLS) was performed with the average scoring (1 to 5 point scale) of the abstract by all the judges as the dependent variable and the above mentioned factors as independent variables. With polytomous variables one of the categories was used as reference category (see results section). Two analyses were performed: one with the scoring form variables only and one with the addition of two other variables, extracted from the general database: the year of the conference (1994: –2, 1995: –1), 2000: +1, 2001: +2, 2002: +3) and the region where the first author of the paper could be located (grouped into the following categories: North-West Europe (Scandinavia, UK, The Netherlands, Ireland), West-Central Europe (Belgium, France, Germany, Switzerland, Austria), Southern Europe (Portugal, Spain, Italy, Greece, Malta), Eastern Europe (Czech/Slovak republic, Baltic states, Romania, Bulgaria, Turkey, former Yugoslavia, Newly Independent States), Non-European countries (USA, Canada, India, Australia, Africa).

Results

Conference location and participation[5]

The first general research question: 'How did the number and origin of the submitted abstracts develop over the period 1994–2002 and what is the relationship between the conference location and the origin of the submitted abstracts?' was specified into the following sub-questions:

1a: To what extent does the place where the conference is held influence the participation from that region in the year of the conference?

1b: In case of a positive relationship between conference venue and participation from the region; does it remain the following year(s)?

---

[5] When we use the term 'participation' we actually mean 'abstract submission'; we do not dispose of detailed information about the conferences' participants.

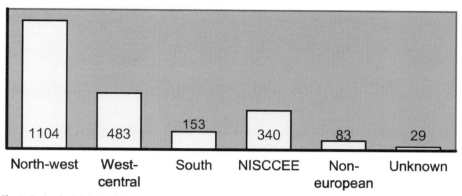

Fig. 2. Regional subdivision of the submitted abstracts over the period 1994–2002

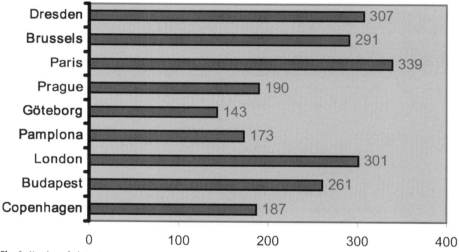

Fig. 3. Number of abstracts per year

A good argument for rotating the conference would be that it stimulates participation from the region; it would even be better if an increased participation would continue in the next or following years. In Graph 2 the regional subdivision of the submitted abstracts over the period 1994–2002 is displayed.

The number of abstracts increased gradually in the years 1994–1996; Pamplona 1997 and Gothenburg 1998 had a lower attractiveness, but the increase started again from 1999 (Prague) till Paris (2000), Brussels (2001) and Dresden (2002) (Graph 3). The influence of the conference venue on the participation is clearly visible; the participation from the host country (Graph 4) is considerably higher in the conference year than before or after. The long(er) term effect of a specific location (as expressed as the percentage of abstracts from a specific host-country) does not seem to be substantial. The effect is limited to the year of the conference.

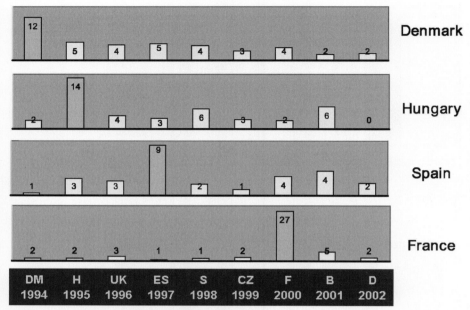

Fig. 4. Participation from countries that hosted the conference

The judgements

Research question 2: 'What is the development in space and time of the average judgements of the conference abstracts?' has been split up into three sub-questions:
2a: Did the average judgements improve over time?
2b: Are there regional differences in the abstracts judgements?
2c: Do the scores of ad hoc judges (recruited annually from the host countries) differ systematically from the scores of the permanent members of the scientific committee?

The overall average of the 2190 abstracts was 3.17; slightly above the mathematical average of a 1 (bad) to 5 (good) scale. In Graph 5 the average over the years is shown. Some conferences receive a higher overall appreciation (Budapest, 1995; Göteborg, 1998) than others (London, 1996; Paris, 2000) but there seems to be no trend in time. The only thing that can be said is that the annual averages regress somewhat to the grand mean.

The geographical spread of the average judgements over Europe is shown on Graph 6 and 7. Countries that had submitted less than 5 abstracts in the period 1994–2002, were left blank.

High averages are found in North-West Europe (with the exception of Ireland and, to some extent, Norway). The lowest rates are found in South-East Europe (Balkan, Turkey). Italy, the Czech Republic have also rather highly rated abstracts. Abstracts from non-European countries like Canada and the USA have high ratings, too. For some countries, that submitted a sufficient number of abstracts (90 abstracts over 9 years), we could see whether there was any progress in the rates (Graph 8). Three patterns could be observed. For some countries (Denmark, Sweden and the United Kingdom) the average rates progressed gradually. For Finland, Germany, Hungary and the Netherlands ratings fluctuated

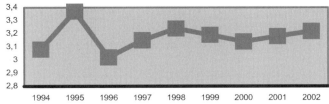

Fig. 5. Mean score per conference, development over time

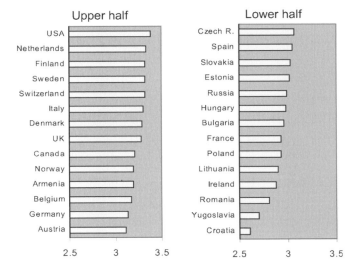

Fig. 6. Mean score of
abstracts per country

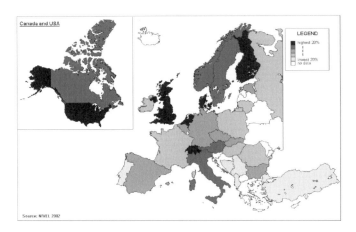

Fig. 7. Map of Europe
with mean scores

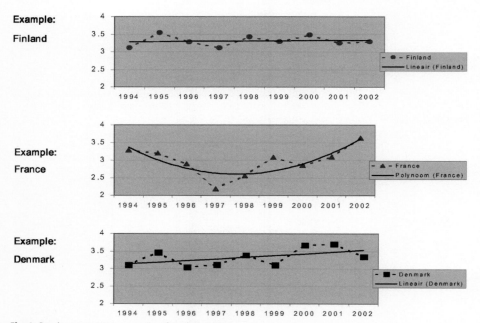

Fig. 8. Development patterns over time for selected countries

slightly (and decreasingly) around the mean while the ratings for France went down in the period 1994–1997 and raised again from 1998 till 2002. For the other countries the number of abstracts submitted over the years was insufficient to calculate a trend.

Topics of the abstracts

Of the 1994, 1995 and 2000–2002 abstracts the topic has been coded in 5 broad categories: (1) health services research (2) epidemiology (public health research), (3) health information, (4) health promotion, and (5) methodology. The distribution of the abstracts over the five topics changed over the years. The conferences started under the 'heading' "Health Services Research" (in 1989); so, it was expected that HSR-abstracts would be more prevalent in the first EUPHA-conferences than in the later years. For epidemiology/public health research we expected that this pattern would be reversed, since EUPHA stands for public health, indicating more emphasis on this subject. Graph 9 shows that this is the case, indeed. The other result worth commenting on is the 'boost' of health information in the last years. The Brussels' conference that had been devoted to this topic is clearly responsible for this result.

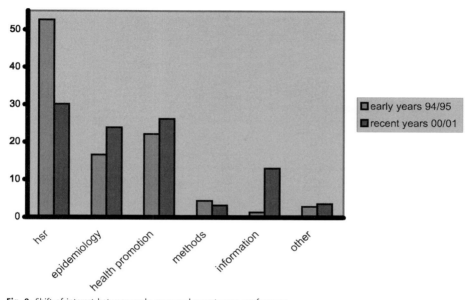

Fig. 9. Shift of interest between early years and recent years conferences

Individual judges

Judges differ characteristically; some are rather mild, some seem to have vinegar in their veins. Some serve long terms, some participate just for a single conference. Most of them judge only a part of the abstracts[6]; some seem to take pride in judging them all (one of our colleagues suggested that this might have a relationship with the quality of the judge's marriage, however, we do not have any information on this).

In order to get an idea, Graph 10. shows the average ratings over the years of a handful of judges, who took part of the jury for at least 5 years.

It is clear that there are mild and strict judges, but the average ratings differ per conference.

There does not seem to be a tendency over time. It is possible that judges adapt their score to the general level of the contributions. Responsiveness is the correct term for this phenomenon. We cannot say much about this responsiveness because we do not have a 'golden standard'; abstracts have not been scored repeatedly by the same judges at different moments in time. There is one question we can answer about the judges. As we explained in the introduction, there are two types of judges: permanent and ad-hoc members of the scientific committee. As the ad hoc members are local, their ratings could differ from the permanent members. In Graph 11 ratings of judges that participated only one year are compared with judges that participated at least five years: the 'old hands'[7].

---

[6] In order to avoid that the first half of the abstracts get more ratings than the last half, the judges are explicitly asked to start judging at a specific abstract number; as the number of abstracts fluctuates between 300 and 400, the total number usually is split into two or three groups; e.g., one third of the judges will start with nr 1, one third will start with nr 150 and one third with nr 300.
[7] We used the number of years as a proxy; one year only for a local member; over four years for an experienced 'permanent' judge.

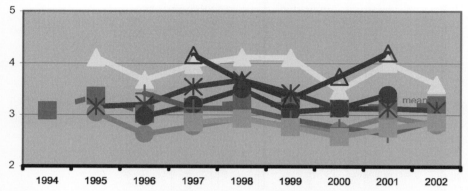

Fig. 10. Scores of several judges that participated in the process for 5 years or more

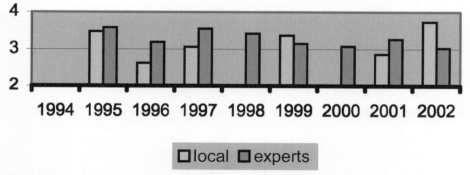

Fig. 11. Differences between local (1 year participation) and experienced (5 years or more) judges

In some cases (the Prague and Dresden conference for instance) the local judges scored more favourably than the experienced judges; in other cases (the Brussels conference is a good example) the opposite happened. The overall result does not allow a clear conclusion; the ratings of local, ad hoc judges do not differ systematically from experienced judges.

Distinguishing 'bad' from 'good' abstracts

For the answer to the last research question "can we answer the question what distinguishes a 'good' from a 'bad' abstract" a selection of the abstracts (all the abstracts of 1994, 1995 and 2000, 2001 and 2002) were rated according to the set of topics described in the method-section of this paper. The ratings related to the general format and structure of the abstract, to the design of the study and to the topic of the study. Two multiple regression analyses were performed (ordinary least squares) both with the average ratings of the abstracts (that is the average of all the judges per abstract) as dependent variable and two sets of predictors. The first set consists of the following abstract characteristics:
1. follows guidelines for structured abstract, yes/no
2. quantitative (ref category), qualitative study or don't know
3. descriptive (ref category), non-systematic comparison, systematic comparison

4. local, national (ref category) or international study
5. fits this year's conference motto (yes/no)
6. fits last year's conference motto (yes/no)
7. topic: health services research (ref category), epidemiology, health promotion, health information or methodology
8. disease related study (yes/no)

Most of the categories are self-evident; some need some further explanation.

Ad 1)   follows guidelines or not; most abstracts follow the 'background-aim-method - result-discussion' scheme, some, however do not.

Ad 2)   Most studies are explicitly quantitative; some are qualitative or a combination of both. In some cases the design could, unfortunately, not be established.

Ad 3)   Research implies comparison (before/after, between subgroups etc.). Many studies are descriptive. Some are systematically comparative, in this case it is known in advance which groups or conditions will be compared. Some studies end up with comparative results (gender differences, SES differences) that were not mentioned in advance. This latter group of design has been dubbed 'non-systematic comparative'.

Ad 4)   The scope of a study (local, national or international) is rather self-evident; some categories of studies (reviews for instance) could not be classified into the local-international continuum.

Ad 5, 6) Self evident.

Ad 7)   Under the topic 'epidemiology' the incidence or prevalence of (self-assessed) health or illness and/or the occurrence of health related risk factors (health determinants) are comprised. Health information includes databases, electronic medical files and health statistics. Health promotion deals with actions to improve health or combat illness. The other factors are self-evident.

Ad 8)   Disease related studies might encompass a specific illness or a group of diseases.

To this set of variables two extra variables were added for the second analysis: the year of the conference (to test whether the average rating increased or decreased over time) and the region (North West (ref category), West central, South, East and non-European). The expectation was that the influence of the variables of the first set would disappear (at least partially) with the introduction of the regional variables. We expected that the higher rates for instance abstracts from North-West Europe was due to the fact that these were more often quantitative, better structured, comparative etc.

The results of the regression analysis are shown in Table 1.

Comparing both analyses it is striking that adding region of the abstract does not alter the results of the first analysis, where region had been left out. Adding year did not change the results and did not contribute to the explained variance. So it is not true that abstracts from North-West Europe get higher scores because they are better structured or less descriptive or quantitative rather than qualitative compared to abstracts from the other regions. The region factor refers to other elements than those already measured. The year of the conference does not matter; abstracts for early conferences do not receive lower or higher marks than abstracts submitted to more recent conferences.

A high scoring abstract
1. follows the guidelines
2. does not follow this year's conference motto but last year's conference motto
3. is quantitative rather than qualitative
4. is internationally comparative and not local
5. is not descriptive but (systematically) comparable

Table 1. Multiple regression analysis of determinants of abstract quality*

Determinants	Model 1			Model 2		
	B	st. error	sign.	B	st.error	sign.
(Constant)	2.83	0.04	0.00	2.98	0.05	0.00
follows guidelines?	0.34	0.03	0.00	0.28	0.03	0.00
MOTTO	0.01	0.02	0.56	−0.01	0.02	0.78
OLDMOTTO	0.25	0.03	0.00	0.24	0.03	0.00
Type of research ref. cat.: quantitative						
Qualitative	−0.09	0.04	0.02	−0.13	0.04	0.00
Combined	0.11	0.06	0.10	0.10	0.06	0.10
Scope of research ref. cat.: National						
Local	−0.15	0.03	0.00	−0.13	0.03	0.00
International	0.29	0.04	0.00	0.27	0.04	0.00
Location not known	−0.08	0.05	0.11	−0.09	0.05	0.08
Design ref. cat.: descriptive						
Non systematic comparison	0.11	0.03	0.00	0.08	0.03	0.00
Systematic comparison	0.21	0.03	0.00	0.18	0.03	0.00
Design not known	−0.08	0.04	0.07	−0.11	0.04	0.01
Subject ref. cat.: HSR						
epidemiology	0.07	0.03	0.01	0.09	0.03	0.00
health promotion	−0.07	0.04	0.07	−0.06	0.04	0.14
methodology	0.07	0.04	0.09	0.05	0.04	0.18
health information	0.06	0.05	0.18	0.11	0.05	0.03
Subject not classifiable	0.06	0.08	0.46	0.07	0.08	0.40
illness specific research	0.03	0.02	0.20	0.04	0.02	0.09
Region ref. cat.: North-West						
West-Central				−0.16	0.03	0.00
South				−0.14	0.05	0.00
NICCCEE				−0.30	0.03	0.00
Non-European				−0.10	0.06	0.06
Adj R2	0.29			0.33		

*) Areas indicate significance levels of $p > 0.05$. Dependent variable is mean score of each abstract.

6. focuses on (determinants of) health rather than health services research
7. is written by a North-West European first author rather than by an Eastern European

Discussion

It seems worthwhile to keep the scoring and submission records of conference abstracts. Even this preliminary analysis gives some quantitative insight in the dynamics of the abstract scoring procedure. It also seems to be worthwhile to score the abstract forms on relevant dimensions; good ratings are, to some extent, predictable.

The quantitative scoring system with multiple judges forms a solid and time saving base for decisions about rejection or acceptance of abstracts. The conference organizers adopted this method from the British Society of Social Medicine in 1991 and it can be recommended to all conference organisers. Although some judges have systematically lower scores than others, the fact that one abstract is scored by about 5 to 10 judges makes the change of only 'sour' judges quite low.

Why this year's motto does not and last year's motto does influence the rating positively, we do not know. A possible explanation could be that criteria for abstracts that are not typical research abstracts are established after the conference organizers are confronted with a substantial set of them. So, the criteria to judge 'health information abstracts' or 'public health practice' abstracts appeared after the Brussels conference of 2001; they were published in the 2002 – call for abstracts. We are also puzzled by the fact that the introduction of the 'region' does not explain away the coefficients in the first analysis. We had expected that abstracts from North-West Europe would have got higher rates because they were better structured, rather quantitative than qualitative, rather comparative than descriptive etc. This does not seem to be the case; introducing the 'region-factor' does not reduce or even alter the previously found coefficients; it adds explained variance of its own.

We do not know which specific predictors hide behind the broad region factor. We have been toying with an idea, but rejected it because of the complex data collection it required; It might be the case that some research received lower rates because it did not add much to the existing knowledge, although the studies might have flawless designs. Some studies show that social health inequalities also exist in Hungary or the Czech republic, because studies were repeated for the first time for these countries. The same goes for smoking prevalence in Georgia or food habits in the Baltics. In our analysis, we did not rate whether a study contributed something new to the domain of research. That would have required a much more complicated data collection.

Limitations of the study

This study is a typical first analysis, driven by curiosity. Literature about quality assessment of research should be included. In fact, a fourth research question should have been added, that reads as follows: 'How valid and reliable is the abstract evaluation process?' Corrections for inter-judge variances could improve real insight into the quality of the abstracts. There might be relevant interactions between year, region and other abstract characteristics, but these were not included in the analysis. The reliability of the ratings of the abstracts by the authors of the paper is not perfect and could have been improved. This may be a recommendation for future research.

The legibility of the abstract was scored low only when it was literally illegible (due to e.g. fax problems) or completely incomprehensible. It may be so that a more refined scale, making a distinction between abstracts in fluent English and those where authors struggled with the language, would contribute to the evaluation of the judges. It would have been nice if lists of conference participants had also been kept and computerized. Now all statements about 'participation' are based on submitted abstracts.

One should notice that the study should not be taken too seriously. It gives an intriguing insight and that is it. Therefore we end with 'lessons for the future'. Based on the results of the regression analysis abstracts can be optimized. The regression analysis provides Hints for an ideal abstract that will be shown below.

Lessons for the future: how to optimize my abstract

Lesson 1: have an author from North-Western Europe as first author; borrow a colleague if you happen to live in the East or South (or organise a fellowship in one of the more favourable countries).

Lesson 2: follow the instructions; use the background, aim, method, results, discussion scheme.

Lesson 3: Have a quantitative design, preferably internationally comparative and not locally.

Lesson 4: Avoid descriptive studies; tell in advance (that is: in the introduction) which groups or situations you are going to compare and why.

Lesson 5: Do a study about health and not about health care (personally the authors would deplore if you did, but it helps a bit if you want to optimize your rate).

Good luck next year!!!!

Other recommendations

In order to promote the scientific development and information exchange from Eastern European countries, the conference might be more often organised in these countries. For instance, the NEWS circulation scheme (see introduction) could be changed in NEWES. Our analyses showed that the conferences lead to a higher participation of those coming from the organizing country.

The fact that the average score of the abstract is around three could interpreted as the outcome of a solid judgement method. However, since the scores are on a 5-point scale, from psychological literature it is known that persons tend to locate their score around the thee. To force judges into a choice for a more positive or negative judgement, a six-point scale could be introduced. (A minor drawback of this is of course that there will be a trend-break in the data, which implies that an analysis like this has to wait another 10 years to be carried out).

Table 2. Scoring form for content analysis

Name of rater	Code	Year	Code	Year	Code	Year	Code	Year
General								
Abstract does not belong to a workshop (0), overall describes a workshop (1), belongs to a workshop (2)								
Does it follow the guidelines?	Yes	No	Yes	No	Yes	No	Yes	No
Is it in English?	Yes	No	Yes	No	Yes	No	Yes	No
Is it legible?	Yes	No	Yes	No	Yes	No	Yes	No
Is it a quantitative (1) or qualitative (2) study? If combined (3), if not applicable (9)								
Type of design: descriptive (1), non-systematic comparison (2), systematic comparison (3), don't know (8), not appl. (9)								
Is it a local (1), national (2) or international (3) study? Don't know (8), not applicable (9)								
Is the topic related to the motto of the conference?	Yes	No	Yes	No	Yes	No	Yes	No
Is the topic related to the motto of last year's conference? Not applicable (9)	Yes	No	Yes	No	Yes	No	Yes	No
Disease(s) under study: Not applicable (0)								
Does it deal with health services/ health systems research?	**Yes**	**No**	**Yes**	**No**	**Yes**	**No**	**Yes**	**No**
Organization (structure, management, planning etc.)	Yes	No	Yes	No	Yes	No	Yes	No
Utilization, supply, demand	Yes	No	Yes	No	Yes	No	Yes	No
Economics (cost, benefit, financing etc.)	Yes	No	Yes	No	Yes	No	Yes	No
Practice and outcome (quality, patient-practitioner-interaction etc.)	Yes	No	Yes	No	Yes	No	Yes	No
Health care policy (laws, regulations, reforms etc.)	Yes	No	Yes	No	Yes	No	Yes	No
Education and training of health service providers	Yes	No	Yes	No	Yes	No	Yes	No
Inpatient care (1) or outpatient care (2), combined (3), not applicable (9)								
Does it deal with epidemiology?	**Yes**	**No**	**Yes**	**No**	**Yes**	**No**	**Yes**	**No**
Mortality	Yes	No	Yes	No	Yes	No	Yes	No
Morbidity (disease focus)	Yes	No	Yes	No	Yes	No	Yes	No
Disability	Yes	No	Yes	No	Yes	No	Yes	No
Health Status (health focus)	Yes	No	Yes	No	Yes	No	Yes	No
Self-assessed health	Yes	No	Yes	No	Yes	No	Yes	No
Variables under study								
Biological	Yes	No	Yes	No	Yes	No	Yes	No
Psychological	Yes	No	Yes	No	Yes	No	Yes	No
Behavioral/life-styles	Yes	No	Yes	No	Yes	No	Yes	No
Socioeconomic	Yes	No	Yes	No	Yes	No	Yes	No
Environmental	Yes	No	Yes	No	Yes	No	Yes	No

Table 2 (continued)

Name of rater	Code	Year	Code	Year	Code	Year	Code	Year
General								
Does it deal with health promotion?	Yes	No	Yes	No	Yes	No	Yes	No
Health education	Yes	No	Yes	No	Yes	No	Yes	No
Public health policy	Yes	No	Yes	No	Yes	No	Yes	No
Does it deal with methods (data collection, measurement, indicators ...)	Yes	No	Yes	No	Yes	No	Yes	No
Does it deal with health information?	Yes	No	Yes	No	Yes	No	Yes	No
Databases	Yes	No	Yes	No	Yes	No	Yes	No
EMD	Yes	No	Yes	No	Yes	No	Yes	No

Other (if the abstract does not fit into one of the above main categories please give a short description, indicate code_year!)

Coding instructions (revised)

▶ Code_Year: If an abstract has the number 11 and belongs to the 1994 abstracts, fill in 11_94 for code_year. Always copy the complete abstract number (e.g. poster 5_94, chr17_95).

▶ Mottos of the conferences:

1994: Epidemiology, Prevention, Health Policy, Health Services Research

1995: Public Health Research, Policy and Practice and Health Care Reforms

2000: Reduction of Health Inequalities. Nutrition and Health

2001: Health Information/Policy

2002: Bridging the gap between research and policy in public health. Information, promotion and training

▶ Please assign one abstract to one of the main categories only (these are: Health Services Research or Epidemiology or Health Promotion or Methods or Health Information or Other). If the abstract seems to belong to two categories, choose the one that it mainly belongs to. Only if no clear decision can be made, it can be assigned to two main categories. This should be the exception however. Please indicate this at the bottom of the form (in the 'other'-field).

▶ If an abstract e.g. makes a comparison between several regions, it should be coded as (1) local instead of (2) national.

▶ Diseases are coded according to the ICD-10. Please fill in the code(s) for the disease(s) as listed below (maximum 3 diseases, separate with commas, if more diseases mentioned: code 99).

1 Certain infectious and parasitic diseases

2 Neoplasms

3 Diseases of the blood and blood forming organs and certain disorders involving the immune mechanism

4 Endocrine, nutritional and metabolic diseases

5 Mental and behavioural disorders

6 Diseases of the nervous system

7 Diseases of the eye and adnexa

8 Diseases of the ear and mastoid process

9 Diseases of the circulatory system

10 Diseases of the respiratory system

Table 3. Themes of the conferences

Location	Year	Theme
Copenhagen	1994	Epidemiology, prevention, health policy, HSR
Budapest	1995	Pub. health research, policy and practice/health care reforms
London	1996	Evidence-based pub. health policy and pract.
Pamplona	1997	Health of the regions
Göteborg	1998	New technology and public health
Prague	1999	A decade of health care reforms
Paris	2000	Reducing inequalities/nutrition & health
Brussels	2001	Health information systems

11 Diseases of the digestive system
12 Diseases of the skin and subcutaneous tissue
13 Diseases of the musculoskeletal system and connective tissue
14 Diseases of the genitourinary system
15 Pregnancy, childbirth and the puerperium
16 Certain conditions originating in the perinatal period
17 Congenital malformations, deformations and chromosomal abnormalities
18 Symptoms, signs and abnormal clinical and laboratory findings, not elsewhere classified
19 Injury, poisoning and certain other consequences of external causes
20 External causes of morbidity and mortality
99 More than three diseases

If the abstract does not deal with a disease, please fill in a for not applicable!

European Journal of Public Health and EUPHA – 10 years on

Martin McKee

Why a European Journal of Public Health?

Anniversaries provide an opportunity for reflection. Where have we come from? Where are we going? And why are we here? My task is to reflect on these questions as they relate to our journal, the European Journal of Public Health.

The first question, where have we come from, is the easiest one to answer. We began as an idea by my predecessor, Per-Gunner Svensson, who identified the need for a public health journal with a particular European focus. Of course there were already many national public health journals, and even some regional ones, such as the excellent Scandinavian Journal of Public Health. At that time the Journal of Epidemiology and Community Health was still largely a British journal, although it has since been transformed under the outstanding editorship of Carlos Alvarez and John Ashton. And of course there were the many more specialised journals in areas such as epidemiology, economics and so on. But at a time when borders were opening all across Europe, whether through the Schengen Agreement within the European Union or the Treaty of Paris, which marked the end of the cold war, there was a clear gap in the market for a specifically European multi-disciplinary perspective.

The rest is history. The journal had predated the creation of EUPHA but once EUPHA was established the benefits of partnership were apparent. The European Journal of Public Health became the official journal of EUPHA. Since then the journal has prospered. While recognising the limits of bibliometric measures, and in particular their inherent bias against non-American journals [15], we can be comfortable, while never complacent about our steadily increasing impact factor. We are also indexed in MEDLINE, bringing our content to a much larger audience.

Adapting to a changing world

The next question is where we are going? This is more difficult to answer. The journal occupies an unusual niche. In an increasingly commercial publishing environment it simply does not fit into the usual mould. By distributing copies to the very large membership of EUPHA it saturates the potential market in Europe. Not unreasonably, many libraries ask why they should subscribe to the journal when they know that they can obtain copies from staff of their institution who are members of EUPHA. This is, of course, great for the journal's ability to reach a wide audience but hopeless for its finances. Although we have a respectable number of subscriptions from universities in other parts of the world, in particular in North America, we have to accept that, in the USA, where the main market for biomedical journals lies, we face a huge barrier simply because of the lack of interest among most Americans in things that take place in other parts of the world [1].

We are also constrained by our method of distribution, with costs borne by the national associations. This means that we cannot easily do what we clearly should if we are to become more timely or to accept a greater number of the many good papers we are now forced to reject. It also makes it difficult to go further beyond the increasingly old-fashioned model of a journal as something that simply publishes those papers that are sent to it, never thinking about what else it can do for its readers by stimulating discussion and debate or bringing them news.

This is why EUPHA is now reassessing the nature of its journal. I am convinced there will always be a case for journals printed on paper, at least until someone develops a light weight computer display that can safely be read in the bath, but we also need to recognise that access to the internet among potential readers is now virtually universal. Ten years ago the idea that someone in Novosibirsk or Kishinev might have easy access to an electronic journal published in the west was unimaginable. Yet increasingly, in countries that missed out on the expansion of static telephone lines during the 1960s, individuals are jumping to new forms of mobile internet access. The world is changing incredibly rapidly and we must ensure that we meet the challenges involved.

The internet offers also offers advantages to those who interact with journals as authors and referees, with an increasing number enabling electronic submission and on-line reviewing. But all of these things cost money, something that we, with our current financial resources, can only dream of.

Yet a paper copy still has many advantages, apart from the ability to read it in the bath. The amount of information available on the internet is immense but how much of it do we ever access? A journal is more than simply an archive of data to be consulted when needed. It also has a role to communicate emerging ideas and prompt debate. If that paper copy no longer drops through our letter box, will we really go to the trouble of looking for it? And what will this mean for the sense of identity that we seek to engender among members of EUPHA, for whom the only connection is often the annual meeting. In other words, how can we grasp the potential advantages of the new technology, without loosing the benefits of the old? Until we answer these questions we can only speculate as to where we will go in the future.

A distinctively European contribution

So we can easily answer the first of our questions, where have we come from? We have more problems with the second one, where are we going? But then, those who predict the future with confidence are often proved wrong [2]. But what of the third question, why we are here?

This is the question that is the most important? What need is there for a distinctive European journal of public health? This apparently simple question raises two issues. One is what it means to be European? The second relates to the nature of public health. We will examine each in turn.

The definition of Europe has long been a subject of exam questions in history and political science. International organisations offer little help. The European Union has expanded from six to the present fifteen countries, and is on the verge of a further expansion that could bring it to 25. This expanded body would include some countries such as Turkey, most of whose territory is in Asia, while excluding countries such as Norway and Switzerland that are clearly European, at least in terms of geography. It also includes places that are geographically very far from Europe, such as French Guiana on the north east coast of South America, and la Reunion, in the Indian Ocean, by virtue of their status as departments outré mer of France, while excluding Danish possessions such as Greenland and British ones such as the Channel Islands. So clearly the European Union cannot take our understanding very much further.

What about WHO? Its European Region inherited the states that constituted the Soviet Union, so it now encompasses countries such as Turkmenistan, with its historical links to Iran, and Tajikistan, which has much in common with Afghanistan. It also includes Israel, but not Lebanon, purely for wider geopolitical reasons.

But maybe this is the wrong paradigm? Maybe Europe is less a geographical expression, as Metternich once disparagingly referred to Italy, but rather it is an idea? Perhaps it is a shorthand for a set of collective values that distinguish those who inhabit a certain piece of this earth from those who inhabit other places? [7]. As the history of Dresden, where this conference is being held, reminds us, this suggestion would have been ridiculed 60 years ago. Then, my country, the United Kingdom, was at war with this one, Germany. Terrible things were done on both sides in the struggle for supremacy of different sets of values and beliefs. This city suffered further over the following 45 years, as the Soviet empire sought to impose its values on this part of a defeated Germany, and on its neighbours to the south and east. Anyone who doubts the benefits of breaking down barriers in Europe should come to Dresden and see why this is important. And it is only since 1990, with the breaking down of the barriers that divided us that we have been able to appreciate what Mikhail Gorbachev referred to as our common European home.

But what does this mean in practice? It is all too apparent that the diversity within Europe is still immense. We speak different languages. We eat different foods. We play different sports, and we find different things amusing. These differences give us a unique advantage as a massive laboratory for understanding the determinants of disease and the effectiveness of different types of policies in tackling them [3]. The observation that heart disease is very much less common in Spain or Italy than it is in Denmark or the UK has led to important insights into the benefits of the Mediterranean diet. One of the greatest contributions that this association has made is to help us come together to look at each other, compare how we share common problems, and learn from our different degrees of success and failure.

For we do have much in common, although often this only becomes clear when we compare ourselves with others. And it is particularly obvious when we compare ourselves with the other major industrialised system, the USA.

This comparison is often particularly difficult for those like myself who live in the United Kingdom. We speak the same language, sort of, even if we pronounce the words differently. The massive penetration of our media by American products, the pervasive presence of American fast-food outlets, and the continuing attempts by some British politicians to win the race with Puerto Rico to become the fifty-first state often causes a crisis of identity, which is especially apparent at times like the present, when Downing Street has reinvented itself as a branch of the State Department.

But we should not allow this to obscure the profound differences, many of which are central to public health. I believe that the journal provides us with a real opportunity to demonstrate our common European values, values that we share with one another regardless of other political differences. One very obvious example is respect for life. All countries in Europe are united in their belief that the state should not deny criminals their right to life. Abolition of the death penalty is a prerequisite for membership of both the European Union and the Council of Europe. It is, fundamentally, a core European value. The USA, in contrast, executes not only those people who are both guilty and aware of what they did, but it is also among the handful of countries to execute those who were teenagers when they committed their crimes, or whose mental capacity was such as to prevent them from understanding what they were doing. A few years ago we published an editorial on the death penalty [14]. But what has this to do with a journal of public health? I believe it has a lot to do with it. It is but one example of where we, as Europeans, have something to say. We can use our journal to draw attention to the injustices that persist because of the retention of the death penalty in some countries.

But Europe is different in other ways. Take health care. All countries in Europe have found some way to ensure universal health care coverage [10]. The way they do it may differ and the fairness with which they redistribute resources may vary. But they still manage to ensure that almost everyone can receive timely and effective health care. This is not the case everywhere else. As a consequence we have published many papers on health and equity and, in particular, we have encouraged studies that have cast light on those who are often least visible in our societies, the migrants who come to our countries fleeing persecution just as many Europeans fled from totalitarian regimes in Europe, seeking refuge in America in previous generations [6].

Taking a wider perspective

We also try to see the big picture. From the earliest days it was recognised that promoting health involves a struggle. This was seen, typically, as our struggle against infections and their vectors. While the poor are disproportionately afflicted by infectious disease, its unpredictability means that everyone is at risk, and it can even bring down political systems. As Lenin noted, "If communism does not destroy the louse, the louse will destroy communism". The struggle between humans and infections is never-ending; the challenge is to keep one step ahead of the microorganisms. This requires constant vigilance and the implementation of policies that tackle the reasons why infections get ahead of the curve. These policies require an international effort and here too we have encouraged papers that look at the scope for collaboration within Europe and world wide [13].

But the leading threats to health are no longer confined to micro-organisms. Death is now being spread by other vectors. Reflecting its role as the leading cause of premature death in Europe, we feature many papers on tobacco. Tobacco is spread by an agent as dangerous as the rats and fleas that brought plague to Europe in the fourteenth century, by an agent, the tobacco industry, that shares many features with the rats that spread plague, although I realise that some rats may resent the comparison.

We became involved with this agent of death a few years ago when we published a paper by an author who, unbeknown to us, while occupying an academic post at a leading Swedish university, was a paid consultant to the tobacco industry [4]. Since then this has become the subject of legal action in Switzerland [11]. As part of this process we have had the privilege of helping to expose the web of secret financial transactions that have allowed the tobacco industry to take advantage of the activities of a small number of academics who continue to seek to discredit the now well-established link between passive smoking and premature death.

Earlier I was somewhat critical of the United States, but this is an issue where we have benefited by learning from our American colleagues, in particular Stan Glantz, at San Francisco, who is one of the true heroes of public health because of his relentless fight against the tobacco industry, regardless of the risk to himself [8]. The work that he and his colleagues did in making available the tobacco industry's internal documents was invaluable to us. Hopefully more researchers in Europe will follow his example, casting light on how the tobacco industry is thinking so that much more effective interventions can be developed to combat them. As the recent article in Stern magazine about the extensive links between the tobacco industry and senior figures in Germany showed [12], there is much to be done on this side of the Atlantic.

Of course some questions have no easy answers. Readers must make up their own minds. But we can try to help by providing the information in a way that facilitates comparison. One recent example, albeit rather technical, was a series of papers that looked at risk adjustment in competing social insurance systems [9]. Another recent commentary looked at the challenges facing epidemiology as it strives to go beyond the relatively easy questions, such as does smoking cause lung cancer to the more difficult ones, where exposures and outcomes are far more difficult to define and where interactions abound [5].

In this article I have argued that the European Journal of Public Health can be more than simply another public health journal. We have sought to ensure that we publish a wide range of original research, from a broad range of disciplines and perspectives, and from a wide range of countries. But we also try to see ourselves as, to some extent, a voice for European public health. However it is our readers who must judge whether we succeed.

Acknowledgements: The success of the journal is a reflection of the dedication of my colleagues on the editorial team: Anita Kallin, Staffan Janson, Carlo La Vecchia, and Johan Mackenbach, as well as Dineke Zeegers-Paget (EUPHA), Claire Saxby (Oxford University Press) and Tineke de Jong-Bijlmer (Z-Stijl).

References

1. Esler G (1998) The United States of Anger: The People and the American Dream. Penguin, Harmandsworth.
2. McKee M (1995) 2020 Vision. J Publ Health Med; 17: 127-31.
3. McKee M (1998) An agenda for public health research in Europe. Eur J Publ Health; 8: 3-7.
4. McKee M (2000) Smoke and mirrors: clearing the air to expose the tactics of the tobacco industry. Eur J Publ Health; 10: 161-163.
5. McKee M (2001) Epidemiology in the 21st century: the challenges ahead. Eur J Publ Health; 11: 241-2.
6. McKee M, Janson S (2001) Forced migration: the need for a public health response. Eur J Publ Health; 11: 361.
7. McKee M (2002) Values, beliefs and implications. In: Marinker M (ed). Health targets in Europe. BMJ Books, London. pp 181-205.
8. Maurice J (2000) Stan Glantz, tobacco warrior. Bull WHO; 78: 947.
9. Saltman RB (2001) EJPH Policy Forum: risk adjustment strategies in three social health insurance countries. Eur J Publ Health; 11: 121.
10. Saltman R, Figueras J (1997) European Health Care reform: Analysis of current strategies. World Health Organization, Copenhagen.
11. URL: http://www.prevention.ch/rylanderpm.htm
12. Wedemeyer G (2002) Kämpfer für den Qualm. Stern, 31 Oct.
13. Weinberg J, Grimaud O, Newton L (1999) Establishing priorities for European collaboration in communicable disease surveillance. Eur J Publ Health; 9: 236-240.
14. Welsh J (2000) The death penalty as a public health issue. Eur J Publ Health 2000; 10: 2-3.
15. Zetterstrom R (2002). Bibliometric data: a disaster for many non-American biomedical journals. Acta Paediatr; 91: 1020-4.

Part II Public Health Research and Practice

Public health and the way forward

GUNNAR TELLNES

Public health is one of the efforts organized by society to protect, promote, and restore people's health. It is the combination of science, skills, and beliefs directed towards the maintenance and improvement of the health of the whole population through collective and social actions [1]. The programs, services, and institutions involved emphasize the prevention of disease and the health needs of the population as a whole. Public health activities change with developing technology and social values, but the goals remain the same: *to reduce the amount of disease, premature death, and disease-produced discomfort, sickness and disability in the population.* Public health is thus a social institution, a discipline, and a practice. The Acheson Report [2] focusing on the future development of public health function in the United Kingdom gave this definition of public health in 1988: "The science and art of preventing disease, prolonging life, and promoting health through organized efforts of society".

Epidemiology and public health in the past

The general concept that the environment influences disease occurrence had its origin in antiquity, and so did a more specific idea that many diseases are contagious [3]. The Hippocratic (app. 460–370 BC) work *On Airs, Waters, and Places* already stressed the importance of considering the variety of environmental influences on diseases in humans.

The question of population health moved from a narrow concern of patrician comfort to political actions to control epidemic disease among the masses [4]. While the rationale for epidemic disease control prevented social disorder, it also stimulated new social concerns about the health and welfare of the poor. From early modern times, disease prevention became increasingly bound to broader issues of social welfare, especially as concerns with health, rather than disease prevention, began to dominate discourses from the nineteenth century. The idea that disease is caused by *contagium vivum*, i.e. a living contagion, necessarily depended upon the development of two other concepts: the specificity of both diseases and their causes, and the existence of harmful organisms [3]. The germ theory competed with the widely accepted ancient miasma theory, which had infective vapours as the central principle. Some practices commonly associated with the germ theory are truly ancient in their origin; for example, the custom of isolating people with contagious diseases is recorded in the Bible and was continued by the Catholic Church during the Middle Ages. And in the mid 1800s, almost 25 years before Pasteur (1822–1895), the *contagium* vivum doctrine was espoused by many European scientists. Indeed, there is evidence that it was the scientific basis for the initiation of the filtration of part of the London water supply in 1829. During this time the contagium vivum theory and the evolving study of epidemiology merged; thus began the current era of epidemiology. The essence of epidemiologic study is the comparison of groups of people with regard to characteristic of in-

terest, i.e. pathological factors more than salutogenic factors as described by Aaron Antonovsky (1923–1994) in his book "Unraveling the mystery of health" from 1987 [5].

However, the earliest recorded account of "an epidemiological comparison study", interestingly enough, is found in the Old Testament in the first chapter of the Book of Daniel.
Daniel asked for vegetarian food to eat and water to drink, and after 10 days his health
was compared to all the youths who had partaken of the food and wine of king Nebuchad-
nezzar. The underlying logic for the modern form of epidemiologic study evolved from
the Scientific Revolution of the 1600s. Francis Bacon at this time (1561–1626) developed
the basis of inductive logic and, with it, the concept of "inductive laws". Many seventeenth
century scientists reasoned that if mathematical relationships could be found to describe,
analyze, and understand the physical universe, then similar relationships, known as "laws
of mortality", must exist in the biological world. In 1747, James Lind (1716–1794) published his hypothesis from epidemiological observations regarding the etiology and treatment of scurvy. From his results, Lind inferred that fruits containing citric acid cured the
scurvy and that this would also provide a means of prevention.

Another epidemiological paper some years later, written by Daniel Bernoulli (1700–
1782) in 1760, had great importance for public health in the years to come [3]. Having
evaluated the available evidence, Bernoulli, a member of the noted European family of
mathematicians, concluded that inoculation protected against smallpox and conferred life-
long immunity. Using a life table, not unlike those of today, he determined that inoculation
at birth would increase life expectancy.

The French Revolution at the end of the eighteenth century stimulated an interest in
public health and preventive medicine, thereby facilitating the development of the epidemiologic approach to disease and public health practice. Furthermore, it permitted several
individuals from the lower classes to assume positions of leadership in medicine. One such
person was Pierre Charles-Alexandre Louis (1787–1872), one of the first modern epide-
miologists. His approach is illustrated by a comment made in 1836: "To determine the
question of tuberculosis (phthisis) satisfactorily, tables of mortality, i.e. life tables, would
be necessary, comparing an equal number of persons born of parents infected by tuberculosis with those in an opposite condition".

In a personal reference to the old epidemic pattern throughout a two-week period in
1849 my great, great grand mother lost her husband, father, and three children in a cholera epidemic on the west coast of Norway. This disaster changed her and the rest of her
family's social life dramatically [6]. One year later, the London Epidemiological Society, organized in 1850, with the initial purpose of determining the etiology of cholera, quickly
expanded its activities. Its report on smallpox vaccination in 1853 was, for example, in
England the main reason for the adoption of the Vaccination Act of the same year, mandating vaccination on a nationwide basis. One of the Society's founding members, John
Snow (1813–1858), conducted a series of classical studies of cholera [7]. His studies comparing two of London's water companies, and his investigation into the Broad Street Pump
cholera outbreak are well known. John Snow's achievement was based on his logical organization of observations, his recognition of a natural experiment, and his quantitative
approach in analysing the occurrence of a disease in a human population. The influence of
his report on Public Health Policy and Practice was more widespread than has been realized. It led for example to legislation mandating that all of the water companies in London
filter their water by 1857, only two years after the report's publication. This example illustrates that the situation is similar in our time, i.e. that there is a fine line between epidemiological science and public health policy and practice [8].

Snow's close friend, Sir Benjamin Ward Richardson (1828–1896) was among the first to
attempt to develop a disease-reporting system and to propose the teaching of preventive
medicine in medical schools. In this context you should notice that it was not until 1883

that Robert Koch identified the cholera *vibrio*. Throughout the 20th century many achievements have been made in the area of Public Health. In this paper, I will not attempt to cover the history of public health. The first part of the 20th century is properly described elsewhere [3, 9, 10]. However, in this context I will mention some examples: Immunisation, motor-vehicle safety, workplace safety, control of infectious diseases, decline in deaths from heart disease and stroke, safer and healthier foods, healthier mothers and babies, family planning, fluoridation, tobacco seen as a health hazard, etc.

Health promotion and the way forward

During the last 15–20 years, however, a modern, international public health movement termed *health promotion* has emerged out of the historical need for a fundamental change in strategy to achieve and maintain health [11]. In former times, social action against principal public health problems consisted largely of erecting physical barriers to the transmission of disease agents and providing immunizations. In the recent history of public health, recognition has grown that the behaviour of individuals in their present milieu and the conditions of life that influence behaviour, constitute a major health issue. The social environment, especially access and encouragement to indulge in tobacco, excessive alcohol, over-eating and too little physical exercise, has become more significant for health than physical environmental hazards. That is the reason for the profound shift in health strategies. The shaping of health promoting settings at work, in hospitals, in schools and in local communities, therefore, has been significantly supported by the World Health Organisation.

Achieving good health is one of the major concerns of contemporary societies. People are now called upon to play their part in creating a "healthier" and more "ecologically sustainable" environment through attention to lifestyle and involvement in collective efforts to manage risk. These strategies are the mainstay of the so-called "new public health" [12].

Today's health care system has mainly focused on pathogenic (illness causing) factors as the basis for treatment. Tomorrow's society probably must focus, to a much greater extent, on that which strengthens health, namely the salutogenic (health causing) factors as described by Antonovsky [5].

Nature-Culture-Health activities:
Creation of a new approach to health promotion

Salutogenic activities raise us and enrich us, build us up and make us more robust, by for instance strengthening the immuno-defense system. Therefore, there is reason to believe that there is an untapped potential for improving public health by employing health-promoting nature and cultural activities. This is also a great challenge to our new multicultural society. The goal is increased ability to cope, productivity and prosperity to *all* people, i.e. not only the affluent members of society, but also the ones who are in danger of becoming permanently incapable of working.

During the last 15 years my own vision has been to create a common arena and forum for wholeness thinking and creativity, i.e. "The Nature-Culture-Health" Interplay (NaCu-Heal), in order to improve people's environment, quality of life and health [13]. The challenge was to get various interest groups, i.e. public agencies, private businesses, voluntary organisations and pioneers, to co-operate in order to develop and bring about its realisation within a health promoting setting.

The NaCuHeal concept

By establishing local meeting places where participants may engage in health promoting nature and cultural activities, we will experience a positive and inclusive community. The activities strengthen the ability to cope, improve quality of life and enable us to deal with everyday life in a positive manner. To encourage Nature-Culture-Health activities, among other things, means emphasizing the positive factors leading to health (salutogenesis). *Health* may in this context be defined as having as little illness as possible while having the energy to cope with the tasks and challenges of everyday life.

Every individual, through the different Nature-Culture-Health activities, for example dance, music, art, physical activity, nature walks, hiking, gardening or contact with pets, will experience the indirect effect of feeling renewed zest for life, inspiration and desire for rehabilitation [13]. For persons certified as sick, this may be a method for returning to work. The direct route through vocational rehabilitation may be of help to some people. For others, however, it may be necessary to take a more indirect and creative route to succeed in their rehabilitation, i.e. to practice and participate in NaCuHeal activities to achieve a more useful and active existence later on. Participating in such creative activities may give each individual a sence of meaning and a desire to act. This "NaCuHeal effect" is for many people the only way to return to a working existence.

Health-promoting NaCuHeal activities and participation in them are becoming an important supplement to today's medicine and health services. All counties and local communities should establish a centre for Nature-Culture-Health, which can work as a catalyst in relation to other institutions within health, culture, outdoor life and schools.

At the National Centre for Nature-Culture-Health in Asker, a municipality west of Oslo, since 1994 there have been several experiments where people on sick leave, in rehabilitation or other social security clients have been helped to find their own talents and capacity for work to maintain function and pleasure in work [14, 15]. The concept of Nature-Culture-Health is based on the idea of stimulating to wholeness thinking and creativity within the Nature-Culture-Health interplay by emphasizing:
► Nature, out-door life, and environmental activities
► Culture, art and physical activity
► Health promotion, prevention and rehabilitation.

At a Nature-Culture-Health centre it is desirable to have positive interactions between persons of all ages, health status, philosophies and social positions. The idea is that such a meeting place between practitioners and theorists, between the presently well and the presently not so well, will be stimulating and enrichening to most people. Through participation in Nature-Culture-Health groups the individual will find the opportunity to bring to life his or her own ideas, for one thing by emphasizing positive and creative activities beyond one self. Persons with different afflictions may forget their health related and social problems for a while. At the same time, NaCuHeal activities may nourish other sides of one's personality that may also need development, attention and strengthening, to prepare for life in the community and new social networks.

400 years of public health services in Norway and future challenges in Europe

In the year 2003, the 400th anniversary of the Norwegian public health services will be celebrated. This commemorates the fact that a medical doctor was paid by public funding in 1603 and has been chosen as a milestone in the public engagement in this field. This appointment was an early example of a growing willingness and ability in Norway to take responsibility for the health of its citizens. It was in Bergen, the city where I grew up and graduated from medical school, that Dr. Villads Nielsen (1564–1616) was first given public funding. This was mainly due to his unique efforts during the plague at the end of the 16th century.

Nowadays, people in Europe live longer and lead healthier lifestyles than ever before. However this does not give grounds for complacency. One in five citizens still dies at an early age, often due to preventable disease, and there are disturbing inequalities in health status between social classes and across geographical areas.

Health systems in Europe are subject to a number of conflicting pressures. So health promotion and prevention is not often given political and economical priority compared to medical treatment. Demographic changes, new technologies and increased public expectations create pressure. Urbanisation, structural reforms and the need to improve the efficiency and effectiveness of health systems create other kinds of challenges for public health in the future.

References

1. Last JM. A Dictionary of Epidemiology: New York: Oxford University Press, 1995.
2. Public Health in England; The report of the Committee of Injury into the Future Development of Public Health Function. Cmnd 289. London: HMSO, 1988.
3. Lilienfeld AM, Lilienfeld DE. Foundations of Epidemiology. 2.ed. New York: Oxford University Press, 1980.
4. Porter D. Health, civilization and state. A history of public health from ancient to modern times. London and New York: Routledge, 1999.
5. Antonovsky A. Unraveling the mystery of health. San Francisco: Jossey-Bass Publishers, 1987.
6. Tellnes G. Slekta vår – ei ættesoge frå Sotra 1600–1979 (Our family history from Sotra 1600–1979). Bergen, Norway: Sotra Trykk, 1979. In Norwegian.
7. Snow J. "On the mode of communication of cholera" In Snow on Cholera. New York: The Commonwealth Fund, 1936; 1–175.
8. Ibrahim MA. Epidemiology and health policy. Rockville, Maryland: An Aspen Publication, 1985.
9. Rosen G. The history of public health. Baltimore: The Johns Hopkins University press, 1993.
10. Larsen Ø (ed). The shaping of a profession. Physicians in Norway, past and present. Canton, MA, USA: Science History Publications, 1996.
11. Bracht N, ed. Health promotion at the community level. New Advances Thousand Oaks, London, New Delhi: SAGE Publications, 1999.
12. Peterson A, Lupton D. The new public health. Health and self in the age of risk. London: SAGE Publications, 1996.
13. Tellnes G. Integration of Nature-Culture-Health as a method of prevention and rehabilitation. In UNESCOs Report from the International Conference on Culture and Health, Oslo, Sept 1995. Oslo: The Norwegian National Committee of the World Decade for Cultural Development, 1996.
14. Pausewang E. Organizing Modern Longings. Paradoxes in the construction of a health promotive community in Norway (Thesis). Oslo: University of Oslo, Institute of Social Anthropology, 1999.
15. Tellnes G. Samspillet natur-kultur-helse ved forebygging i lokalsamfunnet. (The nature-culture-health interplay and community based prevention). In: Larsen Ø, Alvik A, Hagestad K, Nylenna M (ed.). Helse for de mange (Health for the many). Oslo: Gyldendal Akademisk, 2003. (In Norwegian).

Public Health Research Strategies in Europe and the WHO

Godfried Thiers

My starting point for the debate is that Public Health Research (PHR) should sustain Public Health Policy (PHP).

Public Health Policy should intend to avoid or delay death (as long as life has an acceptable quality), to prevent or reduce handicaps, to reduce morbidity, to improve quality of life of diseased and the elderly, to increase capacities of independent life of the elderly and the handicapped. All this should happen with due respect of the freedom of opinion of people about the quality of their life and the acceptability of death.

My experience as director of a National Public Health Institute is that for Health Ministers, the availability of reliable health data is a first priority.

Just to give a single example. At least 2 or 3 times a year there are interpellations in the Belgian Parliament about the so-called high prevalence of certain cancers in some small geographic areas.

It is necessary to be able to respond quickly (max a few weeks) to such questions and to show whether this so-called high prevalence is real or not. A quick and reliable answer of the Minister of Health to such questions, which are often on the front-pages of newspapers, is essential. One needs scientists who are able to make a quick but reliable epidemiological study on this subject. Fortunately, today such quick studies are possible. Ministers will doubt about the importance of PHR if researchers are not able to give, within a short period of time, a clear answer to that type of questions.

I could also give examples of situations where Ministers had difficulties in accepting that certain research projects needed several years before being able to give results.

The major successes of PHR have certainly been in the field of infectious diseases. Just to give a few examples: the eradication of smallpox and the quasi-eradication of poliomyelitis.

This gives, at the same time, a good example of an excellent collaboration between the research community and those responsible for international health policy, i.e. the World Health Organisation (WHO).

Although the WHO is not a research organisation, whenever specific research is needed to sustain its recommendations, WHO makes this public and promotes this type of research (e.g. about the research on smallpox virus needed before the final destruction of the virus). Rather exceptionally the WHO will directly fund research, for example when there is an immediate and important need in a specific field.

An important question – and perhaps a dangerous one to raise in front of Public health researchers – is whether more PHR is needed.

First of all we all know that many scientists conclude their publications telling more research is needed in the field they are dealing with. Politicians do not like to read this, and I can understand that.

There can be no doubt that a lot of research is needed in many new areas, but I have the impression that too many studies just confirm what we know already, without that they have an essential impact on health policies or the outcome of health policies.

This is certainly exact for many studies related to the so-called life-style factors in PHR: smoking, healthy nutrition, obesity, drugs of abuse, AIDS.

Tobacco is an excellent example. We all know what a disaster smoking is for public health. However, non-smokers can hardly escape exposure to this known cancerigen, unless they retire from public life. There is insufficient political will to tackle these problems because there are important economic aspects, including the fact that tobacco taxes bring a lot of money in the public treasury. In Belgium there was recently a violent debate whether there could be tobacco publicity for the Formula 1 championship in Francorchamps. This seems a hypocritical debate. It is forbidden to promote this known cancerigen, but everybody, including children, can freely purchase it.

Do we really need more research on the effects of smoking on health? The answer is no, I think.

Perhaps we need more research on human behaviour and motivation. Which are the fundamental reasons why people want to take risks, accept to live with risks or even love to live with risks.

There are fanatic non-smokers who nevertheless take important other risks in life, like heavy drinking or eating, or exceeding speed limits with their car. Why the human being likes to take risks in life? What are the fundamental reasons for that?

Here we need interdisciplinary research with psychologists and, why not, with those who know to influence behaviour through publicity.

An area where certainly a lot of research should be done is quality of care, in particular at the following 3 levels: general practitioners, specialists, hospital care.

More research should also be done on alternatives of hospitalisation, since the latter is extremely expensive and risky (cfr hospital infections).

In view of one of the major challenges of the coming decennia in Europe, namely the ageing of the population, we need research on how to help people to live independantly and in a good status of mental health, as long as possible, and to reduce the period between this status and death.

Quality in primary health care should also be a priority area for research and the work already done in the field of evidence based medicine is extremely valuable in this respect.

Another area we have to consider as a subject for PHR is, what I will call here "Alternative medicine".

This is an area which has been intentionally neglected by the research community for many years, and this is still the case.

However, we cannot deny that an important fraction of the population, whether we like it or not, has an undeniable confidence in these alternative therapies. The success of the latter has a lot to do with the failures of our classical medicine, not for acute disease, but for certain chronic diseases and suffering, for which classical medicine has no satisfactory responses.

But, times are changing.

In May 2002, WHO launched its first global strategy on traditional medicines. In a declaration it was said: "Traditional or complementary medicine is victim of both uncritical enthusiasts and uninformed sceptics. The new strategy is intended to tap into its real potential for people's health and well-being, while minimising the risks of unproven or misused remedies".

In the issue of October 2002 of the American Journal of Public Health, there is an editorial on "What is the role of Complementary and Alternative Medicine in Public Health", followed by many articles on this subject.

Another point I would like to raise is about the foundations on which PHP is built.

Besides ethical criteria, which have always played a role, there were in the past mainly scientific criteria. They were generally broadly accepted.

We see today two new elements, which play an increasing role in PHP: the precaution-ary principle and some political ideologies.

Risk assessment is one of the important responsibilities of PHR, but more and more, when research does not show significant danger, products are nevertheless not accepted on the basis of this precautionary principle. The principle is already broadly accepted, even at the level of the European Commission.

We must also admit that "green" Ministers take sometimes decisions, which are con-tested by certain scientists on scientific grounds. In my country for example scientists have contested some decisions of a green Minister concerning the acceptability of oral intake of fluoride supplements.

We must admit that Ministers will have more tendency to use irrational arguments when the scientists are uncertain.

Public Health and Public Health Research in the European Union
The need for a new alliance

Hans Stein

The need for cooperation

There can be doubt that there is a very definite need to improve the cooperation and coordination between health policy and health research. We need more research, we need better research and we need research for the right reason. Health Services-, Health-Systems or Public-Health research are all areas, where more and better research is needed very much.

Public Health, as differently as it may be defined in the diverging and at the same time converging health systems in the Member States of the European Union, is not only an academic task, a scientific activity, a research area but at the same time – to my mind possibly even more important – a policy area, a political task calling for political action and not just for scientific analysis and explanation. It is not enough to explain the situation and to analyse the problems, it is necessary to improve it and to find solutions. I sometimes have the feeling, that the policy aspects of Public Health are underestimated, the research part exaggerated. This is also very clearly an area for European cooperation, because many of the problems are similar if not even identical in many countries.

Obviously there is a gap between research and policy. This gap has existed for a long time – and it still exists. The links between the scientific community and the policy decision makers are not as close as they should be. There is a lot of room for improvement. This is the case in many countries and most certainly this is the case in the European Union.

It is the task of research to advice, not to replace policy. Sometimes, possibly very often, researches are disappointed, because their advice is not always asked for, and – if given – not transformed and implemented into action as perfectly and as fast as they would want it to be.

But the laws and realities for policy decision – making are complex and beside needing a sound, possibly data-based "scientific truth" they also have to cope with vested interests, with political pressure, parliamentary majorities, legal issues especially at the European Union level, where the existing competences have to be respected.

"Evidence Based Medicine" may be difficult, "Evidence Based Health Policy" as desirable as it is, is even more difficult. But it helps if policy asks the right questions and research answers them in a way that can be understood.

By working together policy makers and the research community can produce not only more vital knowledge for health but also create a new kind of intersectoral collaboration.

The main objectives of research policies and health policy should be:
▶ to promote a new alliance between the research community and policy makers
▶ to increase the relevance of research projects, designs and reports for political action.

Problems and obstacles

In the past years there has been a gradual but continued process in many countries toward strengthening the scientific and knowledge base for health policy as a whole and health care reform in particular. Many of the new positive developments, be it the rise of "Health Promotion" as the base for a "New Public Health", be it the creation of "evidence based guidelines" to be used in Health Care, be it the establishment and introduction of transparent "quality control measures", to name just a few examples, have been triggered, at least influenced by research. Most certainly they would not have been possible without research. Moreover the wide dissemination of research results has contributed to the creation of a general consensus about the need for reforms, even if the detailed contents of such reforms are presently in the centre of a very controversial political debate. Possibly more research can contribute to making this debate less heated and emotional.

Nevertheless it cannot be said, that research has been the main driving force for change, for social and health reform. It seems that the needed links between reform and progress on the one hand and research and science on the other are much too weak. Because of their different, very often dual roles, scientists and health reformers are quite often fundamentally at odds with each other.

Sometimes the situation reminds me of a three arena circus. In the first arena one finds the policy- and decision-makers, the different stake-holders of the health system. The problems are being thrown at them like balls from the audience. It is this arena that commands the biggest public attention, accompanied by a large media coverage. In the second arena one finds the scientific community and the researchers, their activities getting only limited attention by the crowds and the general media, unless of course if they make some kind of sensational discovery. Nobel prices go to the discoverers of molecular mechanisms and not to those who work out the most cost effective method for treating incontinence. And in the third arena, playing to no spectators at all, one finds those performers who decide research priorities and about financing universities and institutes, most of the time looking for new kinds of research funding and new sponsors. In the present situation of scarce resources it is not surprising that they as well as the general public are preferring classical "discovery" topics of fundamental research and not the less spectacular issues of applied research. The Nobel price is awarded to "Medicine" not to health economics. Different to the circus however, where the 3 arenas are united into one at least in the grande finale, this does not happen in applied health research. There is very little interaction, co-operation and no integration or even "rapprochement" between health policy, research and research funding. The different actors prefer to keep by themselves.

A little booklet published many years ago-in 1994 to be exact-by the WHO/EURO and the Centre for Public Health Research in Karlstadt described the situation as follows- and their findings still apply to-day:

"Traditionally, public health researchers have not been very interested in designing their research to meet the needs of policy makers. Public health research remains centred around traditional health disciplines such as epidemiology, and has not been sufficiently been reoriented towards new emerging priority areas such as programme evaluation including economic evaluation etc. Similarly multidisciplinary and intersectoral research projects are still the exception.

On the one hand, policy-makers and health professionals do not systematically review and use either existing and new knowledge generated by research to support their decisions. On the other hand, many researchers are ignorant of key issues and developments in health policies. Policy makers should point out important topics for research. Researchers should not only study these, but advice policy-makers on their choices, then they should translate those topics into research questions and do the research, but they should not consider their mission completed with the publication of the research results in a scientific journal. Researchers should point out the practical and policy implications of their work and in the case of programme implementation they should not only evaluate the success of the whole strategy, but they should also make plans for the adequate and active dissemination of the relevant information in at least three directions beyond the research community: to decision-makers, to health professionals and to the general population. Finally, policy makers should then use these findings to plan, adjust and run health care systems and services.

Most importantly, what is needed is a new type of alliance between policy-makers and the research community. An effective strategy demands that policy-makers and researchers help each other to fulfil their complementary roles."

These are the necessities. This analysis is still valid today. Progress has been made since 1994, but much still has to be done: What are the chances to improve the situation at the European Union level?

The present situation of Public Health in the European Union

Public Health is up to now not a priority area of European Integration, even if its importance is being realised more and more, even if its included in the European Charter of Fundamental Rights, even if the legal competence basis is being strengthened in the new European Treaty being prepared right now by the Convent for the next Intergovermental Conference, which will take place in 2oo4.

There are a number of reasons for this situation. The main reason seems to me to be that the Member States as well as the health institutions and the health professionals are up to now not really interested in health as a European topic. They as yet see only little value in international cooperation. In line with the principle of subsidiarity they seem to be convinced that health objectives can be fully – and of course a lot better – achieved at a national level. Health is one of the very few policy areas where this kind of "nationalist" thinking still prevails. The problems and opportunities of cross-border cooperation or even globalism for health have not really been discovered yet. However a new line of thinking has been growing for some years now. Influanced by health activities of "non-health" institutions such as the World Bank, the OECD or the Council of Europe (and of course the World Health Organisation) "Internationalism" in health is becoming a reality. One example is a Council of Europe decision "to develop a real European health policy by harmonising the health policies of the member states". The Council of Europe might well make this kind of statement, because just as the other international bodies I have mentioned they – unlike the European Union – lack a binding political power. But their activities have demonstrated the possible scope and purpose as well as the impact of looking beyond national borders in health including health care.

In the European Union the biggest influence towards this change of attitude has to be attributed to the European Court of Justice. In a number of rulings since 1998 the Court by interpreting the Treaty, especially the application and implementation of the fundamental freedoms of movement of people, of goods, services and finances to health has shown, that healthcare is not immune from the influences of EU single market rules. They have shown that they have often indirect and sometimes even unintentional impact on the way healthcare is provided in and by the Member States. Even if the first reactions of the Member States to the now famous "Kohll and Decker cases" were rather negative, because they feared their sole right and responsibility for "the organisation and delivery of health services and medical care" (Art 152 of the Treaty of Amsterdam) were in danger, they today seem to have accepted that Health (and of course healthcare) is a European task, that however the future Health

Strategy of the European Union should shaped by the political decisions of those responsible for health and not by the European Court of Justice. There is nothing wrong with that kind of thinking if they keep to the general lines and principals developed by the Court.

Health Policy in the EU is now entering a new phase of development. It is moving from a series of separate, relatively small scale, quite often unimportant initiatives towards the formation of a more coherent overall policy vision with a clear evidence base. One important driving force for this is the need to respond to the challenges of enlargement and to find effective responses to new threats to health from for example communicable diseases and bio-terrorism.

In this context two activities are especially important:
► The Community Action Programme in the field of Public Health (2oo3–2oo8)
► The Council Report Health Care and care for the elderly: Supporting national strategies for ensuring a high level of social protection.

Both activities contain a number of issues in need of research support.

The Community Action Programme in the field of Public Health (2oo3–2oo8)

This programme was adopted on 23. September 2oo2 by the European Parliament and the Council. It replaced the 8 existing Public Health programs.

The general objectives of this programme are:
a   to improve information and knowledge for the development of public health
b   to enhance the capability of responding rapidly and in a co-ordinated fashion to health threats (including bio-terrorism)
c   to promote health and prevent disease through addressing health determinants across all policies and activities.

The programme shall thereby contribute to:
a   ensuring a high level of human health protection in the definition and implementation of all Community policies through the promotion of an integrated and intersectoral health strategy
b   tackling inequalities in health
c   encouraging cooperation between Member States in all areas of health interest including healthcare especially border-crossing health care issues such as centres of excellence and cooperation in EUREGIOS.

The priority areas for 2oo3 – and most probably for the whole duration of the programme – are going to be:

Cross-cutting themes: Health Impact Assessment; Health in the applicant countries; Tackling inequalities in health; Co-operation between Member States on health services including free movement of patients; Promoting Best Practice and Effectiveness; Aging.

Health Information: Developing and co-ordinating the health information systems; Operating the health monitoring system; reporting and analysis of health issues and producing health reports; Improving access to and transfer of data at EU level; E-Health.

Health Threats: Surveillance; Early warning and response; health Security and preparedness; Safety of blood, tissues and organs; Antimicrobial resistance; Rare diseases.

Health Determinants: Obesity, Tobacco, Environment, Alcohol; Drugs, Mental Health; Sexual Health; Training and Education; Injury; Health Promotion in particular settings (schools, work-sites).

A very important change is that actions under this programme should not be regarded as ends in themselves. Instead they should support and advance policy development in priority areas of the planned New Community health strategy. In this respect the objectives of the actions undertaken to implement this programme are very similar to the aims of applied health research, even if they are not called research. Sometimes it will not be easy to draw the borderline between research and policy action.

Another new key element of the programme is the development of links with other relevant Community programmes and actions in order to promote synergy and to avoid overlaps. In particular this will be done by launching joint strategies and even joint actions to achieve the objectives of the programme. One area where this should happen is of course research. A joint action with the EU research programme is essential – and might be an example of a new kind of alliance between policy and research.

The Commission intends to present a Communication in 2003 concerning the development of a new European Health Strategy. Research should and could play a decisive role in determining its direction and content. It is possibly the first time in history that research is being given such an opportunity.

Council Report on Health Care and Care for the Elderly: Supporting national strategies for ensuring a high level of social protection

This activity is a kind of first joint action between Health, Social Protection and Economic Policy. It was initiated by a Commission Communication in 1999 on "A Concerted Strategy for Modernising Social Protection Ensuring a high quality and sustainable health care" was identified as one of the key issues for closer co-operation among the Member States in the future. This by itself is quite a remarkable situation. At a time when Health policy people were fighting a – loosing – battle of keeping health care out of the European Union influence, other policies were trying to get health care into the European context. And even more important, they received the full blessing of the most important political institution of the EUROPEAN UNION, the summit, where the heads of state meet to set the political priorities. This initiative was indorsed by the Lisbon Council in March 2000, which stressed that the social protection systems need to be reformed, inter alia in order to be able to continue to provide high quality health services in the whole of the European Union. In June 2001 the Gothenburg European Council, in its considerations of what was needed to meet the challenges of an ageing society, asked the Council to take up this topic using the "open method of coordination", a new instrument for Community action in areas where direct EU legislation is not possible. Although there are no rules about the application of this new method, they differ according to the needs of the policy area where they are applied. In general they contain: the setting of targets and objectives, the determination of quantitative and qualitative indicators and benchmarks, the transfer of the targets to national or even regional levels, as well as the monitoring and evaluation of progress, all takes that cannot be done without research.

Having examined the future demographic, technological and financial trends, that present challenges to our future ability to maintain high levels of social protection and health care, it was concluded that three objectives had to be achieved at the same time:

▶ Access for all regardless of income or wealth
▶ A high level of quality of care
▶ Financial sustainability of care systems.

Whereas it was specifically recognised that the organisation and funding of health care systems remain a matter of national competence, it will be a task for the Member States to adapt their very diverse systems to these common identified challenges. A process of mutual learning and co-operative exchange is most certainly going to continue. To start with it will concentrate on the exchange of experiences and best practice, improving in a first step the information base and the development of indicators. All this too is in need of support by research.

The present situation of Public Health Research in the European Union

The history of health research, including Public-Health, Health-Systems and Health Services research is much longer than that of public health policy in the European Union and even a lot more successful, at least up to now. Whereas the first public health programme "Europe against Cancer", a policy initiative without any legal base in the treaty except a so called "catch all phrase", followed by an "European Strategy to fight Aids", Medicine and Health research activities have been going on at the EU level since 1978. It started with the first "Medical and Health Research Programme 1978", which had 4 successors. It was followed by the BIOMED Programme and at present health research is completely integrated into the 6th Framework Programme for Research with its specific programme for research, technical development and demonstration "Integrating and strengthening the European Research Area".

The first Medical Research Programme in 1978 started on a very small scale with a limited budget. Its topics were purely biomedical. From then on the programmes grew very rapidly in size, content and budget. But not only the budget grew. Already 1980, many years before the first health policy activities started, a group "Health Services Research" was established. Since then this kind of policy related research was a part of the EU research effort. With projects like the Atlas "Avoidable Deaths", a kind of forerunner for future Health Status reports, an "Economic Appraisal of Health Technology" or a "Description and Evaluation of Perinatal Care Delivery systems" the foundations were laid for health policy activities. The direct impact of this research on the policy at the EU level of course was very small, partly because for a long time, no health policy existed at the EU level and when it did – starting in the beginning of the 90s – the relations between these two policies were very weak. The biggest impact was probably made by a study "The European Union and Health Services" by the European Health Management Association (EHMA) that was published in 2002 it influenced the development of the EU Health policy strategy to a great extent. It was one of the sources of a policy document "The Internal Market and Health Services" of the so called High Level Committee on Health that influenced Commission and even Member States thinking.

The importance of these research activities is also shown by the fact that long before health care was accepted as EU-topic, it was part and parcel of research activities. It seems that research has much more freedom in choosing its topics, is not eyed with suspicion, does not need a legal base except the one for research. The whole extent of this freedom is shown by the fact, that health services research was not only included as a priority in the fifth Framework Research Programme, but more so by the way its objectives were described in the programme text, namely:

"Improvement of health systems: to improve the health of European citizens and the effectiveness and cost. Effectiveness of health promotion and health care technologies and interventions, to enhance health and safety at work, to evaluate health – care models, to develop evidence base for clinical practice and health policy and to study health variations across Europe."

The Commission made a call for proposals along those lines, but for whatever reason, possibly because there were no good projects, very little research work seems to have been done in that area during the 5th Framework programme. Other reasons are that as in the past the emphasis was put on biomedical not policy related research. And in the evaluation procedures of the proposals made the emphasis is still put on the so called "scientific excellence", less attention being given to the policy relevance, in which the evaluators have little knowledge and interest. The biggest draw back however is the lack of support for health services research from the Member States, who are reluctant to accept that health care issues are being dealt with at EU level. One can only hope that the changing attitudes will also lead to more support for and interest in the necessary research activities.

The new 6th Framework Programme for Research with its priority area 8 "Policy support and anticipating scientific and technological needs" will provide ample opportunities. It contains as a priority area a strand 2 called "Providing health, security and opportunity to the people of Europe". With two priorities:

► Health determinants and the provision of high quality and sustainable health care services and pension systems (in particular in the context of ageing and demographic change)
► Public health issues, including epidemiology contributing to disease prevention and responses to emerging rare and communicable diseases, allergies, procedures for secure blood and organ donations, non-animal test methods.

Their objective is: "Research is needed to deepen understanding and enhance the scientific base for policy on the main determinants of health in the EU and the developments in European health and care services". The first call for proposals made in the beginning of 2003 therefore contains a number of tasks all in direct connection to policy needs. To name just a few examples: establishment of demographic scenarios, investigation of the impact of key lifestyle factors, comparing Member States health costs at individual service level, investigation into different key factors driving health expenditures and in particular their interaction with reference to ageing, the role of the patient in health care systems, performance assessment of health care institutions, strengthening of the surveillance and control of communicable diseases through research networks, development of models on risk assessment including anti-microbial agents etc.

With this new programme and with this call for proposals the EU is making an offer to the research community to engage in research directly connected to planned and ongoing policy activities. It can only be hoped that this offer receives an adequate response and leads to new scientific knowledge needed by policy.

Conclusions

The existing disconnect between research and practice has to and can be overcome. The main obstacles such as funding by different institutions, general directorates or ministries and limited mechanism to transmit policy relevant issues and research questions to research can be solved or at least improved by establishing new procedures for setting priorities in applied and policy related research, by improving problem oriented peer review and evaluation of project proposals and finding new ways of disseminating research results to decision makers.

Priority selection of proposals should use the following criteria:
- needs of society, number of concerned persons
- unserved needs
- economic importance
- relevance for health care system and health care reforms
- scientific and technical innovation
- potential to improve top level research.

In order to apply these criteria a very strong interactive process is needed in which the different needs and interests of science are brought in line with the needs of policy. This could be done by the creation of a system in which:
- Health policy names its needs and defines its issues
- Research responds to the needs and translates them into research
- Policy and research agree on a common strategy including priorities and selection criteria
- Structured links for the implementation are established
- Evaluation of research proposals is done not only on scientific merit but on relevance for policy needs
- Adequate implementation of research results for policy use is assured and
- Evaluation of implementation takes place.

It seems to me that many of these criteria and steps can be implemented in the 6th EU Research Framework Programme.

Moving from research to change is hard and not easy. But it is possible. If we achieve it there is no need to follow a suggestion made in the Lancet some time ago:

"We should stop all research for two years and concentrate instead on implementing what we already know."

Public Health in the Netherlands

ELS BORST-EILERS

Throughout my eight years as Minister of Health of the Netherlands, I spent much time and energy on public health matters. I have always been convinced we can gain more health through public health-measures than through most healthcare provisions.

The article aims to describe the stand of Public Health in Netherlands. First, a few words about the health of our population. The second part describes how the Netherlands is tackling its main health problems and what the successes and failures are. Finally some current issues and dilemmas will be presented.

A brief status report on the health of the Netherlands

An extensive study on this issue was published only last week by the Dutch Institute for Public Health and the Environment. How healthy or unhealthy is today's average Dutch citizen? Generally speaking the Dutch are in good health. They are also living longer than their parents. Men now reach an average age of 75.5 and women of 80.6. Compared with 20 years ago, men have gained 3.1 years of life and women 1.4 years. What's more, people are spending these extra years mostly in good health.

Although we are living longer and healthier, life expectancy among men is not increasing as fast as in most other European Union member states. The increase in life expectancy among women has even come to a standstill. Indeed, we recently dropped into the bottom half of the EU life expectancy table.

As in many other countries in Europe, health is unevenly distributed in the Netherlands. It makes quite a difference to your health whether you are rich or poor, whether you live in a deprived district or in an exclusive residential area or whether you have a low or high level of education.

The key question is: what is causing the stagnation of life expectancy in the Netherlands? It appears that it has little to do with shortages in the healthcare sector. The stagnation stems mainly from our unhealthy lifestyle. I am referring to behaviour like smoking, excessive eating, too many fatty foods, excessive alcohol consumption and too little physical exercise. So it's principally modern health problems that are dragging us down. The recently published World Health Report of the WHO describes many of these problems. When the report was published Director General Gro Harlem Brundtland concluded that "the Western world is living dangerously". The situation in the Netherlands seems tot confirm this. So it's high time for action in the Netherlands. Strengthening public health seems the answer. Public health defined as: to protect and promote health, to prevent disease and to focus on inter-sector health policy and on secondary prevention among the chronically ill.

Health problems and preventive measures

Let me now briefly outline how we are tackling our health problems in the Netherlands and the preventive measures we have taken. I start by mentioning the three pillars of Dutch prevention policy.

The first pillar is Lalonde's model. According to this well-known model, five key factors determine health: (1) personal characteristics, (2) the physical environment, (3) the social environment, (4) lifestyle and (5) healthcare. Each of these factors influences health in its own way. They provide pointers for health policy measures. It has become customary in the Netherlands to set policy targets for health determinants and in particular for lifestyle factors. The targets are expressed in terms of the percentage of smokers and excessive drinkers, and the percentage of people engaging in sport or other active exercise, that we want to reach in a certain year in the future. Such quantitative targets help shaping policy and evaluating policy measures.

The second pillar of Dutch prevention policy is cost-effectiveness. We take the view that the benefits of public health measures must justify the costs. We know what various measures cost in terms of life years gained. These costs vary quite a lot. Most vaccination programmes for children are cost-effective, for example. But not all vaccination programmes. For that reason, we have decided not to vaccinate all newborn babies against hepatitis B. We confine vaccination to the risk group. Another example is the prevention of Legionella disease. The extremely high costs of making the water supply completely free of Legionella outweighs the benefits: it would mean spending many millions of Euros to save one life. But it will be clear that in practice it's not only cost-effectiveness that determines policy. Other arguments play a role, too. For instance the argument of the precautionary principle – meaning you must always limit known risks to the utmost, regardless of the costs. Several left wing politicians in the Netherlands take this view. Another factor one has to reckon with in policymaking is that the "perceived risk" is seldom the same as the "real, objective risk". In the Netherlands, we try to minimize these emotional elements in policy making by a system of rigorous scientific analysis of public health risks. This is done by the Health Council. Since 1902 it has advised the government on health risks and other public health matters. There is yet another obstacle on the road to objective, evidence-based policy-making. I strongly believe that we should make choices not only within healthcare and prevention but also between these two fields. But politicians, parliament and also ordinary Dutch citizens are mainly interested in actual problems in the cure and the care sector, such as waiting lists. Far less attention is given to the long-term effects that preventive measures often yield.

The third pillar of Dutch prevention policy is the idea that promoting and protecting health is not solely a matter for central government. Many parties have a responsibility here: parents and children, schools and pupils, employers and employees, health care insurers and patients. Local governments also bear a special responsibility for the health of their citizens. They must ensure that good quality preventive care facilities are available to every one. Think of such provisions as youth healthcare and clinics for sexually transmittable diseases.

Our successes and our failures

In some areas, we are reasonably successful. For example: we have a good infrastructure in the Netherlands for preventing infectious diseases. You may have heard about our meningitis C vaccination campaign, for instance, a total of 3 million young people up to age 19 have been vaccinated against the disease this year. For such a massive vaccination campaign, you do need an excellent infrastructure. And such an infrastructure is also important in case of a bioterroristic attack with, for instance, smallpox. As important as the availability of enough vaccines. While still Minister, I ordered the production of smallpox vaccine for the entire Dutch population, so we are ready for something that hopefully will never happen.

I believe we may also be proud of our monitoring of food safety. In my last year as Minister, I officially installed the Dutch Food and Non-Food Authority. Its remit is to ensure the safety of our food and all kinds of everyday articles – everything from stepladders to children's toys. The Netherlands is leading in Europe by establishing a food and non-food authority with such a wide range of tasks. I hope others follow this example.

In several other fields, too, health protection in the Netherlands is in good shape. I am referring to such matters as road safety, working conditions and youth healthcare. We have a nationwide system of clinics that see all children periodically. This allows faster identification of problems and timely intervention. Another example is the dramatic reduction of sudden cot death in the Netherlands over the last years, from 1 in 1000 babies to 1 in 8000, one of the lowest rates in Europe. This success is due to careful epidemiological analysis and intensive public education campaigns. We advocated two simple measures: 1) to let the baby sleep on its back and 2) not to cover up the baby, but to use a so-called infant sleeping bag. But there are also many things that we could do better. As Minister, I always advocated closing the gap between prevention and health care. The Dutch healthcare system has far too few incentives for individual prevention. During my term of office, too, we made only very modest progress on that front. Doctors and nurses need to be more aware of the health that can be gained by prevention, integrated in daily health care practice.

Our biggest problem at the moment is the increase in unhealthy lifestyles, that I mentioned earlier. The difficult question here is: how do you get people to change their behaviour? Indeed, Coca Cola and Philip Morris are much better in changing behaviour than we are. Far too many people in the Netherlands continue to smoke despite our restrictions on advertising, a ban on the sale of tobacco products to young people and a continuous public information campaign that includes photos of lungs affected by tar and nicotine.

Ideally, prevention of unhealthy lifestyle should start with young people. Children are being exposed at an increasingly younger age to all kinds of temptations and they often cannot resist these temptations. How do you stop this from happening? This is where we need more research. I will be interested to hear whether you have any experiences from which we in the Netherlands can learn.

Let me mention another of our failures: the health differences between rich and poor. This health divide is a problem many countries face. Our goal is to have increased in 2020 the number of healthy years of life among people in the lowest socio-economic classes from 53 to 56. It will need an integrated effort to reach this target; addressing income, working conditions, living conditions, educational level etc., all at the same time.

Current issues and dilemmas in prevention

One of those dilemmas is: how far can you go in influencing people's behaviour? Should you impose a tax on saturated fats in food – as some experts have suggested – thereby swaying people to adopt a healthier diet? Or should we allow people the freedom to live unhealthily and take the consequences?

Another important current issue is international co-operation. In my opinion: the fight against infectious diseases for instance needs to be organised more internationally. After all, bacteria and viruses do not stop at national frontiers. In the European Union, the Netherlands has always called for a European policy on infectious diseases. We now have a number of dedicated disease networks within the EU. But until recently, there was no formal European programme for combating infectious diseases. The first step in that direction was only taken after September 11 last year. There is now a European action programme aimed specifically at bioterrorism. The Netherlands will seek to expand this into a wider EU structure for combating all major infectious diseases.

A third dilemma is posed by the advance of genetics. Soon, we will be able to predict with growing accuracy whether somebody is likely to be affected in future by a certain disease. On the one hand, this may be seen as a good development from the point of view of prevention. On the other, however, there is the burden of living with the knowledge of a future disease. So: how far should we go with screening programmes? The knowledge of a future incurable disease should never be forced upon people. In the Netherlands, we have, therefore, introduced the Population Screening Act. For certain population screening programmes, you need permission from the Minister of Health.

I hope I have been able to give you a rough picture of the condition of public health in the Netherlands. There is a lot still to be done. In this context the theme of this Meeting: "Bridging the gap between research and policy", is well chosen. To my mind, the most important thing is to put into practice the knowledge that we already possess. Knowledge about health determinants, the causes of unhealthiness and ways of avoiding it. This body of knowledge is growing all the time, but we are doing too little with it.

Therefore and secondly, there should be better interaction between research, policy and practice. We need that interaction to make preventive care more evidence-based and to bring about an alignment with other fields of healthcare. We also need that interaction to get a better picture of the return on preventive interventions, both in terms of health gains and in terms of social and economic returns. Getting that picture will enable us to demonstrate that prevention really does work. In turn, this will raise public health to a higher place on the political agenda.

The third important thing is to do more research, because our knowledge base is still too narrow, particularly on changing behaviour and on risk management. There is hardly any scope for this kind of research in the EU's Sixth Framework Research Programme. Of course, the EU does have a separate public health programme, but that has a budget of only 52 million Euros. In my opinion, the European Public Health Association should try to strengthen the position of public health research in the EU research programme.

Public Health in France

Marc Brodin

Although this seems often to be forgotten, the main role of a health care system is to improve health. It can do so in three main ways. Firstly, it should ensure the delivery of effective health care that meets the needs of the population. Secondly, it should provide both curative and preventive health services. Thirdly, it should, where appropriate, promote actions and policies that address the broader determinants of health. This paper examines the structures and processes that exist within the French health care system that help to take forward this agenda.

Epidemiological facts

The French are in good health; they are healthier than ever before, but ... heavy smoking, alcoholism, adolescent suicide and road accidents are the main causes of premature mortality in our country. The French health system was ranked first by WHO, (a couple years ago) but ... greater emphasis is placed on cure rather than on prevention [1].

Life expectancy currently increases, on the average, by three months each year. Health-adjusted life expectancy has increased even more (68.5 years at birth for men, 72.9 for women; 16.6 years for men and 19.4 for women at 60). The single-disease profile of the less than 60, progressively gives way to multiple and chronic diseases of the elderly. A child born in 2000 should be able to encounter seven generations of his family; this interaction between at least four generations at one time is a major new phenomenon in the history of humanity.

Among the most noticeable epidemiological facts reported, in the January 2002 High Committee for Public Health report, we can note the following (Table 1).

▶ For the younger group (one to fourteen), the incidence of allergies, asthma and overweight or obesity has been increasing steadily over the years. Asthma now affects more than ten percent of the young.

Table 1. Main health problems

(1–14)	Injuries, Cancer, **Allergies and Asthma, Overweight**
(15–44)	**Violent deaths (traffic injuries, suicide)** Occupational injuries, Alcoholism, Cancer, Reproductive Health, STDs, Mental Health
(45–74)	**Cancer (lungs, digestive, beast)** Cardiovascular diseases, Mental Health Menopause-related disorders
(> 75)	Cardiovascular diseases, Cancer **Neurological deterioration (dementia)** Sensorial impairment Osteoporosis, degenerative arthritis

Table 2. Premature deaths (1 to 64). % total number of years of life lost

► Cancer	25%
Men: Lung + upper airways and digestive tract (10%)	
Women: breast cancer (9%)	
► Cardiovascular diseases	11%
► Violent deaths	35%
Road injuries (11%)	
Suicide (11%)	
► Alcohol-related diseases	5%
► AIDS	5%
► Other causes	19%
avoidable mortality ∼ 20% of overall mortality	

► Violent deaths or handicaps resulting from traffic-related injuries, suicide or occupational injuries are the key factors impairing health between fifteen and forty-four.

► Cardiovascular diseases and cancer become the major causes of death after 45, whereas their incidence may be associated with behavioural and environmental factors from earlier periods of life.

► Neurological impairment (dementia), sensorial deficiencies and osteoarthritis are among the main chronic diseases afflicting quality of life beyond 75.

► Once the French reach the age of 65, their life expectancy is one of the best in Europe. However, the mortality before sixty-five is one of the worse in Europe. At the age of 25, young French are at least twice more likely to die violently than young people from Northern Europe.

► Life expectancy is also seven to eight years longer for women than for men. Similar disparities are also seen between regions (North versus South) (2) and between socio-economic groups (3). Even though health has improved across all socio-economic groups, differentials seem to be increasing.

► Avoidable mortality before 65 accounts for about 20% of total mortality. This avoidable mortality may first be due to behavioural risk factors (road injuries, suicide, lung cancer, cancer of the digestive tract, AIDS, STDs,...), and to insufficient access to preventive care (early diagnosis of breast cancer,...) (Table 2).

The health care system

Three pillars support the French public health system:
► National authorities are in charge of quality, safety, access and redistribution
► The Social health insurance system is in charge of financing health care
► Local authorities are in charge of social aid funded through general taxes.

National authorities

The national government is responsible for setting policy and regulating the system

The national government has overall responsibility for the public health system, with input from various advisory councils and an increasing number of specialized technical agencies.

The ministry of health must ensure the harmonious development of the health system, the efficient use of resources, and their equitable repartition between regions. Legislation

Table 3. Specialized safety agencies. Specialized safety agencies (under MOH oversight)

> ▶ AFSSAPS (Pharmaceutical and health products safety)
> ▶ AFSSA (Food safety)
> ▶ ANAES (Accreditation and evaluation)
> ▶ EFS (Blood products)
> ▶ EFG (Transplantation)
> ▶ INPES (Prevention and health education)
> ▶ InVS (Epidemiological surveillance)
> ▶ AFSSE (Environment)
> ...

gives the ministry of health total control over the deployment of high technology equipments, and over the number of beds authorized in public and private hospitals. There are numerous controls over training and registration of health personnel.

The government also initiates national programs addressing major public health problems. Assessing needs and setting public health targets are Ministry of Health (MOH) responsibilities at the national level. MOH decentralized offices are responsible for implementing public health programs and ensuring the safety of health facilities.

Several agencies have been put in charge of specific responsibilities, ranging from the safety of pharmaceutical and health products, to health surveillance and to the implementation of health promotion and health education programs. Their development over the past decade underlines the growing importance given to behavioural, environmental or care-related health factors (Table 3).

The main responsibility for regulation and for setting national quality and safety standards lies at the central level. The National Agency for Accreditation and Evaluation in Health (ANAES) is responsible for conducting the accreditation process of health facilities and developing clinical guidelines, health technology assessments and economic evaluations of diagnostic and therapeutic strategies based on systematic reviews and expertise.

There are also numerous controls over pharmaceutical goods. Beyond the assessment of toxicity and efficacy that is part of the regulatory pre-marketing evaluation process, pharmaceutical drugs are evaluated in terms of medical service rendered, based on expert judgment regarding their benefits in clinical practice, including a comparison with alternative treatments. Both are conducted under the authority of the National Agency for the Sanitary Safety of Health Products (AFSSAPS), whose remit was extended in 1998 to include all health and cosmetic products, as well as post-marketing control and surveillance.

The Parliament

Since 1996, an annual Social Security Financing Bill (PLFSS) setting *a national objective for sickness funds expenditures* (ONDAM) is submitted to the Parliament by the government. However, this bill funds broad sectors and types of expenses rather than plans or programs addressing health priorities. Following the recent (March 2002) bill on *patients' rights and the quality of the health system*, a specific report on public health policy should now be submitted by the government to the Parliament before the debate on the PLFSS.

A new bill defining 5-year (required time perspective) public health strategies (health problems and populations; risk factors and health determinants; coordinated and integrated sets of actions and services; specific quantified or qualified objectives) is currently under preparation, to be discussed in the Parliament. We have not had any such law since about 30 years. Its stated objectives are the following:

- ▶ To reduce health inequalities,
- ▶ To prevent avoidable morbidity and mortality
- ▶ To preserve quality of life and autonomy
- ▶ To balance and coordinate health care, individual and collective prevention
- ▶ To "enable people to increase control over, and to improve, their health".

High Committee on Public Health and National Health Council

Since 1994, [4] the High Committee on Public Health (HCSP) has published three well-documented reports on *Health in France* (the last in March 2002) [5], as well as numerous specific reports. According to the recent law, the HCSP should evolve into an independent expert advisory panel providing assistance to the Minister of Health in defining public health priorities, and issuing a yearly report to Parliament evaluating the implementation of public health policies.

The National Health Council (CNS) was established in 1996, comprising representatives from the health care professions, public and private institutions, regional health councils and qualified persons. Its missions were to consider available evidence and propose public health policy priorities and health care management orientations in an annual report.

Regional public health structures and interventions

Regional Health Councils were established in 1996. They include representatives from the MOH decentralized offices, regional hospital care agencies, local governments, regional sickness funds, health and social professionals and institutions, and patients' associations. These meet annually to identify regional public health priorities that could be addressed by regional health programmes under the authority of the MOH decentralized offices.

Regional health priorities identified by Regional Health Councils have included prenatal health care networks, dependence in the elderly, cancer screening and prevention, mental health and suicide, school failure, alcoholism, road traffic injuries, housing improvement (lead poisoning prevention), access to health care and prevention. They should now evolve into more permanent formations, while bringing together various regional advisory committees that were established over the years to address specific health system issues.

Specific Regional Programmes for Access to Prevention and Care were instituted in 1998 to coordinate public efforts by national government offices, local governments and sickness funds so as to improve access to and utilisation of appropriate health care for all segments of the population. Their effectiveness has not yet been evaluated.

Under the authority of the MOH, Regional Hospital Care Agencies (ARH) regulate hospital care facilities. The deployment of major equipment has been regulated since 1970. Regional five year Schemes for Health Care Organization (SROS) were instituted in by a 1991 bill to coordinate the redeployment of private and public hospital facilities and to improve their integration in addressing major regional health problems. ARHs control the allocation of funds to hospital facilities within regional budgets set by the MOH, and are mandated to set up contractual arrangements with private and public hospitals to provide services according to the SROS.

Sickness funds and health care

The more recent development of health services' financing can be traced back to 1945, when the first social security law was enacted. Health care provision followed the German

Bismarckian model, which provided cover to the employed population and their dependants through social security and sickness funds [6]. This model relies on shared financial coverage, abundant supply of services, state controlled private and public sectors, free choice of provider and free prescriptions. Cover was at first limited to industrial workers; other sectors of the workforce and their dependants were added through extensions to social security coverage.

This social welfare system is mainly financed by compulsory contributions shared between employees and employers. In the past ten years, additional resources have come from taxes (especially income taxes of retired persons); taxes now represent 40% of the resources for health care.

Sickness funds are managed by elected representatives of employers and trade unions under the authority of the MOH. They mostly channel funds to health care providers. Funds are disbursed to public and private hospitals, as well as individual patients in reimbursement of services provided by private health professionals. Sickness funds also manage a "National Fund for Prevention, Education and Health Information" (FNPEIS) to finance prevention and health promotion activities, mostly revolving around clinical care and addressing diseases associated with high expenditures (diabetes, high blood pressure).

Private health professionals provide most ambulatory care, under fees schedules contracted with sickness funds, regardless of the actual content of the consultation. The dominant model for private ambulatory practices remains one of individual entrepreneurs, although the number of group practices has grown regularly. Public teaching hospitals provide increasingly specialized care, and also, more and more frequently, primary care through their emergency departments. Local public hospitals provide mostly non-specialized acute and long-term care. Private hospitals provide a significant part of surgical and obstetric care, and some specialized medical care.

The distribution of services between public and private hospitals has been influenced largely by differences between their funding schemes, under capped budgets for public hospitals and fee-for-service agreements for the private sector. Local networks that brought together varied health and social professionals to address the needs of specific vulnerable groups (e.g. elderly) traditionally were organized quite informally, often around family practices. Co-ordinated networks of health professionals have developed on a voluntary basis, responding to different needs and pursuing different objectives.

Currently, patients may choose freely where and when they access the health care system. Services provided are covered regardless of need or effectiveness criteria. Co-payment has been used extensively as an incentive to curb demand for *unnecessary* care, while full coverage was ensured for major interventions and a limited set of chronic conditions associated with significant expenses. Different reimbursement rates are applied to prescription drugs according to an assessment of their actual therapeutic value.

This national social health insurance system covers about 75% of health care expenses: overall, coverage is close to 100% for hospital stays and around 50% for ambulatory care. Patients cover the shortfall, although 80% retain additional coverage through mutual funds or private insurance. Mutual funds and private insurance companies provide complementary coverage and also develop health promotion and education programs.

However, several studies have documented that patients with limited resources gave up necessary care for financial reasons. Universal Medical Coverage (CMU) was instated in 2000 to provide shared complementary coverage to patients in severely precarious conditions. Recent evidence suggests that this scheme has helped its intended beneficiaries in securing basic and/or complementary coverage, and in increasing health care utilisation. About 10% of the population still may have difficulty obtaining care for financial reasons: being unable to afford complementary insurance but earning too much to be entitled to CMU (Fig. 1).

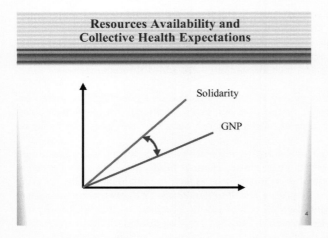

Fig. 1. Resources Availability and Collective Health Expectations

Local governments

Local governments, at communal or district level, are mostly in charge of preventive and social aid programs. They are responsible for social and medico-social interventions, such as planning the distribution of social and medico-social institutions, or regulating fees for social services (district-level regulation for social aid).

Together with mutual funds and non-governmental organizations they run a limited number of local health centres providing primary care to the general population, in some cases for specific affections (e.g. cancer or STDs), or preventive care to pregnant women and children under 7, including free prenatal care and children immunizations.

In 2001, funds allocated to district-level social aid programs amounted to a total of 10.7 billion Euros, to be compared to the 127.8 billion Euros allocated to Health care expenses. These funds went to the following social and medico-social areas:

► 47% to social aid programs for children (education, institutional placement)
► 29% to handicapped persons (housing, pensions for handicapped adults, compensating pensions)
► 17% to the elderly (housing, home aids, autonomy support funds)
► 7% to the unemployed (Minimum insertion income).

Environmental hygiene is the responsibility primarily of city or communal councils, with varying degrees of involvement. Some have developed very active communal hygiene, safety offices and programs.

While screening programs are, by law, the responsibility of district-level elected councils, national screening programs for major life-threatening diseases (e.g. cancer) can be set up under the authority of the Ministry of Health, following recommendations from the National Health Council.

Sources of health information and public health expertise

Numerous sources of health information are available in the diverse institutions involved in health care, financing, administration or research. These are, however, largely uncoordinated. Several disease-specific registers have been set up over the past decades. The data collected by the sickness funds in the course of the patients' reimbursement process and the DRG based system set up to improve hospitals resource allocation may also provide some information regarding the amount and type of care received by patients.

Population based registers include the national analysis of death certificates and regular surveys conducted by the National Institute for Statistics and Economic Studies (INSEE), the Research and Studies Centre in Health Economics (CREDES), and the National Institute for Prevention and Health Education (INPES). Regional Observatories of Health were set up in the 1980s (the earliest in the 1970s) as non-governmental organizations funded by subventions from or contracts with national and local authorities to develop regional health information systems. Their reports outline regional health needs, and an assessment of the implementation and effectiveness of health policies [7].

While public health expertise is available increasingly in the universities and national research institutes, its activity has traditionally been channelled toward biomedical or theoretical research. Efforts to improve this situation include the development of specialized agencies with appropriate technical expertise (e.g. the Research and Studies Centre in Health Economics (CREDES), mostly funded by national sickness funds), the creation, in 1998, of a Directorate for Research, Evaluation and Statistics (DREES) at the MOH and, in 1992, of the National Institute for Health Surveillance (InVS), expanding on the National Network for Public Health established in 1999 to develop epidemiological interventions. But significant additional efforts are needed to develop a consistent base of public health and health services research expertise.

Conclusions

The French health care system can be characterised by fragmentation of functions, many actors pursuing disconnected goals [8]. This makes it very difficult to develop the integrated responses that increasingly are needed to address the challenges of the future, as chronic diseases become more important and new therapeutic options make the health care responses ever more complex.

The development of consumers' expectations (following patients' duties and users' rights), new information technologies and the unavoidable international comparisons within Europe, have recently raised growing interrogations. New demands emerge from multiple sources, including biomedical researchers (research on human embryos), public health experts (asbestos), patients' associations (informed consent, access to information), relayed by the new information media, and sometimes sanctioned by landmark decisions from judicial courts. The march 2002 bill creates regional mediation structures with the authority to set up financial compensations.

In the context of European harmonization, there is a plurality of cultures and values. Liberal economic driving forces within the European Market unsettle national solidarity mechanisms organized by each state. Key values of the French Republic are under tension: Equality vs. equity, Freedom vs. liberalism, Fraternity vs. solidarity [9]. Respect for individual rights and privacy conflicts with open processes of collective institutional management, commercial interests and marketing approaches (Fig. 2).

While the focus has remained on health care financing and control rather than patients and public health outcomes, and on curative care rather than health promotion, some important developments are beginning to address these challenges. Increasing efforts have been made in the past decade to support responsible health policy choices with both expert advice and preliminary debates among major interest groups. Over recent years, both the High Committee for Public Health and the National Health Council have been promoting the use of explicit effectiveness and efficiency criteria to fund a combination of preven-

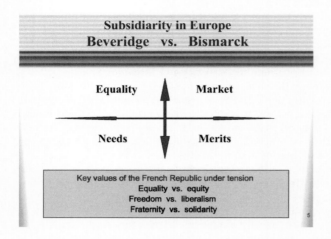

Fig. 2. Subsidiarity in Europe

tive, curative and rehabilitation services addressing identified health priorities. The combination of regional public health structures and hospital agencies provide a mechanism by which coordinated policies addressing the health needs of the population can be developed and implemented.

There is a need to extend the scope of public health activities and to develop more comprehensive public health policies including significant prevention components at the individual and collective levels. Resources available should be balanced against collective health expectations. The rules governing resource allocation should evolve from the reimbursement of health products and services to coordinated health programs, that is from market-driven individual choices for immediate results, to collective investments in health care and promotion in the long term.

References

1. Rapport sur la santé dans le monde 2000 Ed: OMS, Genève, juin 2000.
2. Gérard Salem, Stéphane Rican, Eric Jougla, Atlas de la santé en France, les causes de décès Ed: John Libbey Eurotext, vol 1, Paris 1999.
3. Annette Leclerc, Didier Fassin, Hélène Granjean, Monique Kaminski, Thierry Lang, Les Inégalités sociales de santé Collection "Recherches" - Ed: la découverte/Inserm, octobre 2000.
4. Health in France 1994–1998, High committee on public health – Ed: John Libbey Eurotext, Paris, Novembre 1998.
5. La santé en France 2002 , Haut Comité de la Santé Publique – Ed: La documentation Française, Paris, Février 2002.
6. Richard B. Saltman & Josep Figueras, European Health Care Reform, Analysis of current strategies - World Health Organisation, Regional Office for Europe Ed: WHO Regional Publications, European Series, n° 72, Copenhagen 1997.
7. La santé observée dans les régions de France, actualisations et analyses – les études du réseau de la fédération nationale des observatoires régionaux de santé, novembre 2000.
8. Dominique Polton, Quel système de santé à l'horizon 2020? Rapport préparatoire au schéma de services collectifs sanitaires – Ed: la documentation française, janvier 2001, Paris.
9. Nicole Questiaux & Axel Kahn, Progrès technique, santé et modèle de société: la dimension éthique des choix collectifs – Ed: Comité consultatif national d'éthique pour les sciences de la vie et de la santé, N° 57, 20 mars 1998, Paris.

Public Health in Germany

Friedrich W. Schwartz · M. Wismar · Ulla Walter · Marie-Luise Dierks

The context for Public Health:
prevention and Health Care in Germany

Modern health systems are extremely complex and expensive. This is true for Germany too. Germany's total health expenditure, expressed as a part of the domestic economic product is the third largest worldwide. In contrast to this top position in terms of expenditure our rank in life expectancy for adult men or women is disappointingly low [29].

Our perinatal indicators are excellent, oral health has improved substantially but a lot of severe threats and risk constellations are not tackled adequately. Preventive care, curative and rehabilitative services are lacking timely organisational structures and efficient management [17–19].

At the moment, the core of our health care system, our statutory health insurance, our pride since Bismarck's times over 120 years, is hit by an acute financial crisis. The political decision makers have ignored the signs of overloading this subsystem with many social task, which seemed to be financed so easily by wage depending contributions.

But the long standing weakness of our labour market produced an ongoing erosion of the financial basis of this wage depending insurance system. This had been aggravated by faults in economic integration in our national unification process and by weak efforts to integrate our immigrant population groups adequately. On the side of expenditure of our health care system we observe – following the patterns of western medicine – an stupendous overuse of diagnostic and acute care services contrasting with a neglect of many aspects of the care for the chronically ill. In spite of a complex system of 900 institutions (Fig. 1) with tasks in the preventive sector we observe almost the absence of structured national preventive activities beyond classical hygiene politics, or classical health protection at the working place or technical, or legislative and educational efforts in traffic safety. Yet, there are positive preventive efforts: 10 years ago the unified Germany started an intensified child and youth dental health programme, which raised the formerly very low oral health status in children to an extend, that oral health in German children is now among the best in Europe – one of our few new preventive success stories.

The German physicians in ambulatory care also offer broad flowering bouquets in medical screening for our population where the results show a mixed picture: good results in the nearly eradication of cervix carcinoma, unsatisfying results after three decades of occult blood screening in colon carcinoma finding, a nearly disastrous result after three decades of grey or wild screening for mamma carcinoma with high costs and an unacceptable overload of false positive declared cases [19]. The medical screening and care for pregnant women and for child development seems to be effective for good direct perinatal outcomes but widely ineffective in initiating good health behaviour patterns for young mothers regarding nutrition and smoking.

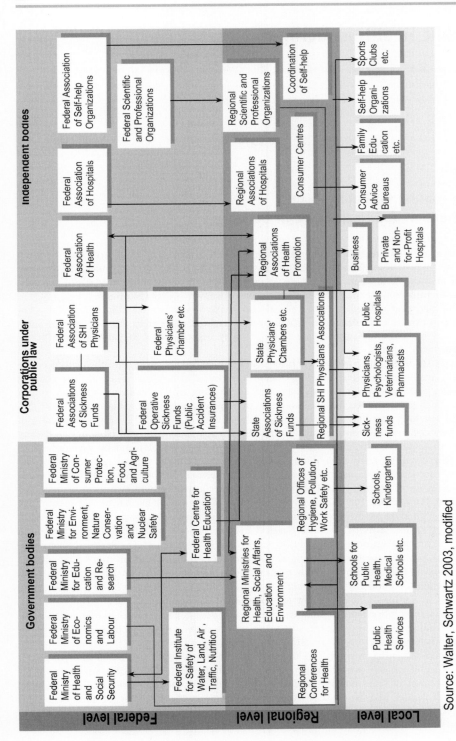

Fig. 1. Institutions and structures of disease prevention and health promotion at federal, regional and local level (Source: Walter, Schwartz 2003, modified)

Source: Walter, Schwartz 2003, modified

The child development screening programme from birth to youth is intensive and expensive but with a lot of scientific doubtful elements. In all those programmes we miss a strict and useful ongoing evaluation. Our physicians in the ambulatory sector offer a screening programme for some renal and circulation diseases, but its scientific background and its health impact is so doubtful that there is much discussion to de-list it. Instead we need a functioning and intensive prevention programme to roll-back our killer No. 1 in the middle aged population, the coronary heart disease. This prevention programme must be implemented both on the micro- and national level.

Our Federal Council for Health Care (Sachverständigenrat) voted strongly for this programme and also for a national anti tobacco campaign [19]. In the pre-election time this summer all German political parties did support these ideas strongly, and our red-green government announced national coordination efforts in all preventive activities. But currently, the overwhelming flood of acute financial calamities in the German social system could be a risk for more investment in prevention.

And the bureau of our chancellor – the chancellor himself is a well-known smoker – just recently voted – together with Austria and Luxembourg – against the anti-tobacco-advertising-decisions of the European Commission.

It is the Public Health community in Germany, which had and has to monitor these developments, to analyse the failures and the successes and to motivate and guide the politicians to move towards a healthier society and towards a cost effective health care system.

What is – after this short picture of the status of the German health system – the background and the near future of our Public Health community in Germany?

Public Health training programmes in Germany

Using qualification models in Great Britain, Scandinavia and the United States, post-graduate courses in Public Health were established in Germany between 1989 and 1995 at nine locations; in order of their founding dates: Bielefeld, Hannover, Heidelberg, Düsseldorf, Dresden, Berlin, München, Ulm and Bremen. In addition, Dr. PH or PhD programmes in Public Health had been established in some locations.

At the present time approximately 300 student places per year are offered on a university level. Nearly all programmes provide the opportunity to combine the study with a part-time job. According to the database at the German Coordinating Agency for Public Health, around 1200 candidates had successfully graduated until the end of the year 2001. [1]

Additionally to the university-based Public Health programmes, many other programmes or courses, focussing on Public-Health topics as Health Economics, Health Prevention, Epidemiology as well as full Public Health courses are running on a bachelor-level, some of them are distance-learning programmes. At present about 280 of these courses are offered.

The objective of the Master of Public Health programmes on the university level was and still is to train experts for management and decision-making processes within the public health service, legal sickness funds, associations of physicians and in public private mix-programmes, also specialists for the development, implementation and evaluation of health-promoting and preventive programmes and experts for research and teaching and partly also for the industry.

---

[1] Deutsche Koordinierungsstelle für Gesundheitswissenschaften [German Coordinating Agency for Public Health], oral communication.

New fields of activities, i.e. in Health Technology Assessment, evidence-based medicine, integrated or managed care or disease management, become increasingly interesting, both on the side of health care providers and of the public and private sickness insurances.

To ensure a high quality level of the teaching process, the German Association for Public Health established a multi-level process for a nationwide core curriculum, which serves as a minimum standard for all teaching programmes (http://www.mh-hannover.de/institute/epi/public-health-studium/index.htm). German Public Health programmes are therefore quite similar in their basic training (i.e. in the first year), but they differ – i.e. according to their research activities – within the range of the specialization courses.

Public Health programmes in Germany put high effort in the process of international co-operation and international perspectives by involvement in the European masters programme, by special courses in international and European health and health management or by international student courses, running on a complete international basis.

The actual employment opportunities for our graduates is positive, and the future developments as well. This is underlined by the results of surveys in 1996 and 2000: One third of the respondents were working in Public Health research, 20 % were employed in the Public Health services, 10% at sickness funds and physicians associations, 4% in national and international institutions of development and co-operation and 4% in the pharmaceutical industry [7, 11].

On the other side, it is remarkable that after more than 10 years of a successful development process the Public Health training programmes are so far still unknown by 40% of the potential employers if we include hospitals, pharmaceutical companies and business consultancies [21].

The future of Public Health in Germany

The context

The future of Public Health in Germany and Europe goes far beyond the compensation of health related social inequalities. Public Health emerges as an important force shaping our society towards better health for all.

There is clear evidence that the future of Public Health in Germany is inseparably linked to the international perspective. Not only science has become an international business more than ever before. Also health policy is certainly co-determined by policy transfer and policy diffusion from abroad [3]. Moreover, the impact of European integration both on health services [4] and Public Health – with threats and opportunities inherent in it – [2] should not be underestimated. Yet, there is a growing national and international perception of the social and health impact of global markets, well illustrated by recent activities and studies of the WTO (World Trade Organisation) [5, 8, 30].

To develop a vision on the future role and significance of Public Health in Germany, we can do this in cautious optimism which is grounded in the astonishing developments taking place during the last decade: A university based Public Health structure in Germany was successfully established as an academic discipline [25], a political practice and a social reality [9, 24]. These developments, can be best understood as a delayed modernisation [22]. They had been financed by a ten-year promotion programme of our Federal Ministry of Research. A good indicator is the rise of the science impact of German publication in this area and programme (Fig. 2). Starting from scratch and catching up at least partly with some of the leading nations in such a short time endows us with good faith in our abilities to meet the challenges lying before us – and they are numerous [1, 13–17, 19, 20].

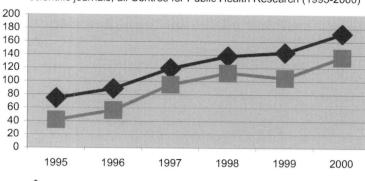

Fig. 2. Evaluation of the German Centres for Public Health Research (2001)

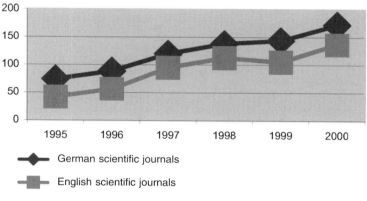

Fig. 3. Evaluation of the German Centres for Public Health Research (2001)

Yet, in comparison to clinical medicine our scientific infrastructure is still very limited. There is almost no funding by the industry. And the federal state has delegated so many tasks to the self-governing bodies of the health care system that funding of Public Health research that contributes to capacity building is permanently insecure.

The policy impact of Public Health in Germany is striking, taking into account that Public Health has been established very recently. A limited but highly relevant number of examples shall illustrate the importance of Public Health in Germany.

► In all-important national and regional advisory boards and councils in German health policy, Public Health scientist or people with Public Health background play a dominant role.

▶ The Federal Committees of Physicians and Sickness Funds, and of Dentists and Sickness Funds and the Federal Hospital Committee have the task to assess all new and existing medical technologies according to their effectiveness, efficiency, ethical issues and so on. This task would have been impossible without the methods and the practice of Health Technology Assessment. Health Technology Assessment was introduced and carried out during the last 5 years by Public Health experts and is now by and large accepted by all key actors in the health policy arena [14].

▶ Public Health has put a lot of effort into establishing an outcome-orientation in health care. This was long denied as impractical. Today, disease-management programmes in Germany are in implementation, which define outcome-oriented targets for patients.

▶ The fortunes of health promotion and prevention have changed considerably during the last 13 years. Yet, a lot of evidence has been produced and compiled by Public Health research to underline, that health promotion and prevention can be effective and efficient [17, 19, 23]. In the 2002 election campaign in Germany all political parties explicitly put health promotion and prevention on the political agenda for the next four years.

▶ Germany is underway to define health targets on the national level (www.gesundheits-ziele.de). These targets are not defined by a handful of Public Health enthusiasts, on the very contrary Public Health thinking has spread and broadened into the health policy arena. More then 70 key institutions and almost 200 experts including members of patient organisations are involved in the effort [12].

▶ German scientists have played a remarkable role in evaluating the impact of European integration (4, 29). The Council, the Commission and the British Government have drawn on these findings.

A list of wishes for Public Health in Germany

Nevertheless, if we would be asked to write a list of yet unfulfilled wishes for Public Health in Germany, you would find some of the following phrases on it:

▶ Public Health requirements are considered as an essential horizontal policy across all government ministries.

▶ The value and the instruments of Public Health are understood by the population.

▶ Concerns of patients, citizens, insures and consumers are taken into account, also shared decision making and the representation of patients.

▶ A firm evidence base for health promotion and prevention also for secondary prevention and rehabilitation has been established by Public Health research.

▶ The instruments of evidence based health care are fully established which includes a long time research programme for health services and health system research.

▶ Health promotion and prevention are institutionalised and adequately financed (including and effective tobacco control policy).

▶ Multi sectoral health policies are standard overcoming boundaries between health promotion and prevention on one side, and diagnostics, therapy and rehabilitation and long time care on the other.

The future development of Public Health in Germany can build on a number of well established academic approaches ranging from epidemiology to health economics and from research into children to the aged (for an overview see [6, 27]). Moreover, the public health community has produced a growing experience in participating in the political process.

The future of Public Health in Europe

But wishes for Germany are not enough: The Constitutional Treaty of the European Union, which is currently drafted by the European Convention should established Public Health as a specific policy area alongside with social policy, consumer protection, and environmental policies. Despite current plans to designate Public Health a subordinated constitutional status as an area where the European Union may take supporting action, Public Health shall be acknowledged to be of high relevance on the European level.

▶ Seamless cross-border healthcare delivery is one of the areas in which the values and advantages of European citizenship could be easily understood and realized by the populations in the member states as patients, citizens and consumers.
▶ The European social model has to be reconfirmed. This should not only be a reconfirmation of the financial basis but it should strengthen the incentives and structures for prevention and Public Health in general towards more health for all.
▶ The integration of health requirements into all community policies is of overall importance especially in the areas of agriculture, trade, research and environment.
▶ The European Union should become a major player in trade related Public Health initiatives such as curbing the tobacco epidemic.
▶ The European member states should start an open and transparent benchmarking process for the best public and individual health care system.
▶ The European level should act as a clearing house both for the development of methods and empirical results in the discipline of health impact assessment and should be a responsible "laboratory" for creative experimental solutions in achieving better health.

Public Health – the global challenge

The future of Public Health will transcendent borders. Not only the border of the nation state but also those of the European Union. According to article 25 Declaration of Human Rights of the United Nations "everyone has the right to a standard of living adequate for the health and well-being [...] and medical care [...]". To bring this normative assumption to reality is in the well-understood self-interest of Germany and Europe. The campaigns to eradicate polio and measles, the attempts to curb the global tobacco epidemic [26] are good examples for the necessity to think global. Moreover, the prevention of wars, civil wars and economic catastrophes from which uncontrollable migration and Public Health disasters results – with severe repercussions on all industrialized countries   must be in the self-interest of Europe.

The emergence and regulation of global markets fostered by the World Trade Organization (WTO) will be having a growing impact on Public Health issues. Public Health issues will need to be integrated. First, the General Agreement on Trade in Services (GATS) currently under negotiation at the WTO in Geneva – should balance the opportunities of trading health services against the risks of liberalising health care systems. The movement of patients and of professionals will due to good governance in the health sector enhance the effectiveness of health care and satisfy the interests and ambitions of patients and of many doctors and nurses. Second, the General Agreement on Tariffs and Trade (GATT), which governs world trade, leads to concerns about the health impact of worldwide traded goods. The introduction of evidence based Public Health standards could have good influence on the game. It is a win-win-situation for both producers and consumers. Finally, the Trade Related Intellectual Property Rights (TRIPS) should enable also developing countries to offer the best health care to their people. International organisations and private enterprises can support the national authorities trying to reach that goal [30].

References

1. Abel-Smith B, Figueras J, Holland W, McKee M, Mossialos E. Choices in health policy: an agenda for the European Union, 1995. Dartmouth: Aldershot/Brookfield USA.
2. Bellach B-M, Stein H. The new Public Health Policy of the European Union. Past Experience, Present Needs, Future Perspectives, 1999. Urban und Vogel: München.
3. Bennett CJ. Review Article: What is policy convergence and what causes it? British Journal of Political Science 1991;21.
4. Busse R, Wismar M, Berman PC. The European Union and Health Services: The Impact of the Single European Market on Member States, 2002. IOS Press: Amsterdam.
5. Cornia GA. Globalization and health: results and options Bulletin of the World Health Organization 2001;79:834–841.
6. Deutsche Gesellschaft für Public Health e.V. Public-Health-Forschung in Deutschland, 1999. Huber: Bern.
7. Dierks M-L, Flaschka C, Frühbuß J, Hagedorn C, Weitkunat R. Berufsfelder und Karriereperspektiven für Absolventen der universitären Postgraduiertenstudiengänge "Public Health". In: Kälble K, von Troschke J (eds) Aus- und Weiterbildung in den Gesundheitswissenschaften/Public Health. Deutsche Koordinierungsstelle für Gesundheitswissenschaften: Freiburg. 1997:68–82.
8. Drager N, Beaglehole R. Globalization: changing the public health landscape Bulletin of the World Health Organization 2001;79:803.
9. Fälker M, Lange P. Haben sich Ihre Erwartungen an Public Health erfüllt? Was erwarten Sie von der Zukunft? Public Health Forum 2002;36:13–4.
10. Gesellschaft für Versicherungswissenschaft und -gestaltung (GVG) e.V. Gesundheitsziele.de – Forum Gesundheitsziele Deutschland. Gesundheitsziele für Deutschland: Entwicklung, Ausrichtung, Konzepte, 2002. AKA: Berlin.
11. Lorenz H, Pundt J. Verbleibsforschung von Absolventen des Berliner Postgradualen Studiengangs Public Health Das Gesundheitswesen 2000;62:A89.
12. Perleth M, Jakubowski E, Busse R. "Best Practice" im Gesundheitswesen – oder warum wir evidenzbasierte Medizin, Leitlinien und Health Technology Assessment brauchen Zeitschrift für ärztliche Fortbildung und Qualitätssicherung 2000;94:741–744.
13. Sachverständigenrat für die Konzertierte Aktion im Gesundheitswesen. Jahresgutachten 91 – Das Gesundheitswesen im vereinten Deutschland, 1991. Nomos Verlagsgesellschaft: Baden-Baden.
14. Sachverständigenrat für die Konzertierte Aktion im Gesundheitswesen. Gesundheitswesen in Deutschland: Kostenfaktor und Zukunftsbranche. Band I: Demographie, Morbidität, Wirtschaftlichkeitsreserven und Beschäftigung; Sondergutachten 1996. Nomos Verlagsgesellschaft: Baden-Baden.
15. Sachverständigenrat für die Konzertierte Aktion im Gesundheitswesen. Gesundheitswesen in Deutschland Kostenfaktor und Zukunftsbranche. Band II Fortschritt Wachstumsmärkte Finanzierung und Vergütung. Sondergutachten 1997, 1998. Nomos Verlagsgesellschaft: Baden-Baden.
16. Sachverständigenrat für die Konzertierte Aktion im Gesundheitswesen. Bedarfsgerechtigkeit und Wirtschaftlichkeit, 2001.
17. Sachverständigenrat für die Konzertierte Aktion im Gesundheitswesen. Bedarfsgerechtigkeit und Wirtschaftlichkeit. Band I: Zielbildung, Prävention, Nutzerorientierung und Partizipation. Sondergutachten 2000/2001, 2001. Nomos Verlagsgesellschaft: Baden-Baden.
18. Sachverständigenrat für die Konzertierte Aktion im Gesundheitswesen. Bedarfsgerechtigkeit und Wirtschaftlichkeit. Band II Qualitätsentwicklung in Medizin und Pflege. Sondergutachten 200/2001, 2001. Nomos Verlagsgesellschaft: Baden-Baden.
19. Sachverständigenrat für die Konzertierte Aktion im Gesundheitswesen. Bedarfsgerechtigkeit und Wirtschaftlichkeit. Band III: Über-, Unter- und Fehlversorgung. Gutachten 2000/2001. Ausführliche Zusammenfassung, 2001.
20. Saltman RB, Figueras J. European Health Care Reform: Analysis of current Strategies, 1997. World Health Organization Regional Office for Europe: Copenhagen.
21. Schienkiewitz A, Lotz E, Hofmann W, Dierks ML. Post-Graduate Public-Health-Programmes in Germany. Z f Gesundheitswiss 2002 (10):345–356.
22. Schwartz FW. Public Health: Zugang zu Gesundheit und Krankheit der Bevölkerung, Analysen für effektive und effiziente Lösungsansätze. In: Schwartz FW, Badura B, Leidl R, Raspe H, Siegrist J editors. Das Public-Health-Buch. Gesundheit und Gesundheitswesen. Urban und Schwarzenberg: München. 1998:2–5.
23. Schwartz FW, Bitzer EM, Dörning H, Grobe T, Krauth C, Schlaud M, Schmidt T, Zielke M. Gutachten Gesundheitsausgaben für chronische Krankheit in Deutschland: Krankheitskostenlast und Reduktionspotentiale durch verhaltensbezogene Risikomodifikation, 2000. Pabst: Lengerich.

24. Schwartz FW, von Troschke J, Walter U. Entwicklung der Forschungslandschaft Public Health in Deutschland. In: Public-Health-Forschungsverbünde in der Deutschen Gesellschaft für Public Health e.V. editor. Public-Health-Forschung in Deutschland. Huber: Bern. 1999:23–32.
25. Siegrist J. Was wurde erreicht? – Evaluation der Public-Health-Forschungsverbände Public Health Forum 2002:10:8–9.
26. The World Bank. Curbing the Epidemic. Governments and the Economics of Tobacco Control, 1999. The World Bank: Washington, D.C.
27. Walter U, Paris W. Public Health; Gesundheit im Mittelpunkt, 1996. Alfred & Söhne: Meran.
28. Wismar M, Busse R. Europa Ante Portas Gesellschaftspolitische Kommentare 2001;42:14–18.
29. World Health Organization. World Health Report 2000. Health Systems: Improving Performance, 2000.
30. World Health Organization, World Trade Organization. WTO Agreements & Public Health. A joint study by the WHO and WTO Secretariat, 2002. Word Trade Organization: Geneva

Ageing and Health Policy

Margot Fälker

Demographic change – how can we save solidarity?

The Problem

The demographic picture in many countries, including Germany, is rapidly changing. There is a growing percentage of people over 60 or 65 years of age. The entire population is shrinking, and the number of working people in relationship to the number of children and retired people is decreasing, as you can easily see from the table. The two models, with different retirement ages and assumptions for the annual number of immigrants, show the consequences of this trend. The "ratio of burden" in the first model exceeds 100 percent in the long-range and in the second model the ratio of burden nearly remains at the current level [1].

Population development, employment ratio, burden ratio

The reason for this development is triple ageing, meaning that three factors are responsible for this progression and its velocity.

First, life-expectancy is growing. Today the average life-expectancy for women is 81 years, and for men 75 years. At the beginning of the century life-expectancy was about 30 years less than it is today.

Table 1. Development of Population, Ratio of Employment, Ratio of Burden

| Year | Immigration 100 000 persons p.a. Retirement age 60 years | | | Immigration 200 000 persons p.a. Retirement age 65 years | | |
	Population in 1000	Percentage of employed 20 to 60 years	Ratio of burden*	Population in 1000	Percentage of employed 20 to 65 years	Ratio of burden*
1999	82 037.0	56.2	78.0	82 037.0	62.6	59.6
2010	81 085.9	55.6	79.9	81 497.3	60.9	64.1
2020	78 791.8	53.6	86.5	80 339.1	61.0	63.9
2030	75 186.6	48.0	108.2	77 976.9	57.1	75.1
2040	70 457.2	47.5	110.4	74 545.6	54.6	83.2
2050	64 973.3	46.7	114.0	70 381.4	55.0	81.7

* Ratio of population under 20 and above 60 years per 100 persons between 20 and 60 years.

Secondly, the percentage of elderly is growing as a consequence of a cohort effect. In the 1950s and 1960s Germany experienced a baby boom. These age groups will begin to reach retirement age from 2010 onwards.

The **third** factor we can identify is low fertility rates of 1.4 children per woman during the last 10 years. These rates are too low to keep the population size at its current level.

Effect on health care systems

Though ageing isn't equivalent to sickness and disability, experience shows that health care needs and expenditures increase with age at the micro and macro level. According to the thesis of compression of morbidity, on the macro level health care expenses don't increase automatically or linearly with ageing. Instead, expenditures accelerate with proximity to death, and death at a younger age is much more expensive than death at an older age [2]. Experts estimate that the isolated effect of ageing on health care expenditures is only about 3 to 4 percent of the expected growth rate. Macroeconomic forecasts for the next 40 to 50 years based on different implications to internal and external factors (employment-rate, especially of women; fertility-rate; number of immigrants; general economic development; the development and cost of medical and technical innovation) estimate contribution rates between 16 and 30 percent [3]. From international comparative data we can see that nearly all industrial nations might reach their limits of affordability in capacity planning and financing health care according to ageing, as well as medical and technological innovations.

Financing problem in social health insurance schemes based on solidarity

Financing of the German social health insurance is based on the principle of solidarity with income related contribution rates up to a threshold limit (3375 Euro per month, 2002). As a consequence of this financing structure it is necessary to maintain a balance between contributions and expenses to avoid additional burdens to employers and employees, who each finance 50% of the contributions. In past years general economic growth rates were very low and Germany had a high rate of unemployment. As a consequence, the health insurance revenue base was weak and at the same time, expenditures, especially for drugs, increased. In addition to these problems, offering and organizing adequate health care provision according to the needs of the population, and especially the needs of the elderly, is in general a policy challenge.

In addition to these economic problems the Advisory Council for the Concerted Action in Health Care presented a report in which the following deficits of the German health care system were identified [4].

Deficits of the German health care system

▶ The German health care system belongs to the most expensive ones in the world, but it doesn't belong to the most effective ones according to commonly used outcome-parameters like life-expectancy or disability-free life-expectancy.
▶ There is a respectable amount of over-, under- and misuse, especially in the field of drug treatment.

▶ In particular, the treatment of chronic diseases is inefficient. The structures of the system are oriented to acute care and the treatment of organic disorders.
▶ There is a lack of patient-, target- and preventive orientation according to the special needs and the individual social situation of the chronically ill.
▶ There are too many interfaces between inpatient and outpatient care, prevention and rehabilitation.
▶ Treatment is insufficiently oriented on evidence-based guidelines or other models of best practice.

Solutions: How can we solve the above mentioned problems? How can we meet the challenge?

International discussion and comparative studies [5] show a range of options between spending more and more money for health care services and cost-containment policies. On one side are national health services with target oriented policy programs and rationing of the benefit packages, and on the other side are highly competitive systems with a comprehensive medical supply where the ability to get adequate care highly depends on the individual economic capacity. For Germany solidarity and equivalence in the access of a comprehensive benefit package are central principles in providing and financing health care. With the aim of improving quality, reorganizing the system in the direction the Advisory Council proposed and enhancing efficiency, the Federal Ministry of health introduced several bills [6] in the last legislative period.

Selected health care acts in the 14th legislative period

▶ Reform of the Risk Compensation Scheme
▶ The Act on Diagnosis-Related Flat Rates in Hospitals
▶ The Drug Replacement Act
▶ The Act to Limit Pharmaceutical Expenditure
▶ Other Bills

Age-related burdens of chronic disease and the main deficits mentioned by the Advisory Council should be met largely with the Risk Compensation Scheme Reform.

Central elements of the reform of the Risk Compensation Scheme Reform

▶ With the introduction of financial incentives health insurance funds are motivated to develop disease management programs for important chronic diseases. The financial compensation health insurance funds receive for patients enrolled in these programs abolishes undesired incentives for risk selection.
▶ The introduction of a high-risk-pool for patients with expensive benefits. Above the threshold value of 20 450 Euro per year, 60% of the expenses are compensated via the risk pool.
▶ Introduction of a morbidity oriented risk equalisation structure in 2007.

Within the disease-management-programs the application of evidence-based guidelines is foreseen, and the pilot function of the general practitioner and the interlinking of services are strengthened. The programs include preventive care and patient-education for better self-management of disorders. Further, health care providers have to document treatments and outcome-parameters of the patients regularly to enhance quality assurance.

With the Drug Budget Replacement Act the pharmaceutical budget and the collective liability of health care providers included therein were abolished. Further, measures in this act were designed to improve quality and contain costs in the pharmaceutical sector. Against the background of constantly increasing drug expenses, and the fact that agreements on an expenditure volume and cost efficiency targets of the self-administration don't work, additional regulations in this field are necessary.

The Act to stabilize Contribution Rates currently is in the parliamentary process [7]. Due to the weak revenue base and running expenses the act includes a bunch of regulations in different areas of the health care system to secure its affordability.

Structural reforms shall follow next spring. Additionally, the Minister appointed a new Advisory Council [8] with a focus on age-related challenges. This Council shall discuss reform options and give restructuring recommendations to the pension insurance system and the health care insurance system.

Scope of reform options

As I already mentioned, in national and international discussions there are a wide variety of reform options that meet different targets. Possible reform target could be:

Reform targets

- ▶ Cost-containment to keep health care expenses low
- ▶ Adequate health care provision for the whole population according to needs
- ▶ Equal access to health care services and equality in treatment
- ▶ Equal distribution of health care financing
- ▶ Discharge auxiliary labour costs to improve the competitive situation of Germany in global markets.

Examples of options to meet this targets

Financing

- ▶ Enhancing the threshold limit
- ▶ Extension of the revenue base to all kinds of income
- ▶ Inclusion of the whole population in mandatory contribution payments
- ▶ Introduction of individual risk-adjusted premiums with tax transfers for people with lower incomes
- ▶ Introduction of sectoral or global budgets
- ▶ Tax-financing for co-insured without own income.

Reduction of expenses

- ▶ Rationing or exclusion of benefits and services
- ▶ Enlarging co-payments.

Structural measures

▶ Enhancing competition between health funds through more flexibility in individual contracting with health care providers
▶ Enhancing competition based on quality between health care providers
▶ Changing reimbursement schemes and schedules
▶ Mobilizing efficiency reserves by avoiding of over-, under- and misuse
▶ Developing new models of health care provision (e.g. health centres) and new interlinking structures between inpatient and outpatient care, rehabilitation and nursing care
▶ Capacity planning.

The above mentioned possibilities are only some of the models that have been discussed recently or have been published in scientific literature [9]. There is a large number of other measures and combinations of the above mentioned options. A quick glance at international comparative data shows advantages and disadvantages of certain combinations [10].

International comparison of health care expenditures

As you can easily see health care expenditures in the USA – a highly competitive health care system based on principles of individual risk and ability to pay – are much higher than in any other system.

On the contrary, a tax financed system like the UK is much cheaper, however it has trouble providing its population with the necessary services and is characterized by explicit rationing.

A few years ago Switzerland introduced mandatory health insurance for the whole population. Financing is based on per capita premiums and transfer payments for people with lower incomes. Managed care structures should improve the efficiency of health care provision. Nevertheless, expenses are increasing in Switzerland more rapidly than in Germany.

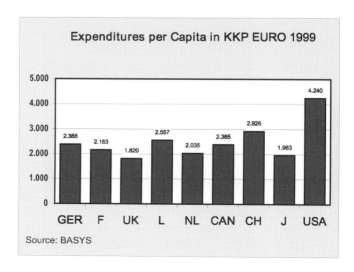

Fig. 1. Expenditures per Capita in KKP EURO 1999

Source: BASYS

Against the background of the problem's complexity and the respectable number of options in scientific and political discussion, the propositions and recommendations of the Advisory Council for age-related questions can be expected with great interest.

Conclusion

Finally, I would like to make a few short remarks on general tendencies that contribute solutions to age-related problems in the financing and provision of health care, and that could save solidarity.

First of all, increasing employment rates usually strengthen the revenue base for the statutory health insurance. Though the effects of the proposals from the Hartz-Commission are not exactly quantifiable a favourable influence from higher employment rates on the statutory health insurance revenue base can be expected.

Further, it has to be mentioned that during the last few years the employment-rate of women grew continuously to about 60 percent and contributed to a stabilization of the revenue base in all insurance schemes [11]. A new, family friendly policy can give incentives for women to enter or return to the labour market after having children. The French example, with a comprehensive supply of full-time kindergartens and schools, shows that such incentives work. Employment of women is not only important for the labour market in general, but is especially important for the health care market because 70 percent of care givers and nurses are women.

With respect to the fact that the imbalance between working people and the volume of retired people will increase in the next 20 years, immigration may weaken the problems in the social insurance schemes. International comparative data show that immigrants help to establish new and prospering markets. At the same time the age structure (mixture of children, people of employment age and retired people) of the whole population will change so that solidarity between young and old people, healthy and sick and employed and retired reaches a new balance.

Recent analysis estimates that between 40 and 60 percent of all diseases are chronic diseases and shows the percentage increases with ageing. Beyond the above mentioned measures to enhance the revenue base and provide people with adequate health care services, it is necessary to strengthen health care prevention to avoid diseases, particularly chronic diseases, that cause individual and collective burden. This burden can be reduced if acute disability periods and treatment needs could be diminished.

Until now, there is no other health care system or country that has found a probable solution for the above mentioned challenges to age-related questions concerning the health care system. Reforms in Germany will have to take into account the traditional and historical background of the current German health care system, the new coalition agreements on further health care reforms, requirements and liabilities to the integration process of the European Union and the already existing options and recommendations concerning the search for a new balance between competition and solidarity.

How can we save solidarity?

- ▶ Enhancing of the revenue base for contribution by
- ▶ Enhancing general employment rates
- ▶ Improving the conditions for employment of women
- ▶ Immigration

► Avoiding over-, under- and misuse in health care provision
► Enhancing quality orientation and effectiveness of health care provision
► Giving new incentives to health insurance funds and health care providers
► Enhancing health care prevention to avoid diseases, particularly chronic diseases.

References

1. Statistisches Bundesamt, Wiesbaden 2000, Bevölkerungsentwicklung Deutschlands bis zum Jahr 2050
2. Zweifel P., Felder, S., Meier, M. Baden-Baden 1996, Demographische Alterung und Gesundheitskosten: Eine Fehlinterpretation, in: P. Oberender (Ed), Alter und Gesundheit. Sachverständigenrat für die Konzertierte Aktion im Gesundheitswesen Sondergutachten 1996, Gesundheitswesen in Deutschland – Kostenfaktor und Zukunftsbranche, Bd. 1: Demographie, Morbidität, Wirtschaftlichkeitsreserven und Beschäftigung. Brockmann, Hilke 2002, Health Treatment for the Elderly, MPI for Demographic Research, Rostock, Germany
3. Ulrich, Volker, Medizinisch-technischer Fortschritt, Demographische Alterung und Wachstum der Gesundheitsausgaben: Was sind die treibenden Faktoren in: Zeitschrift für Gesundheitsökonomie und Qualitätsmanagement 5/6, 2000 (163–172)
4. Sachverständigenrat für die Konzertierte Aktion im Gesundheitswesen, Gutachten 2000/2001, Baden-Baden, Bedarfsgerechtigkeit und Wirtschaftlichkeit. Stellungnahme des Bundesministeriums zum Gutachten des Sachverständigenrates für die Konzertierte Aktion im Gesundheitswesen „Bedarfsgerechtigkeit und Wirtschaftlichkeit", BT-DRS: 14/9885 vom 21.08.2002
5. OECD, Horizontal Project on Ageing Related Diseases, Ottawa 2001
6. Gesetz zur Reform des Risikostrukturausgleichs 2001; Gesetz zur Einführung des diagnoseorientierten Fallpauschalensystems für Krankenhäuser (Fallpauschalengesetz) 2002; Arzneimittelausgaben-Begrenzungsgesetz (AABG.) 2002; Arneimittelbudget-Ablösungsgesetz (ABAG.) 2002
7. Beitragssicherungsgesetz 2002
8. Pressemitteilung des BMG Nr. 179 vom 12. Nov. 2002 Kommission für die Nachhaltigkeit in der Finanzierung der Sozialen Sicherungssysteme
9. Klose, J., Schellschmidt, H., Bonn 2001, WIDO 45, Finanzierung und Leistungen der Gesetzlichen Krankenversicherung. Pfaff, Anita u.a. Kostendämpfung in der gesetzlichen Krankenversicherung, Frankfurt 1994. Wille, E. /Igl,Ch. Köln 2002, Zur Reform der Beitragsgestaltung, insbesondere der Pflichtversicherungsgrenze in der gesetzlichen Krankenversicherung
10. Statistisches Bundesamt, Wiesbaden 2002, Gesundheit Ausgaben 1992–2000; Schneider, Markus, u.a. BASYS, Gesundheitssysteme im internationalen Vergleich, unveröffentlichter Bericht
11. Enquete-Kommission Demographischer Wandel, Berlin 2002, Herausforderungen unserer älter werdenden Gesellschaft an den Einzelnen und die Politik, Deutscher Bundestag

Ferenc Bojan Memorial Lecture – the meaning of life expectancy for the individual, for Public Health and for Social Security Systems

CHRISTIAN VON FERBER

Life expectancy a promising but neglected field of research

Figures about the life expectancy of various populations are a regular part of official statistics. The continuous publication of death tables fulfils an important function in public health reporting for the purposes of formulating and implementing health and social policies. Those figures from official statistics are of great use to the population and health sciences for two reasons:
1. They provide reliable if highly condensed information about mortality rates in a given sample. As such they are a record of real events in the observed population.
2. Within the context of research, they become a framework for testing hypotheses. The information, which was primarily collected for official purposes, finds a secondary use within a system of theoretical assumptions.

The step from empirical statements about the mortality rates in a given population to the modelling of indicators for the testing of theories in the health sciences has several advantages, though these are not always sufficiently acknowledged. However, it must also be said that the secondary use of data from official statistics as indicators for theory-based research requires constant checking in order to avoid false inferences.

Research using indicators touches on a core question about methods in the health sciences. That is why I would like to make it the subject of my Ferenc Bojan memorial lecture. In one of his last publications: "Avoidable mortality. Is it an indicator of quality of medical care in Eastern European countries?" of 1991 [1], Bojan had used data about the differences in mortality between Eastern and Western European countries. Life expectancy, as found in official statistics, however, is not just an indicator for the quality of medical care but also for the general state of health of the population. As the end point of an individual life the time of death says something about an individual's biography; but it also tells about some of the general conditions, which according to the health sciences, either promote health or advance fatal diseases. For the investigation of this basic problem in the health sciences the secondary use of official statistics has the following advantages:
1. The official statistics provide comprehensive and continuous data that could never be compiled from a primary health science survey. Investigations about mortality or life expectancy are without doubt the domain of research based on secondary data. That type of research takes data from official statistics compiled, for example, for insurers [2] or health departments, reorganises them in view of the research problem and evaluates them with respect to certain hypotheses [3, 4]. Unlike in primary surveys the research design has no influence on the data collection; it is focussed solely on the interpretative framework.
2. The collection of data about mortality and life expectancy is similar in almost every country. As a standard, the data are arranged by sex and age groups. The WHO has

made enormous efforts to foster the continuous collection of internationally comparable data, especially about mortality rates [5, 6]. This has given the health sciences the opportunity to undertake international comparative research. Such research is highly relevant for the modelling of hypotheses about the influence of economic and social factors on the general state of health of populations.

3. In many countries data arranged by regions are also available. Based on regional differences and/or social indicators inferences can be drawn about economic and social factors that influence life expectancy. Such regional or sub-regional data are a unique opportunity for social epidemiology to test its hypotheses on real socio-ecological settings [7, 8]. Surprisingly, the socio-ecological approach involves a methodology, which had been developed in the context of social hygiene for the investigation of the causes of communicable diseases [9]. Naturally, the search for characteristics related to a person's individual biography and biology dominates the investigation of the causes of non-communicable diseases. Mortality rates of populations defined by their socio-geographical background, however, allow researchers to take into account again settings and contexts. They are a bridge to the reality of life styles and dying when interpreting the data. For people live within such settings: they frame their daily lives, challenge them, bind them, and sometimes overwhelm them. A setting can literally materialise, e.g. as the level of pollution to which people are subjected. Settings become effective in the social connections of everyday life, in what sociologists illustratively call "milieu" or "community" and town planners refer to when they characterise a suburban area.

4. Variations in life expectancy: over time, between the sexes, between countries and regions, or based on socio-economic indicators can be observed and evaluated as in a "natural experiment". By "natural experiment" I mean transformations in the situation of a population caused by environmental changes and/or political decisions. What interests the health sciences are the resulting changes to the general state of health. "Natural experiments" are to be distinguished from interventions based on health policy decisions and aimed at an improvement in the general state of health of a population. Such directed interventions are open to evaluation. "Natural experiments", on the other hand, require interpretation in order to draw any inferences from them. This is a real challenge to any research using secondary data.

Three "natural experiments" that are accompanied by striking changes and variations are currently receiving special attention in the health sciences.

a   Statistics suggest an increase in life expectancy in all countries and across all age groups. Its long-term effects on the population and social structure are called "demographic change". That change calls for a fundamental reorientation of our social security systems (pensions and health services) – a new "contract between the generations". The current political task becomes even more pressing as the increase in life expectancy is accompanied by a tendency to call into question conventional views about the biological limits of the maximum age we can attain [10, 11]. With that demographic change we encounter long-term changes in the structure of our population; we do not sufficiently understand their causes, yet we already have to consider their consequences for social and health policy [12].

b   The collapse of the Soviet Union and its economic and social order has caused dramatic changes in life expectancy, especially for people of working age: in particular, the difference in life expectancy between men and women has grown in favour of the latter (Table 1) [13].

c   Sub-regional differences in life expectancy remain stable within larger regional or national economic or social units even if the general life expectancy increases [7, 8]. That observation poses a fundamental question for the formulation and propagation of health goals within social security systems. Can such systems, like the model ones in Western and Central Europe, limit themselves to offering equal access to up-to-date health services for all citizens? Or do they have to extend the notion of equality to the results of their health services, and how could these be guaranteed? That is not just a question of policy but also a challenge to the health sciences to investigate how far claims of equality match reality. A first step is an investigation of the causes of "inequality before dying and death". Health science research into poverty and inequality has produced important results in that respect, not least on the basis of data from official statistics. At the same time it has produced a controversy over the interpretation of its results. Such controversy is to be expected not only because of competing hypotheses – that would be no different from the usual critical reception of research results. The controversy results from the use of data collected primarily for health report purposes as indicators: as such these data are subject to a far larger number of possible differing explanatory uses, even in research conducted outside the health sciences. Secondary data research has more leeway in the interpretation of such indicators than research using primary data. That is an opportunity for the health sciences because it can employ the variety of its special disciplines. It is also an opportunity for health policy because it can draw on a wider range of options for intervention and their public justification. Yet it is also a serious danger – the danger of drifting into the speculative and politically utopian.

Table 1. Age-Adjusted Mortality Rates and Life Expectancy, Russia and United States, 1990 and 1994

	Age-Adjusted Mortality Rate			Life Expectancy at Birth		
	1990	1994	Percent Change	1990	1994	Change, y
Russia						
Total	1192.7	1581.6	32.6	69.2	64.1	–5.2
Male	1688.4	2290.5	26.7	63.8	57.7	–6.1
Female	892.2	1098.4	23.1	74.4	71.2	–3.2
United States						
Total	803.4	784.7	–2.3	75.4	75.7	0.3
Male	1035.3	996.4	–3.8	71.8	72.4	0.6
Female	628.8	621.8	–1.1	78.8	79.0	0.2

Francis C. Notzon et al. JAMA Vol. 279 (1998) p.795

To summarise our deliberations thus far: the official mortality statistics provide unique data for the health sciences. They can be considered as comprehensive surveys. They reach back uninterrupted far in time and are secure for the foreseeable future. Their reliability is being continuously improved, not just for scientific purposes. The surveys are comparable across countries and supported by international organisations. They are geographically structured to a depth of several layers. The data for individuals as well as populations can be utilised for the research purposes of various disciplines: medicine, economics, social sciences, town and regional planning. Accordingly, the results of such multidisciplinary research are of interest to a broad spectrum of policy making such as health and social policy, economic policy or policies for regional development.

Such an advantageous situation poses two challenges for the health sciences.
1. The health sciences claim to be interdisciplinary. They support the demand to integrate different scientific methods.
Unlike in the fundamental sciences, however, this is not a goal in itself.
2. From their predecessors, social hygiene and social medicine, the health sciences have accepted the function of giving policy advice. Their support at the universities is not least based on the political expectations that go along with that role.

Both these challenges mean that the clarification of controversial interpretations of changes and variations in life expectancy between societies and regions is of vital importance to the health sciences. Let me try and explicate this problem with respect to the rival interpretations of the dramatic reduction in life expectancy in Russia after the collapse of the Soviet empire, as they, too, are intended to draw inferences from this "natural experiment" for the development of the health system.

Does life expectancy indicate the effects of "natural experiments"? Methodological and theoretical implications

With the political and economic changes in Russia after 1989/90 the life expectancy decreased, especially for the 35–55 age group and particularly for men. That development was particularly dramatic in Russia, but it affected also the Eastern and South-Eastern European countries of the former Soviet empire, though not the former Soviet republics of Central Asia [14, 15].

There is now a large number of studies that attempt to explain those events. They agree in the global assessment that the decline in life expectancy and the economic and social upheaval in the former Soviet empire are not just accidentally connected but that there is a causal relationship, which is yet to be explained. The suggestive retort that the decrease is nothing but a statistical artefact because the figures about life expectancy before Gorbatchov's glasnost were manufactured does not stand up to scrutiny [13, 14].

An analysis of the causes of death shows that there is no increase in the number of deaths from cancer if one disregards those caused by the abuse of alcohol or nicotine [16]. Even the claim that the regions with high environmental pollution are responsible for the overall increase in mortality is not supported by the data [14, 16].

The influence of alcohol and tobacco abuse, however, is supported. It shows not just an increase in deaths caused by diseases that are causally related to the consumption of these substances such as cirrhoses of the liver or lung cancer. There is also a surprising incidence of alcohol related fatal accidents or violence as well as deaths from hypothermia [13]. The Gorbatchov-initiated campaign against alcohol abuse, for example, clearly showed successful epidemiological results (Fig. 1).

With the above mentioned analysis of the data the health sciences find themselves on the firm ground of mono-causal explanations. However, they explain only a part of the entire mortality increase in Russia at the beginning of the 1990s, and as far as alcohol and tobacco abuse are concerned only the clinically documented final phase. An investigation of which conditions of the fundamental social and economic transformation lead to the leaping and lasting changes in the habitual consumption of cigarettes and alcohol is not part of that analysis.

Uncertainty and controversy result for those reasons of deaths that are multi-causal and can be influenced both by medical treatment as well as health conscious behaviour and health promotion. Those reasons account for the majority of the increase in mortality. As a consequence, the framework for investigation must be extended beyond clinical medicine and epidemiology. We have to look for conditions that can both explain the sudden increase in mortality and are strongly influenced by political, economic and social change. It is evident that this is a real challenge to the health sciences, and that they must find convincing extensions to the biomedical paradigm and suggest measures for intervention, which promise real success.

An analysis of the available theories shows that the health sciences have met this challenge with great enterprise and exemplary to rigour. There is a remarkable plurality of re-

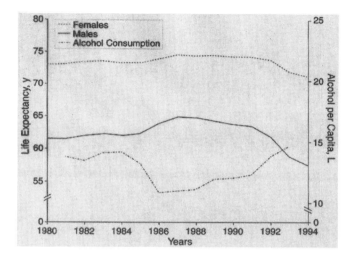

Fig. 1. Life expectancy – alcohol per capita. Source: Notzon et al. JAMA, March 11, 1998 – Vol. 279, No. 10 p 794

search concepts employed to explain the dramatic increase in mortality in Russia during the 1990s. I will first give an overview of the most influential contributions and then draw some conclusions:

1. It is obvious to look at the role of the Soviet or Russian health system first. Were the events too much for the health system? Did a system that had been neglected for decades buckle under a situation of increasing shortages?

That analysis is supported by the following considerations:

a The life expectancy of the people in the Soviet Union had been falling behind that of the Western countries since the 1960s [13].

b The Soviet Union did not adjust its strategies and concepts for prevention to the increasing importance of non-communicable diseases. Centralistic structures and sweeping state controls militated against the introduction of decentralised health promotion and the transfer of responsibility to the individual [14].

That same analysis, however, is put into question by the following considerations:

a Long-term deficits can, if at all, only partly explain dramatic changes in life expectancy.

b Staffing levels within the Soviet health system were good compared to Western countries. Its deficits related more to qualifications and performance incentives. Remuneration levels were significantly below those of jobs in the productive sectors.

c The increase in mortality affected mainly people of working age, not so much children and the aged.

There is thus a consensus that the level of health services cannot be regarded as one of the major causes for the decline in life expectancy in Russia [13, 14, 16].

2. What effect did the collapse of the economy have? Can the loss of purchasing power and the increase in poverty among wide sections of the society explain the increase in mortality? This analysis is based on economic indicators, which could be observed parallel to the increase in mortality: the reduction in real incomes and the resulting increase in the proportion of income spent on food. Those indicators have the advantage that there are a number of reliable sources of data for them. Yet they have the disadvantage that they are immediately related to only very few causes of death.

According to the available data the average per capita income in Russia declined by two thirds between 1990 and 1995 [16]. In 1995 about half the households lived below the poverty line. From 1987/88 to 1993, i.e. within a five-year-period, the percentage of households below the poverty line increased from 2 per cent to 38 per cent. Thus it is not an exaggeration to speak of a dramatic change in people's lives. Whilst in 1991 the average proportion of expenditure for food was 28 per cent of household income, in 1994 that had increased to 40 per cent [16].

A convincing inference from these indicators to an increase in mortality, however, can be drawn only for a few causes, which account for less than 5 percent of deaths. In addition, regions of greater poverty are not necessarily regions of greater mortality. And the regional differences in the proportion of poor households are considerable; they vary from 10 per cent in Moscow to 70 per cent in the Altai region [16].

All explanations thus far have been based on the available data about changes to social security services with a direct or indirect effect on the preservation of health. They do not take into account the individual resources of the people and their possible failure to cope with the upheaval. For the collapse of a social system that did not only look after people's material needs but also tried to control their thinking must affect the personality of these people. Unlike the systems in the West the Soviet system claimed a state monopoly on economic control as well as the control of people's thinking and feeling. The claim for control was matched by a guarantee of security with respect to people's material needs. The health sciences thus cannot satisfactorily explain the effects of the collapse of such a system by just looking at the decline of services.

Unfortunately, there are only few studies about the influence of power structures on personality development [18, 19]. However, they do justify the hypothesis that the collapse of the Soviet system did not only result in declining services but also caused deep personal and social upheaval bringing about a massive loss of personal resources. Yet such personal resources make an important contribution to the way people cope with the symptoms of disease and the preservation of health [16, 20, 21] – which brings us back onto safe ground in health science research about how people cope with illness and crises in their lives.

That approach can be found in three explanatory concepts employed in studies about the mortality increase in Russia at the beginning of the 1990s:

▶ The stress concept. It appears to be apt to explain the increase and the quantitative contribution of cardiovascular causes of death in the 35–65 age group. That concept is made operational by a hypothesis that lifestyle changes largely account for the increase in mortality [14].

▶ The concept of the social status. The relevance of this concept is underlined by the differences in mortality among status groups – differences that despite the radical changes at that time remained or even grew [16].

▶ The socio-ecological concept. That concept combines the data about regional differences in mortality with indicators about the structure and situation of the population in sub-regional health reporting [7, 8].

Perspectives for future research

There is a lack of reliable and sufficiently comprehensive data to support any of the three concepts and the hypotheses derived from them. Thus we can discuss them here only in two respects:

a Are the concepts justified and rich enough for the problem at hand?
b Do they suggest health policies that can be implemented?

Stress concepts can be made operational and applied only to certain types of settings and contexts such as organisations or small groups. They fail in view of upheaval experienced by people through the collapse of an entire social system.

Lifestyle concepts explain poverty through the concept of impoverishment (pauvreté). But they cannot explain why Russia experienced a decline in behavioural attitudes to health.

The social status concept reproduces the result, known from Western countries, that social status and mortality are related to each other in reverse proportion. It leaves unexplained why in Russia the status related differences in mortality rates appear to be growing, not only because there is a lack of data about the social structure, its changes and the relevant mortality rates, but also because that concept lacks theories and hypotheses that relate the social status to health conscious behaviour and milieu. Without knowledge about the personality structures that go with the primary and secondary socialisation into a social status position, the concept lacks the explanatory power that it claims to have.

Socio-ecological concepts promise more success, not least with respect to policy implementation. Unfortunately though, as far as Russia is concerned, the necessary data are lacking [16]. In order to demonstrate the advantages of this explanatory approach I will therefore introduce the exemplary research that Gerhard Meinlschmidt and his group at the Centre for Public Health in Berlin have undertaken in that city-state after reunification. Their analysis combines the data about life expectancy with a complex set of information about the socio-economic situation of the people in different suburbs (Stadtbezirken). The socio-economic situation is operationalised in a "social index". It consists of a number of variables about "population and household structure", "education and work", "income, jobs, unemployment and social security payments" as well as "health".

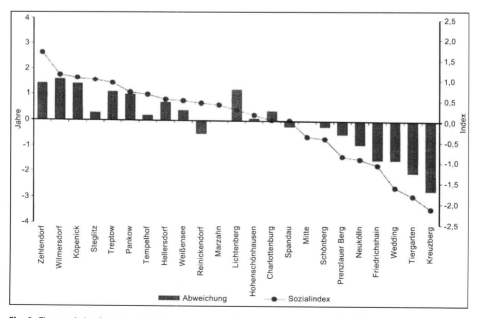

Fig. 2. The correlation between social characteristics and life expectancy for men 1997–1999 (comprehensively) in the suburban districts ("Stadtbezirke") of Berlin – Deviation (in years) from the average in Berlin (74.1 years)

Looking at the "social index" for the Berlin suburbs over a five-year-period we discover a high degree of stability. The social index shows a significant correlation with life expectancy and other indicators of "early mortality" or "causes of death that can be influenced by medical treatment" [7] (Fig. 2).

The advantages of combining data about mortality rates with socio-ecological indicators are apparent. I conclude with naming three of them:

1. The socio-ecological approach relates data about the mortality within a population to those aspects of the population's social situation, which are important for the individual and at the same time, characterise a setting, context or milieu of social relationships for the population as a whole, i.e. what sociologists call a community.
2. Since the "social index" includes characteristics such as education and degrees gained, the influence of the social situation on the mortality can be differentiated into "social" and "personal" resources. This opens a way to distinguish between environmental conditions within the community and personal resources for the analysis of mortality rates. I consider such differentiation necessary if a health system aims to achieve not only equal access to health services but also equal results from them. As the analysis of the Centre for Public Health in Berlin shows, the combination of social index and personal resources – called status index – is not the same for all Berlin suburbs. If we employ a factor analysis we can see that the status index explains 22 percent of the total variability among the 23 Berlin suburbs.
3. Unlike the other explanatory concepts only the socio-ecological approach promises a way to distinguish, for the purposes of intervention, between avoidable, conditionally avoidable and unavoidable causes of death and to justify appropriate health measures accordingly. In this respect the approach bridges the gap between research and policy in public health. In view of the future perspectives for Public Health it is my wish that the analytical approaches developed by the Centre in Berlin will be widely applied in other *Länder*.

References

1. Bojan, F.; Hajdu P.; Belicza E. (1991) Avoidable mortality. Is it an indicator of quality of medical care in Eastern European countries? Quality assurance in health care. 3: 191–203
2. Ihle, P.; Köster, I.; Schubert, I.; von Ferber, Chr.; von Ferber, L.; (1999) Versichertenstichprobe der Gesetzlichen Krankenversicherung. Wirtschaft und Statistik 9/1999:742–749
3. von Ferber, L.; Behrens, J. (Hg.) (1997) Public Health Forschung mit Gesundheits- und Sozialdaten – Stand und Perspektiven. Sankt Augustin (Asgard)
4. von Ferber, L. (Hg.) (1994) Häufigkeit und Verteilung von Erkrankungen und ihre ärztliche Behandlung. Köln und Leipzig (ISAB)
5. WHO. World Health Report 2000 (2000) Geneva: WHO
6. Mathers C.D.; Sadana R.; Salomon J.A.; Murray Ch.J.L.; Lopez A.D. (2001) Healthy life expectancy in 191 countries, 1999 Lancet. 357: 1685–1691
7. Lebenserwartung in Berlin 1986–1994 – Trends und regionale Unterschiede. Diskussionspapier 29 (1997) herausgegeben von der Senatsverwaltung für Gesundheit und Soziales Berlin
8. Borrell C.; Arias A (1995) Socioeconomic factors and mortality in urban settings: the case of Barcelona Spain In: Journal of Epidemiology and Community Health 49:460–465
9. Mosse, M.; Tugendreich, G. (1913) Krankheit und Soziale Lage München (J.F. Lehmann).
10. Oeppen J.; Vaupel J.W. (2002) Broken limits to life expectancy: Science. 296, 2002 (www.sciencemag.org)
11. Tuljapurkar S.; Li N.; Boe C. (2000) A universal pattern of mortality decline in G7 countries Nature. 405 (www.nature.com)
12. Bickel H. (2001) Lebenserwartung und Pflegebedürftigkeit in Deutschland. Gesundheitswesen 63:9–14

13. Notzon F.C.; Komarov Y.M.; Ermakov S.P.; Sempos Ch. T.; Marks J.S.; Sempos E. V. (1998) Causes of declining life expectancy in Russia. JAMA 279:793–800
14. Cockerham W.C. (1997) The social determinants of the decline of life expectancy in Russia and Eastern Europe : A lifestyle explanation. Journal of Health and Social Behaviour. 38:117–130
15. Reamy J.; Dreskovic St. (1999) Life expectancy in Central and Eastern European Countries and Newly Independent States of the former Soviet Union: Changes by gender. Croatian Medical Journal 40:237–243
16. Chen L.C.; Wittgenstein F.; McKeon E. (1996) The upsurge of mortality in Russia: Causes and policy implications. Population and Development Review 22:517–530
17. Velkova A.; Wolleswinkel- van den Bosch J.H.; Mackenbach J.P. (1997) The East-West life expectancy gap: Differences in mortality from conditions amenable to medical intervention. International Journal of Epidemiology. 26:75–84
18. Elias N. (1939, 2. Aufl. 1969) Über den Prozeß der Zivilisation. 1. Bd. Wandlungen des Verhaltens in den weltlichen Oberschichten des Abendlandes; Bd. 2. Wandlungen der Gesellschaft. Entwurf zu einer Theorie der Zivilisation. Basel (Francke)
19. Steinkamp G. (1993) Soziale Ungleichheit, Erkrankungsrisiko und Lebenserwartung. Kritik der sozialepidemiologischen Ungleichheitsforschung. Sozial- und Präventivmedizin 38:111–122
20. Badura B. (Hg.) (1981) Soziale Unterstützung und chronische Krankheit. Zum Stand sozialepidemiologischer Forschung Frankfurt (Suhrkamp)
21. Badura B.; Kaufhold G.; Lehmann H.; Pfaff H.; Richter R.; Schott T.; Waltz M. (1987) Leben mit dem Herzinfarkt. Eine sozialepidemiologische Studie. Berlin

The significance of drug utilization for Public Health

Liselotte von Ferber · Hugh McGavock · Ingrid Schubert
Robert H. Vander Stichele · Emilio J. Sanz

The frame of reference of the workshop

Liselotte von Ferber

Public Health aims at improving the health of populations by prevention. It is seldom considered in this frame of prevention that drug use, besides its desired effects, has adverse drug reactions and interactions that may result in iatrogenic ailments, illnesses and even deaths. Inadequate drug prescribing by the physician and inadequate drug use by the patient therefore minimize the desired effect but not necessarily the adverse effects. As a result, the cost utility outcome is in iatrogenic illness and death. Prevention of this iatrogenic morbidity and mortality has to be achieved by monitoring and promoting the quality of drug use. This is the unifying core of the contributions by which drug utilization research and – based on this research – the policy of drug use will supports Public Health in its strategic planning.

To achieve its preventive targets Public Health mostly makes use of population management approaches and organisational measures. Drug utilization research and policies on the other hand are mainly located at the micro level. Drug utilization research assesses the drug use of the patients and drug prescribing of the physician or the drug counselling of the pharmacist. As a result of this research, policy in drug use proposes strategies to optimise drug prescribing and counselling of patients with respect to drug safety, and to improve the quality and cost effectiveness of drug utilization by information and education of patients as well as of physicians and pharmacists. Focussing on the micro level of interactions between doctors and patients, between pharmacists and consumers as well as on information networks for patients', drug utilization research is confronts many different settings of drug use and a broad spectrum of the needs of patients. Drug utilization research therefore relies on multidisciplinary approaches. This is a challenge for research as well as an opportunity for drug policy making. Research offers many and different opportunities for interventions. We will characterize this special situation of drug utilization research and policy in the framework of public health by four essential settings of prevention. There are different options to optimise the quality of drug therapy and drug use. The four most important settings to improve drug utilization are presented below. In contrast to the mainstream of Public Health, these are bottom – up strategies, bridging the gap between research and policy.

The contribution of H. McGavock deals with the setting of prescribing by the doctor. This contribution shows the avoidable risks of illness, emergency hospital admissions and even hospital deaths attributable to prescribed medication. It was drug utilization research, which showed that this iatrogenic morbidity and mortality is mostly caused by sub-standard medical care, i. e. malpractice of prescribing which, in the avoidable cases, is the consequence of a knowledge deficit. Strategies for promoting quality prescribing in primary care are the bridge between research and policy to reduce the pandemic of prescription-related morbidity and mortality.

The contribution of J. Schubert deals with the setting of counselling by the pharmacist. Preventing the pandemic of drug-induced morbidity is an important, but underestimated goal of public health oriented prevention. Public health methodology offers five major functional steps to optimise population health: assessment, problem identification, policy development, implementation and evaluation. These have to be adopted to optimise the everyday task of the pharmacist, counselling the patient on his/her drug use. This is an important task of the pharmacist, as will be shown. This counselling of the patient concerning the right indication, the right dosage and possible adverse drug reactions and drug interactions may help to reduce the pandemic of drug-induced morbidity. This drug utilization concept aims especially at patients with self-medication, e. g. pain relievers, and elderly multimorbid patients receiveing polypharmacy with great risks of interaction.

The contribution of R. Vander Stichele deals with providing the patients with information and supporting their competence. This contribution stresses the crucial but up to now neglected significance of the patient's behaviour for the outcome and effectiveness of his/her treatment. It draws attention to some deficiencies of drug utilization research itself: drug monitoring needs patient-related data collection and methods of clinical psychology and medical sociology to analyse it, and must therefore combine quantitative and qualitative research methods. One bridge between research and policy in this field is the provision of objective, independent results of drug utilization research to health care professionals and patients. For example, are current package inserts optimal for delivering objective, relevant and independent information to the patient?

The fourth contribution deals with settings where an especially vulnerable group – the children are treated. Prevention has to consider groups with special problems, particularly. This contribution shows that the doctor does not usually communicate with the child patient but with its parents, since parents are responsible for and may interfere with the treatment. To optimise drug use, the children themselves must be addressed. As a prerequisite for prevention of iatrogenic illness in children, they should be educated in their knowledge and attitude towards their illness and their medication.

In remarkable contrast to the fact that children belong to a group of vulnerable subjects, is the lack of clinical studies, which evaluate drug safety in children. As a result, off-label and unlicensed drug use in children is very common. Prevention of avoidable iatrogenic morbidity and mortality therefore needs clinical as well as drug utilization studies, under adequate legal and ethical controls.

Strategies for promoting cost-effectiveness in primary care prescribing and for reducing the pandemic of prescription-related morbidity and mortality

HUGH MC GAVOCK

As the title indicates, this presentation introduces two overlapping topics to the work shop.

Prescription-related disease

The most reliable quantification of this worldwide problem is the incidence of acute (emergency) hospital admissions attributable to prescribed medication, excluding para-sui-cide. Approximately 5% of acute admissions in all age-groups are due to this cause, rising to between 10% and 12% in the elderly (over 70) [50, 76]. Similar figures have resulted from studies in the USA [30] and UK. A recent Norwegian study [18] showed that 18% of all hospital deaths of elderly patients were drug-related, half of them assessed as "avoid-able". Since public health administrators are most strongly motivated by quality research data from their own region, it is strongly recommended that priority be given to investiga-tion of prescription-related morbidity and mortality in each country and region.

There are at least four perceived reasons for these statistics:

1. The un-necessary use of drugs leads to 100% risk and zero benefit, e.g. peripheral va-sodilator drugs for end-stage ischaemia of the limbs; pharmacologically-active cough medicines; high-potency steroids for mild eczema; omeprazole for mild dyspepsia; dia-zepam for mild anxiety and antibiotics for viral respiratory tract infections. Research examples of these were given [15].

2. Imprecise diagnosis – often unavoidable in general practice, leading to equally-im-precise use of drugs. Research examples, in which doctors recorded their diagnostic "label", their certainty and their prescribing response were presented [77].

3. Inadequate teaching of the pharmacological basis of therapeutics in UK medical schools, leading to a lifetime's inadequate knowledge of the causes of risk, benefit, ad-verse drug reactions and especially, adverse drug interactions. This betrayal of medical training is compounded by the superb innovation of the drug industry over the past 40 years, producing hundreds of new, more powerful drugs, which require a high level of scientific understanding for their safe and effective use.

4. The advent of "evidence-based medicine". It is probable that the strict, undiscriminat-ing application of evidence-based treatment is contributing to the pandemic of iatro-genic disease in the elderly. The example of a 75-year old patient with low-grade left ventricular dysfunction, arterial fibrillation, hypertension, osteo-arthritis of the hips and early Parkinson's disease was presented as an illustration, for discussion. Such a case requires the most careful judgement as to which evidence-based treatment is un-avoidable and which can be discarded – the re-appearance of the art of medicine, com-promise.

Promoting cost-effective prescribing (a) methods, (b) barriers

▶ Many studies across the developed world have shown how responsive general practitioners are to scientific and economic logic in prescribing (i. e. cost-effectiveness). Examples include:
1. Germany   the "Pharmacotherapeutic Circles" or study groups in the Hess region: 100 GPs saved DM 4.5 m (Euro 2.25 m) in one year compared to GPs in the then BRD and improved their quality of prescribing [21].
2. The "DATIS" academic drug detailing program in South Australia" – 10% of drug budget saved with improved safety [39].
3. The MEDICAID "COMPASS" program in the USA – major improvements in safety and economy [61].
4. The Northern and Southern Ireland "Best Buys" program, saving over £ 10 m yearly in each state [44]. Potential saving was £ 40 m for a population of 1.6 m people.
5. The UK-wide "Fund-holding" scheme average prescribing economies of c. £ 50 000 per practice [51], = £ 500 m yearly (10 000 fundholders).

▶ Barriers to the promotion of cost-effective prescribing.
1. Drug marketing. Skilful marketing of new products to doctors, whose knowledge of pharmacology is inadequate, with many inducements, is perfectly legal. Those concerned with promoting cost-effective prescribing will always have an uphill struggle against this reality [40].
2. The reluctance of governments with large drug manufacturing interests, to harm industrial profitability. A good example is any country, whose government or statutory health insurance is almost a monopoly buyer, but which allows the drug industry to make annual profits well above the rate of inflation.
3. The EU has been a major barrier to those new members whose new drugs licensing policy demanded proof of superiority (rather than non-inferiority) such as Sweden and Iceland, which are now flooded with "me-too" drugs, like the rest of Europe.

The future

The following recommendations were put to the workshop.
1. Undergraduate and postgraduate medical education should contain pharmacology and therapeutics as major elements, including professional examinations for all specialities, and regular life-long revision.
2. All doctors should receive yearly feed-back of their prescribing, with analysis and recommendations for improvement.
3. Doctors should be indirectly rewarded for achieving optimal cost-effectiveness, year by year.
4. Governments should restrict excessive drug industry prices and profits. As health service budgets become more strained, this is likely to occur.

All hospitals with emergency departments should be required to record their iatrogenic (prescription-related) admission rate, which should slowly decrease if (1) to (3) above are implemented.

How pharmacists might use methodologies of drug utilization research and public health research to improve their services

INGRID SCHUBERT

That the use of drugs is an issue of public health relevance was a terrible lesson of the thalidomide catastrophe. Even now, the public health relevance of drug use is demonstrated by the fact that avoidable and preventable adverse events, over- and underuse of drugs, still occur. Further, we face rising drug costs but we do not know for sure whether they are proportionate to the achieved health outcomes. Therefore it is not surprising that we find drug related projects within public health research programs and within public health conferences. As one factor, the quality of the drug use process can be influenced by the work of the pharmacist. Therefore it might be justified to have a look at the profession and its understanding of its central professional task.

Handling drugs is an everyday task of pharmacists. During the second half of the last century, almost all over the world, the profession started to change its technical and drug-centred orientation towards a more patient-oriented perspective. In Germany, the first step had been to introduce pharmacology into the profession's curriculum at the beginning of the seventies. After a long intra-professional debate [58], the pharmacists adopted the new task of drug counselling as part of their professional identity, for example, by embodying it into their occupational statutes and into continuing educational programs during the 80s of the last century. This service orientation has been supported by changes within the health care system and by the growing market share of OTC drugs. Professional tasks are, for example, to make sure that the patient/client chooses the appropriate OTC-drug for his/her complaints or that different drugs (from different GPs or due to self-medication) do not interact with each other. But to have an occupational statute does not mean that this task is always fulfilled. Consumer organisations criticise pharmacists for not counselling patients sufficiently; further, they judge the drugs recommended as not being first choice drugs. One professional strategy – besides others-, has therefore been to implement quality assurance instruments and improve counselling activities. The Saxonys Chamber of Pharmacists was the first to introduce the concept of quality circles for pharmacists in Germany. An example will be given of the successful application of public health research methodology [33].

The critique of consumer organisations and others underlines the necessity and the benefit of a person-related service, which in turn gives pharmacists the opportunity to reinforce their patient-centred orientation. By integrating a new pharmaceutical discipline – clinical pharmacy – into the pharmacy curriculum in the late 90s, they expanded the scientific knowledge of the profession. This is an important tool and resource for inter-professional jurisdictional debate as it allows us to define new problems and solving strategies and to present them as belonging to the core tasks of the profession [1]. This professional "competition" for new tasks will be even more successful when problems are addressed that are mostly neglected by other professions in the field. The optimisation of the drug use process is one such topic. The pharmacists took up a public health perspective by proposing to accept responsibility for improving the health outcomes of patients (their quality of life) by detecting and preventing drug-related health problems. This new professional orientation was introduced in the early nineties as "pharmaceutical care". Again the Saxonys Chamber of Pharmacists initiated a project to develop a pharmaceutical care program for patients suffering from chronic pain [34].

In the following projects, patients with pain have been chosen as a focus, due to the fact that pain-relievers are one of the most widely used drug groups. In Germany they rank first according to the number of prescribed packages and it is estimated that about three quarters of pain-relievers are purchased for self-medication. On the other hand, we know that adverse effects concerning gastrointestinal problems are mainly due to acetylsalicylic acid and NSAIDs (nonsteroidal antiinflammatory drugs) and often lead to hospital admission [29].

Example 1. To improve a service requires first an analysis of deficiencies. This in turn demands instruments and strategies, both to get feed-back on routine procedures and to make use of this information for continuing education. To achieve these goals, the pharmacists implemented a data-based quality circle. This concept – primarily developed and tested by L.v. Ferber et al. [22, 23] to improve the prescribing habits of GPs – adopts the three major functions of public health for the research process: 1. assessment and problem identification; 2. policy development; and 3. assurance and evaluation [31].

The assessment of the counselling activities of pharmacists was achieved with a short-documentation (generating data by self-report of the pharmacist); the quality of the drug selection could be assessed with the help of the pharmacy computer system. The learning process followed the PDCA-Cycle (Plan-Do-Check-Act) addressing the questions: What are we doing? What do we want to improve? How do we want to act? What barriers do we have to face? And finally – did we improve? The learning process was stimulated by an anonymised comparison of the counselling activities between the pharmacies, the opportunity for an exchange of experience during the circle meetings and the joint development of counselling contents and strategies. Following the public health view that there are vulnerable groups which need special attention and further that resources are limited, the pharmacists recommended focussing the counselling efforts on special patient groups: older people with polypharmacy, patients purchasing two different kinds of pain relievers or large packages, and children. The results are summarized in Table 1.

Example 2. The aim of the second project was to develop a pharmaceutical care program for patients with chronic pain. According to Hepler and Strand "Pharmaceutical care is the responsible provision of drug therapy for the purpose of achieving definite outcomes that improve a patient's quality of life. These outcomes are 1. cure of a disease; 2. elimination or reduction of a patient's symptomatology; 3. arresting or slowing of a disease process; or 4. preventing a disease or symptomatology" [28]. In order to achieve the above listed outcomes the pharmacist has to co-operate with the patient and other health professionals (and vice versa). New instruments have to be developed and abilities to be acquired

Table 1. Evaluation of the quality circle for pharmacists: pre-post comparison of the counselling activity

	Pre-Intervention (1998) 1285 patients [%]	Post-Intervention (2000) 930 patients [%]
Patients with...		
...counselling	44	61*
Children/adolescents (< 20y) with counselling	64	90
Elderly patients (> 60y) with counselling	42	53
...counselling initiated by the staff actively	40	50
...pain reliefer as single ingredient drug	38	53

Source: Krappweis, Schubert et al. 2000; * $p > 0.001$, χ^2 Test.

in order to (i) identify potential and actual drug-related problems; (ii) resolve actual drug-related problems; and (iii) prevent drug-related problems [28].

With these three main functions of pharmaceutical care mentioned by Hepler and Strand, the close relation to drug utilization research and its contribution to public health is clear: A structured interview with the patients, a medication profile and an analysis of the subjective and objective data collected, form the basis for developing a pharmaceutical care plan. Drug related problems are detected with the help of a retrospective medication review. The leading question is *"Does the right patient receive the right drug with proper dosage and suitable application form for the correct indication?"* With other words: "Are we doing the right things right?" which is a phrase well known in quality assurance and health care research.

Considering patients with pain, the pharmacists identified the following problems [34]:

- Inappropriate drug combination: e.g. two different NSAIDs at the same time, inappropriate use of a fixed-dose combination
- Inappropriate use by the patient concerning the frequency of use (too often, too seldom)
- Inappropriate dosage (e.g. overdosage of ibuprofen, underdosage of acetylsalicylic acid)
- Potential interaction (e.g. triptane with ergotamine)
- Adverse events (e.g. drug addiction; fear of adverse events of the patients concerning opioids and corticosteroids, gastrointestinal problems caused by NSAID, ergotamineinduced headache)
- Inadequate effect of the drug (patient is dissatisfied with pain management)
- Discontinuing therapy (patient stopped taking drug)
- Therapeutic problems (drug regime not according to guideline; i.e. lack of prokinetic drug for migraine patient; anti-emetic drug for opioid patient, insufficient pain therapy).

Although the number of patients sureyed was very small, the project demonstrated that quite a spectrum of different drug-related problems and information needs occur, even when patients have long experience of their symptoms.

Discussion and conclusion for future public health policy

Both examples given here demonstrate that the instruments and working procedures of public health science and drug utilization research can be successfully applied by pharmacists to improve the professional service: We found that the quality circle work stimulated the pharmacy team to improve counselling activities and we received feed-back from participating pharmacists that the delivery of pharmaceutical care (including drug monitoring and drug utilization review), contributed to the pharmacist's professional satisfaction, an aspect that is difficult to quantify but that should not be neglected or underestimated. But we also have to note that the new working procedures (data-based quality circle work and drug utilization reviews as a central element of pharmaceutical care) has not spread very much within the professional community of pharmacists until now. One reason is that they are time-consuming (for example the documentation of patient interaction, providing pharmaceutical care) and they are not remunerated (for example pharmaceutical care). Furthermore, pharmacists have to note that in general, patients/consumers have not been informed about the new service and are not used to the pharmacist as a person taking over responsibilities for the drug use process. Therefore they do not ask as actively for information or further care as pharmacists would expect them to do. Besides, pharmacists face new competitors in the form of managed health care organisations and call centres who claim to be in charge of the patients' compliance and health behaviour. In order to further establish and improve pharmacists' contribution to prevent drug related morbidity and to optimise drug utilisation some changes concerning education, remuneration and co-operation and information exchange with other health professionals have to take place. The following activities and strategies – some of them started already – might help to achieve these aims:

▶ To translate the curriculum for pharmacology and clinical pharmacy into action in all pharmacy departments at university,

▶ to intensify the public health aspects of the pharmacists work in continuing education,

▶ to implement working routines for the pharmacy team in order to address patients in special need of information (e.g. pharmacy based training how to counsel, what to focus on, whom to offer pharmaceutical care),

▶ to implement a quality assurance system that enables each pharmacy to analyse, evaluate and improve its services (e.g. data based quality circles, peer review),

▶ to set up interprofessional discussion groups (GPs, Pharmacists, community nurses) in order to exchange profession specific knowledge (e.g. on new drugs) or patient related problems (compliance, perceived effect of drug),

▶ to establish a tool for information exchange concerning the drug use and diseases/indication between patient, physician and pharmacists (e.g. smart cards),

▶ to use pharmacists as a source for monitoring new drugs or screening for special drug related problems (e.g. indication for prescribing, documentation of side effects),

▶ to communicate the drug and health related services of the pharmacist to patients and other health professionals in order to sensitise for drug related problems (cf. the statements of McGavock in this paper).

▶ Last but not least, to implement an adequate remuneration system for pharmacists who contribute to public health concerns by counselling the patient intensively, by accompanying the drug use process of the patient and by informing physicians systematically about drugs or patient problems.

Bridging the gap between research and policy in public health regarding pharmaceuticals. Focusing on the patient

ROBERT H. VANDER STICHELE

Introduction

Within the health care system, pharmaceuticals are probably among the most cost-effective interventions, with high standards in research and development of new therapeutic compounds. The cost of innovation is however of major concern, due to raising expenditures and questions about appropriateness and effectiveness of drug utilization. In clinical trials and pharmaco-economic studies, efficacy, safety and cost-effectiveness of new pharmaceutical interventions are thoroughly assessed in a difficult process of health technology assessment. The majority of systematic reviews in the Cochrane Library deal with clinical questions related to the use of medicines. Yet, most of this evidence has been collected in the framework of rigorous clinical trials, where patients are expected (after informed consent) to execute treatments faithfully, and are rigorously supervised for that purpose.

In real life, things are different. Patients are free to choose among treatments and to continue or discontinue the chosen treatment. In the drug distribution system, many prescribing errors and dispensing errors are made, sometimes, but not always spotted or corrected by attentive patients [9, 19, 32, 46]. Patients make errors. Patients do not comply with prescribed regimens, sometimes rightly and sometimes to their own detriment. It is only recently that the human factor, the patient factor, has been taken into account, when assessing the outcome of therapy and the effectiveness of treatments. The problem is that the borderline positive evaluations of cost-effectiveness of interventions coming from clinical trials change to neutral or negative when the human factor is taken into account.

A central role for patients' preferences

Public health policy has become a quest to find the best available interventions, applied in the best possible way [55]. In the new paradigm of Evidence-Based Medicine, medical decision-making becomes a triangular process:

The new but crucial element of the preference of the patient has been introduced for several reasons. First, science has not yet found ways to weigh objective but separate measurements of risk and benefit, and this is then left to the patient, the recipient of the intervention. Secondly, the historical evolution of 'consumerism' and the ethical principles of patient autonomy have transformed the doctor-patient relationship into a therapeutic partnership. For the correct execution of the intervention, the acceptance and co-operation of the patient has become crucial [59]. Objective information is one way to achieve this, in the hope that the information will be convincing enough for a rational person, pursuing his/her optimal health status. Furthermore, informing the patient objectively has become an ethical duty by the principle of informed consent [48]. Persuading patients to accept treatment with emotional arguments alone or bullying is no longer an option. Enforcing health policies with drill, coercion, or indoctrination is outdated.

Three implications for the field of pharmaco-epidemiology and drug utilization research

Firstly, the monitoring of utilization of drugs should become more patient-oriented, instead of drug-oriented. Many countries are still struggling to put up traditional continuous monitoring systems, based on administrative databases of drug dispensing (either through the wholesalers, the pharmacies or the insurers). Despite privacy problems, the future is however with clinical data collecting systems at the micro-level of physician-patient interaction (or pharmacist-patient interaction), combining registration of the morbidity and prescription.

Secondly, measurement of patient compliance with new precise techniques (electronic monitoring) is crucial, in the research setting and in the clinical setting, especially in situations where an exact knowledge of compliance patterns is necessary to correctly appraise the relation between intervention and effect. Continued application of crude, invalid measurement methods such as pill count and questionnaires will lead to failure to choose the best drug therapies and to failure to detect non-compliance and its consequences [71, 72].

Thirdly, drug utilization research must evolve from a quantitative, number-crunching science to incorporate various methodological approaches to the measurement of the subjective values, opinions, preferences and attitudes of patients. This means extension into the field of clinical psychology, medical sociology and even anthropology. It necessitates the ability to combine quantitative and qualitative research methods.

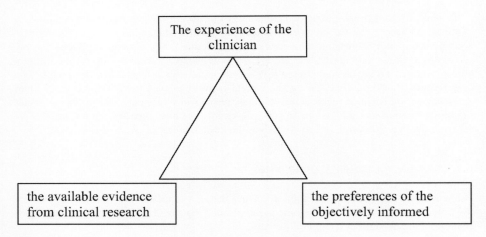

Fig. 1

The eclectic discipline of drug utilization research can help to bridge the gap between research and health policy with regard to pharmaceuticals, by identifying special target groups, by monitoring the effects of pharmaceutical policy measures, and thereby generate findings that can help to design effective implementation programs to foster the appropriate use of effective drugs.

Focus on the provision of objective, independent, drug information to health care workers, health care policy-makers and patients

Objective, independent drug information is the tool par excellence to bridge the gap between the available evidence on pharmaceuticals on the one hand, and the dispenser, prescriber and patients, all making decision as to drug choice, on the other.

Assuring the availability of objective information should be the responsibility of the health authorities. One can argue that it is the task of the health care provider to take all the necessary steps to be able to have access to valuable sources of information at the point of care. But it seems wise for health care policy-makers to take a more organizational approach and to invest in the logistics of providing independent information to health care workers (and the professional civil servants and decision-makers who work inside the health care policy departments).

Independent drug information for the health care professional

Almost every country has a national Drug Information Center (DIC), related in various degrees to health authorities and academic clinical pharmacologists, editing physician-desk reference books and drug bulletins [43]. One aspect of policy is to stimulate these centres, provide them with the modern means of communication through print, web, personal digital assistants and medical record software, to enable the messages of independent drug information to flow more freely.

(Note: Drug utilization researchers should cooperate with these centres, who are often the national keepers of the list of licensed medicines, which are currently available on the market. This is a valuable tool needed for valid cross-national monitoring of drug consumption. On the other hand, drug utilization researchers can help the DICs by providing priority lists for topics of drug information.)

Since the development of the Cochrane Collaboration, the advent of the Evidence-Based Medicine movement and publications like Clinical Evidence, health care workers now have access to valuable sources of point-of-care information, brought to them by new communication technologies (IT).

Here is a chance to break the traditional isolation of health care workers, at the coal face of the health care system (general practice and peripheral hospitals), who do not have access to the scientific library system, at least not as medical students and health care workers in academic clinics do.

A number of countries or health care areas are now envisaging the purchase of national licences for these information sources and the installation of a virtual medical library with essential information sources, available to all health care workers in their own language [35, 68].

Independent drug information for patients

In the Evidence-Based Medicine paradigm, the objective information of a well-informed patient is crucial.

The Cochrane Collaboration has embarked on simplification of the abstracts of the more then 2000 systematic reviews it is maintaining, to make them accessible to patients. Health authorities have set up web sites with independent health and drug information, some with limited patient counselling, and are regulating patient information more intensely [46].

With regard to pharmaceuticals, the European Union has a policy of patient package inserts, to be distributed with every packet dispensed. This authoritive document should reflect the official information of the Summary of Product Characteristics, produced and accepted at the registration of the drug and updated thereafter.

This is one of the few examples where an industry is legally obliged to communicate in an understandable way with its clients (patients).

There is room for improvement in the quality of this important medium. Research into patients preferences should pave the way for the development of sound theoretical models and communication strategies to be incorporated in the editing of these inserts. The inserts are currently mainly oriented towards risk information (side-effects and contra-indications, interactions). There is considerable need for positive messages in this document [73]. Qualitative drug utilization research, focusing on the impact of the patient package inserts could provide important information for the optimal production of this invaluable vehicle of understandable, but valid, objective and balanced drug information at the point of care.

Evidence-based drug information and/or direct-to-consumer advertising?

In the May 2002 report of the High Level Group on innovation and provision of medicines (European Union and G10 Group) carried a recommendation (number 10) with regard to patient information on pharmaceuticals. It called for a reviewing of patient package inserts taking into account views of users. Furthermore, it called for regulation of pharmaceutical advertising and enhanced information for patients in a public-private partnership (http://Pharmacos.eudra.org./F3/g10/g10home.htm).

A power struggle is developing at the European level around Direct-to-Consumer Advertising [41, 53]. Will pharmaceutical companies be allowed to address the patient directly, either by short promotional messages or by extensive information of varying degrees of objectivity, even for prescription-only medicines? On October 23, 2002, the European Parliament rejected a proposal to relax the ban on advertising for prescription drugs (in the field of AIDS, asthma, and diabetes) by 434 against 42.

Meanwhile, in cyberspace, pharmaceutical companies have not waited to take up the opportunities of the Internet to establish relationships with the patients consuming their medicines.

Health Authorities face a historic choice to invest or not to invest in the extension of objective, independent drug information to the patients in the new media. The cost of this investment would be relatively low. The Drug Information Centres, now serving the health care professionals, could be called upon to develop expertise to extend their activities towards the general public, making maximum use of the wonders of the new media.

Drug Utilization Research has been the witness of the lost battles and victories in the fight between commercial information and independent drug information. This struggle has been going on for a long time, it is continuing in cyberspace, but this time with a fairer chance for providers of objective, independent information to reach effectively larger audiences and to make a difference with regard to the rational prescribing and rational use of drugs.

Drug utilization in children: Are there more benefits than risks?

EMILIO J. SANZ

Drug utilization as a part of both clinical pharmacology/pharmacy and epidemiology constitutes a field of work closely related to public health. In Europe, drug utilization research is developing in the framework of public health and thus is related, but with a different "'emphasis", than the more American approach to pharmacoepidemiology. In this latter approach, efficacy and safety are the key, together with some economical evaluations (normally in order to probe that "this new drug" is worthwhile). From the "'European drug utilization" concept the emphasis is more on effectiveness and efficiency; that is, the way drugs should be used to better achieve their health potential, more than to improve their business profit or cost/benefit analysis.

Another important aspect of drug utilisation in relation to the "rational use of drugs" is whether targeting the individual is more relevant and useful than targeting the structures, or vice versa. Both prescribers and patients have many hidden agenda when dealing with drugs. As social tokens, drugs are not merely used for the relief of symptoms or the treatment of diseases, but they are also used as identifiers of care, means to achieve "the privileges of illness", grounding reputations (of a caring or compliant persons, for example), or by reverting to the "magical". Such a complex network of interactions very seldom reacts to structural and organizational changes, but very rapidly changes when an individual, personally relevant and adequately implemented action occurs. A typical example might be the sharp drop in sales or prescription after scandalous press campaigns, about a drug. Targeting the education, and which is more important, the values – explicit and implicit – of both prescribers and patients, is the key to long-lasting changes in trends.

The use of drugs in children may be seen as a particular field in which both technical and societal issues are at work, and constitutes a good example of these types of interaction.

Children as "methodological and therapeutical" orphans

Despite the increase in research and knowledge about drugs, children are often "methodo-logically and therapeutically orphans". They are normally healthier than adults, use fewer drugs, have a lower rate of admission to hospitals, and despite the number of visits to the general practitioner or "general paediatrician", present a smaller number of diagnoses than adults. Apart from this, children normally show a very good recovery from non-serious diseases, and are probably better psychologically adapted to disease than adults; possibly because they don't fully understand the long-term consequences of disease, have less preju-dices (and less experience), and normally have greater support by others. But, when they are seriously ill, they need effective and safe drugs in appropriate dosages, sometimes with imperfectly recognized genetic factors and peculiarities on the progression of the disease or the pharmacodynamics and pharmacokinetics of the drugs.

What do we know about this situation?

There is a substantial lack of systematic attention to this area of drug epidemiology: drug use in children is a 'hidden' reality in the literature; the wealth of methodological develop-ments that have taken place in the general field of drug use monitoring has barely reached children. Children can still be considered "methodological orphans" with respect to the transferable knowledge of the benefit/risk profile of therapies they receive [8].

Drug utilisation in children is a relatively poorly understood area of Clinical Pharma-cology in these days (56). There are too few studies that analyse diagnoses and drug pre-scription patterns. A lot of them are based on sales data and not on diagnoses [4, 12]. Lack of information is especially due to the unavailability of databases containing informa-tion about the more frequent diagnoses in each area, as well as the indications for the pre-scriptions written. Most of the available studies are based on data collected from only one country, without comparisons with other locations [3, 13, 27, 38, 45, 54, 60, 62, 75], or are dedicated to pharmacological treatments of specific diagnosis [6, 37, 47, 52], or therapeutic groups [11, 42, 49, 74].

The necessity for a wider range of knowledge about these aspects, and the possibility of comparing data from different world areas prompted the EURO-DURG to start, in 1997, a project based on drug prescribing in children (CHILDURG). From a descriptive angle, CHILDURG is intended to detect possible areas of improvement in the outpatient prescrib-ing to children by comparing the different variables analysed.

In the CHILDURG study, a randomly selected sample of 12 264 paediatric outpatients seen in consultation rooms of urban and rural areas and attended by the paediatricians or general practitioners of the seven participating locations (Tenerife, Valencia and Barcelona (Spain), Toulouse (France), Sofia (Bulgaria), Slovakia and Russia) was analysed. Data on patient demographic information, diagnosis and pharmacological treatment, were collected on pre-designed forms. Diagnoses were coded using the ICD-9 and drugs according to the WHO-ATC classification.

The average number of diagnoses per child varied slightly, from 1.1 in Russia to 1.5 in Slovakia. In the ten most common diagnoses, URTI (urinary tract infections) are in the first position in all locations; asthma prevalence is greatest in Tenerife (8.4%), whereas it accounts for only 1.6% in Bulgaria, and is not present in the top-ten diagnoses in Slovakia or Russia. Tonsillitis, otitis, bronchitis and dermatological affections are common diag-noses in all locations. Pneumonia is only recorded in Sofia (3.8%) and Russia (2.3%). The average number of drugs prescribed per child varies from 1.3 in Barcelona to 2.9 in Rus-sia.

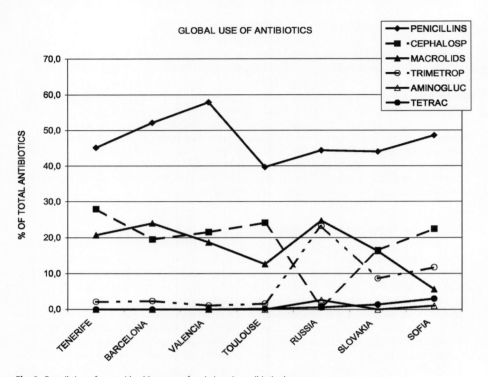

Fig. 2. Describtion of a considerable range of variations in antibiotic therapy

There are no great differences in the proportion of pharmacological groups prescribed, but a considerable range of variations in antibiotic therapy is observed as described in Fig. 2.

Visits for check-up are not recorded in Russia or Slovakia whereas in Toulouse these visits account for 16.2% and in the other locations the percentage varies from 6.1% (Tenerife) to 1.9% (Sofia). Homeopathic treatments are registered only in Toulouse. As a general comment, except in asthma prevalence, there are no great differences in the diagnostic patterns between locations but the variation in the number of drugs prescribed per child and the pattern of antibiotic therapies are much greater than expected from the pure morbidity patterns. There are several other areas for improvement that have been identified in this study [57].

Apart from prescriptions, a large number of children are also exposed to various home remedies, and the "home modification" of therapeutic regimens. In the study by Trott, Z. [67] 1750 questionnaires (anonymous inquiry) were given to parents of children at four schools in Bavaria. On average, each child took 3.17 drugs per year, mainly for respiratory infections, fever, pain and gastrointestinal symptoms. Analgesics, nasal preparations, cough medicines, gastrointestinal medications and antibiotics were used frequently and psychotropic drugs only rarely (rank 20). Overall, drugs and home remedies were used with almost equal frequency (1.23:1). Of the parents who responded, 79.3% were satisfied with the prescribed drugs; but 9.1% stated that they changed the dosage of the prescribed drugs. So much for the use of drugs in children; it seems that children use fewer drugs, they have fewer side effects but the use of antibiotics is still very high nowadays.

Table 2. Off-label and unlicensed drug use in paediatrics

		Unlicensed %	Off-label %	Total observed
Outpatients	Gavrilov 2000	8	26	132
Neonatal Intensive Care	Avenel 2000	10	62	40
Neonatal Intensive Care	Conroy 1999	10	54.7	70
Paediatric wards	Conroy 2000	7.3	38.6	624
Paediatric wards	Turner 1998	6.9	18.2	609

But even when drugs are correctly used, the knowledge we have about them is very limited. There are too few clinical trials of drugs in children and that prevent prescribers from having the requisite knowledge for the correct use of a medication in children. Why is this so? There could be several causes. First, pharmacokinetics and pharmacodynamics in children are different from those in adults, particularly in certain developmental stages, and there is a lack of controlled clinical trials, which sufficiently evaluate the efficacy, and safety of most drugs in children [2]; this results in the off-label use of drugs for children. Secondly, children are the "third partners" in the doctor-patient relationship, with their parents (mostly their mothers) acting as the interface between the clinician and the treatment. This creates difficulties in recognizing and describing symptoms and arriving at the correct diagnosis, apart from the issue of "maternal transferred self-medication", which is all too common. For the same reason, the use of medication must take into account not only the clinical value and parental convenience, but children's preferences as well (route, taste, etc.). Finally children are normally seen as passive recipients of clinical care and not expected (or obliged) to intervene in the control of their own medication, even when they become older.

The result is an enormous **"off-label"** and **"unlicensed"** use of drugs in paediatrics. The first reports on the extent of the problem appeared in 1992 [5] and then J. Collier highlighted this in an editorial in Br J Clin Pharmacol [14]. The first study on the extent of the problem in children was by Gavrilov in 2000 (24). In this study, out of 222 prescriptions issued in the general paediatric ambulatory unit of a Hospital, 8% were unlicensed and 26% off-label. Since then a number of other papers [7, 16, 17, 69, 70] have analysed the problem in several settings, as it is shown in Table 2.

This is a problem for two reasons: the first is that valid and useful drugs are used in children without the safety requirements and the adequate knowledge to get optimal use of them. Secondly, the incidence of ADRs may be increased. Nevertheless ADRs are less often reported in children than in adults, and there is no easy explanation of that fact. Less morbidity, less intensive use of drugs, more difficulties in finding the causal relationship; so, have ADRs in children a lower prevalence or are they under-reported?

The health policy issue here is how to promote clinical research with children. The need for further studies is clear. On the one hand we need more clinical and research data. Clinical trials are very seldom performed in children, mainly due to issues of costs and responsibilities and to regulations, which frequently result in major obstacles. On the other hand one might ask: Is it ethical? Is it advisable? According to the last revision of the Helsinki declaration, "Vulnerable subjects need special protection of their rights and welfare to ensure that they do not bear more than their fair share of the burden of participation in research" (Art. 27), but also add in the same article that "The inclusion of vulnerable subjects in biomedical research is most readily justified in the context of research designed to develop new diagnostic, prophylactic or therapeutic modalities for classes of vulnerable subjects (e.g., children or persons with mental diseases) or the basic knowledge upon which such developments can be based; such research must necessarily involve members of the relevant vulnerable groups as subjects".

On ethics, there is the additional requirement of informed consent. So, it is primarily a problem of satisfying legal and ethical conditions of the trials. In this sense, the new FDA regulation promoting research in children is to be encouraged and imitated [20] (The new proposed pediatric labelling legislation, promoting new studies on (old and new) drug use in children would grant six months of market exclusivity to medicines that have undergone pediatric studies.) Clinical trials in children must be supported by paying particular attention to the ethical issues, the methodological problems and the relevance of the knowledge to be obtained. The N-of-1 trials [25] are probably a reliable alternative, especially in the first stages of developing a new drug. In conclusion, as several authors stated in BMJ recently "Support for studies in paediatric medicine is needed [36]."

Finally, another point needs to be addressed. How do the children themselves see their medicines and the risk of side-effects?

In the study by Hamm et al. [26] they showed that a patient's satisfaction did not depend on whether they received a prescription for antibiotics or not, but rather on the time the doctor spent with them in the consultation room. Children are often neglected during pediatric consultation and communication (most of it is between doctors and parents) and their knowledge about medicines and their autonomy in medicine use is systematically underestimated (USP Open Conference. Children and medicines: Information isn't just for grownups. September 29-October 1, 1996. Reston. Virginia and USP Ad-hoc advisory panel on children and medicines: The "Ten Guiding principles for teaching children about medicines". USP, Washington 1998 (available at www.usp.org; last accession January 23, 2003)). During the last ten years, a multidisciplinary team of social scientists, pediatricians and clinical pharmacologists has been involved in the study of childrens' knowledge, perceptions and attitudes to health, disease and medicine use in several European countries [10, 65, 66]. Presently the team is investigating children with asthma under the auspices of the European Commission's BIOMED (Directorate General XII). The research includes the exploration of children's perceptions and comprehension of asthma, the role of the disease and its medication in their lives [64], and childrens' and parents' perceived needs for information about the care and management of asthma [63].

Many children have clear explanations about concepts regarding their status of health and disease, many have good knowledge about drugs, and when using a chronic treatment (anti-asthmatic for example) show a great amount of autonomy (both perceived and granted by the parents). There is a very good ground for health education in the actual knowledge and attitudes of the children. Their perception of the efficacy and risk of medicines is, in general more adequate and safe than the knowledge and attitudes of many adults.

In conclusion for Public Health policy makers

▶ Clinical Trials in children should be encouraged and promoted despite the difficulties and peculiarities. Governmental regulations should change to promote it.

▶ At the same time, more intensive post-marketing surveillance and Drug Utilisation Studies are needed in order to identify the critical points of the current use of drugs and to promote a better use of them.

▶ Prospective surveys of off-label use and unlicensed use of drugs in children is an issue that is closely related to the lack of clinical trials but that must be addressed soon with innovative methods.

▶ State sponsored health education programs are essential to optimize the use of health resources when dealing with children and especially to achieve the "informed" over-the-counter use of medicines both to children and their parents.

▶ More research on the efficacy and safety of drugs used in children is needed.

Acknowledgement

We are grateful to the Fritz and Hildegard Berg-Stiftung im Stifterverband der Deutschen Wissenschaft, who sponsored this international and interdisciplinary workshop. The participants formulated recommendations for the future Public Health policy of drug utilisation and will have to work at their realization.

References

1. Abbott A (1988) The System of Professions. An Essay on the Division of Expert Labor. Chicago and London: The University of Chicago Press
2. ADEC (Australian Drug Evaluation Committee) (1997). Report of the working party on the registration of drugs for use in children. Published 1-10-1997. (Available ADEC Secretariat: brenley.milsom@health.gov.au)
3. Ahmad SR, Bhutta ZA (1990) A survey of paediatric prescribing and dispensing in Karachi. J Pak Med Assoc 40:126–130
4. Andrew M (1990) Toverud EL. [Prescription of drugs in Norway to children aged 0–12 years]. Tidsskr Nor Laegeforen 110:3215–3219
5. Anonimous (1992) Prescribing unlicensed drugs or using drugs for unlicensed indications. Drug Ther Bull 30:97–99
6. Arnold SR, Allen UD, Al Zahrani M, Tan DH, Wang EE (1999) Antibiotic prescribing by pediatricians for respiratory tract infection in children. Clin Infect Dis 29:312–317
7. Avenel S, Bomkratz A, Dassieu G, Janaud JC, Danan C (2000) [The incidence of prescriptions without marketing product license in a neonatal intensive care unit]. Arch Pediatr 7:143–147
8. Bonati M (1994) Epidemiologic evaluation of drug use in children. J Clin Pharmacol 34:300–305
9. Bootman JL, Harrison D, Cox E (1997) The Healthcare Cost of Drug-Related Morbidity and Mortality in Nursing Facilities. Arch Int Med, 157:2089–2096
10. Bush PJ, Trakas DJ, Sanz EJ, Wirsing RL, Vaskilampi T, Prout A (1996) Children, medicines, and culture. New York: Pharmaceutical Products Press
11. Cars H, Hakansson A (1997) Prescriptions of antibiotics for children. Prescribing habits of district, hospital, and private physicians. Scand J Prim Health Care 15:22–25
12. Catford JC (1980) Quality of prescribing for children in general practice. Br Med J 280(6229):1435–1437
13. Collet JP, Bossard N, Floret D, Gillet J, Honegger D, Boissel JP (1991) Drug prescription in young children: results of a survey in France. Epicreche Research Group. Eur J Clin Pharmacol 41:489–491
14. Collier J (1999) Paediatric prescribing: using unlicensed drugs and medicines outside their licensed indications [editorial]. Br J Clin Pharmacol 48:5–8
15. Connolly JP, Mc Gavock H (1999) Antibiotic prescribing for respiratory tract infections in general practice. Pharmacoepidem. Drug Safety 8:95–104
16. Conroy S, Choonara I, Impicciatore P, Mohn A, Arnell H, Rane A et al. (2000) Survey of unlicensed and off label drug use in paediatric wards in European countries. European Network for Drug Investigation in Children. BMJ 320(7227):79–82
17. Conroy S, McIntyre J, Choonara I (1999) Unlicensed and off label drug use in neonates Arch Dis Child Fetal Neonatal Ed 80:142–144
18. Ebbeson J, Buajordet I, Erikssen J et al. (2001) Drug related deaths in a department of internal medicine. Arch Intern Med. 161:2317–2323
19. Edgell ET, Summers KH, Hylan TR, Ober J, Bootman JL (1999) A framework for drug utilization evaluation in depression: insights from outcomes research. Med Care 37(4 Suppl):AS67–76
20. FDA (1997) Pediatric patients; regulations requiring manufacturers to assess the safety and effectiveness of new drugs and biological products; proposed rule. Federal Register 62(158):43889–43916

21. Ferber L von (1997) Evaluation der Pharmakotherapiezirkel in der KV Hessen 1995/96. Qualitätssicherung durch Pharmakotherapiezirkel, Evaluation von 8 Pharmakotherapiezirkeln der KVH 1995/1996. QualiMed 5 97/3:2734
22. Ferber L von, Bausch J, Köster I, Schubert I, Ihle P (1999a) Pharmacotherapeutic Circles. Results of an 18-Month Peer-Review Prescribing-Improvement-Programme for General Practitioners. Pharmacoeconomics: 273–283
23. Ferber L von, Köster I, Schubert I, Ihle P (1999b) How to set up and run prescribing quality study groups for general practitioners including problems and outcomes. In: Handbook of Drug Use Research Methodology edited by Hugh McGavock. The United Kingdom Drug Utilisation Research Group, New Castle upon Tyne, pp 197–215
24. Gavrilov V, Lifshitz M, Levy J, Gorodischer R (2000) Unlicensed and off-label medication use in a general pediatrics ambulatory hospital unit in Israel. Isr Med Assoc J 2:595–597
25. Guyatt G, Sackett D, Adachi J, Roberts R, Chong J, Rosenbloom D et al. (1988) A clinician's guide for conducting randomized trials in individual patients. CMAJ 139:497–503
26. Hamm RM, Hicks RJ, Bemben DA (1996) Antibiotics and respiratory infections: are patients more satisfied when expectations are met? J Fam Pract 43:56–62
27. Hawkins N, Golding J (1995) A survey of the administration of drugs to young infants. The Alspac Survey Team. Avon Longitudinal Study of Pregnancy and Childhood. Br J Clin Pharmacol 40:79–82
28. Hepler DD, Strand LM (1989) "Opportunities and Responsibilities in Pharmaceutical Care", Am.J. Pharm.Educ., 53, 7S–15S
29. Hoffmann A, Hippius M, Sicker T (1998) Adverse drug reaction monitoring in Jena – experiences of a regionalized pharmacovigilance centre Toxic. Pathol. 50, pp 453–457
30. Huang B, Bachmann KA, He X et al. (2002) Inappropriate prescriptions for the ageing population of the United States: an analysis of the National Ambulatory Medical Care Survey, 1997. Pharmacoepidem. Drug Safety 11:127134
31. Institute of Medicine, Committee for the Study of the Future of Public Health. Division of Health Care Services (1988) The Future of Public Health, National Academy Press, Washington, DC
32. Johnson JA, Bootman JL (1997) Drug-related morbidity and mortality and the economic impact of pharmaceutical care. Am J Health Syst Pharm 54:554–558
33. Krappweis J, Schubert I, Krappweis B (2000) Qualitätssicherung der Beratung der Schmerzpatient in der Apotheke. Abschlussbericht.
34. Krappweis J, Schubert I (2002) Pharmazeutische Betreuung von Patienten mit chronischen Schmerzen in sächsischen Apotheken, Abschlussbericht des Projektes für SLAK und Förderinitiative Pharmazeutische Betreuung e.V.
35. Lacroix EM, Mehnert R (2002) The US National Library of Medicine in the 21st century: expanding collections, nontraditional formats, new audiences. Health Info Libr J. 19:126–132
36. Lennon R, Quinn M, Collard K (2000) Support for studies in paediatric medicine is needed. BMJ 321(7270):1228
37. Mainous AG, III, Hueston WJ, Love MM (1998). Antibiotics for colds in children: who are the high prescribers? Arch Pediatr Adolesc Med 152:349–352
38. Massele AY, Ofori-Adjei D, Laing RO (1993) A study of prescribing patterns with special reference to drug use indicators in Dar es Salaam Region, Tanzania. Trop Doct 23:104–107
39. May F, Rowett D (2000) DATIS Academic drug detailing to general practitioners – techniques, problems and outcomes. In: Handbook of Drug Use Research Methodology. UK Drug Utilization Research Group, pp 178–196
40. Mc Gavock H, Webb CH, Johnston GD, Milligan E (1993) Market penetration of new drugs in one U.K. region – implication for GPs and administration. BMJ 307:11181120
41. Mintzes B (2002) For and against: Direct to consumer advertising is medicalising normal human experience: For BMJ 324:908–909
42. Molstad S, Hovelius B, Kroon L, Melander A (1990) Prescription of antibiotics to out-patients in hospital clinics, community health centres and private practice. Eur J Clin Pharmacol 39:9–12
43. Mullerova H, Vlcek J (1998) European drug information centres – survey of activities. Pharm World Sci. 20:131–135
44. Needham R (1987) Ministerial letter of thanks to Northern Irish GPs on cost-effective prescribing. Department of Health and social Services, Northern Ireland, pp 5
45. Niclasen BV, Moller SM, Christensen RB (1995) Drug prescription to children living in the Arctic. An investigation from Nuuk, Greenland. Arctic Med Res 54 Suppl 1:95–100
46. Nightingale SL, McGinnis TJ (1997) The role of the US Food and Drug Administration's patient information initiative in cost-effective drug therapy. Pharmacoeconomics 11:119–125
47. Nyquist AC, Gonzales R, Steiner JF, Sande MA (1998) Antibiotic prescribing for children with colds, upper respiratory tract infections, and bronchitis. JAMA 279:875–877

48. Oxman AD, Chalmers I, Sackett DL (2001) A practical guide to informed consent to treatment. BMJ Dec 22–29 323(7327):1464–1466
49. Pennie RA (1998) Prospective study of antibiotic prescribing for children. Can Fam Physician 44:1850–1856
50. Pirohamed M, Breckenridge AM, Kitteringham NR et al. (1968). Adverse drug reactions. BMJ 316: 1295–1298
51. Rafferty T, Wilson-Davis K, Mc Gavock H (1997) How has fundholding in Northern Ireland affected prescribing patterns? BMJ 315:166–170
52. Resnick SD, Hornung R, Konrad TR (1996) A comparison of dermatologists and generalists. Management of childhood atopic dermatitis. Arch Dermatol 132(9):1047–1052
53. Rosenthal MB, Berndt ER, Donohue JM, Frank RG, Epstein AM (2002) Promotion of prescription drugs to consumers. N Engl J Med. 346:498–505
54. Rylance GW, Woods CG, Cullen RE, Rylance ME (1988) Use of drugs by children. BMJ 297(6646):445–447
55. Sackett DL, Rosenberg WM, Gray JA, Haynes RB, Richardson WS (1996) Evidence based medicine: what it is and what it isn't. BMJ 312:71–72
56. Sanz EJ (1998) Drug prescribing for children in general practice. Acta Paediatr 87:489–490
57. Sanz E, Hernandez MA, Ratchina S, Stratchounsky L, Peire MA, Lapeyre-Mestre M et al. (2002) Drug utilization in outpatient children. A comparison between Tenerife, Barcelona and Valencia (Spain), Toulouse (France), Sofia (Bulgaria), Slovakia and Russia. (Submitted)
58. Schubert I (1994) Apotheker – wozu? Eine Studie zur Berufsentwicklung des Apothekerberufs in der Bundesrepublik. Deutscher Apotheker Verlag Stuttgart
59. Stevenson FA, Barry CA, Britten N, Barber N, Bradley CP (2000) Doctor-patient communication about drugs: the evidence for shared decision making. Soc Sci Med. 50:829–840
60. Straand J, Rokstad K, Heggedal U (1998) Drug prescribing for children in general practice. A report from the More & Romsdal Prescription Study. Acta Paediatr 87:218
61. Strom BL, Morse ML (1988) Use of computerized databases to survey drug utilization in relation to diagnoses. Acta. Med. Scand. Suppl. 721:1320
62. Tomson G, Diwan V, Angunawela I (1990) Paediatric prescribing in out-patient care. An example from Sri Lanka. Eur J Clin Pharmacol 39:469–473
63. Trakas D (2000) Living with asthma in childhood. ASPRO II. Contract Number HBM4-CT96-0266. European Commission GDXII. Health Services Research. BIOMED2
64. Trakas D (1997) The pharmacological and socio-cultural management of childhood asthma. ASPRO I. Contract Number BMH1-CT94-1399. European Commission GDXII. Health Services Research
65. Trakas DJ, Sanz E (1996) Childhood and medicine use in a cross-cultural perspective: A European concerted action. European Commission Directorate-General XII Science, Research and Development
66. Trakas DJ, Sanz EJ (1992) Studying Childhood and Medicine Use: A Multidisciplinary Approach. 1 ed. Athens: ZHTA
67. Trott GE, Wirth S, Badura F, Friese HJ, Nissen G. (1993) [Drug treatment of 7- to 14-year-old children. Results of a parent survey]. Z Kinder Jugendpsychiatr 21:148–155
68. Turner A, Fraser V, Muir Gray JA, Toth B (2002) A first class knowledge service: developing the National electronic Library for Health. Health Info Libr J. 19:133–145
69. Turner S, Longworth A, Nunn AJ, Choonara I (1998) Unlicensed and off label drug use in paediatric wards: prospective study. BMJ 316(7128):343–345
70. Turner S, Nunn AJ, Fielding K, Choonara I (1999) Adverse drug reactions to unlicensed and off-label drugs on paediatric wards: a prospective study. Acta Paediatr 88:965–968
71. Urquhart J (2001) Some economic consequences of noncompliance. Curr Hypertens Rep 3:473–480
72. Urquhart J (1999) Pharmacoeconomic consequences of variable patient compliance with prescribed drug regimens. Pharmacoeconomics 15:217–228
73. Vander Stichele RH, Van Dierendonck A, De Vooght G, Reynvoet B, Lammertyn J (2002) Impact of benefit messages in patient package inserts on subjective drug perception. Drug Inf J 26:201–208
74. Wang EE, Einarson TR, Kellner JD, Conly JM (1999) Antibiotic prescribing for Canadian preschool children: evidence of overprescribing for viral respiratory infections. Clin Infect Dis 29:155–160
75. Wessling A, Soderman P, Boethius G. (1991) Monitoring of drug prescriptions for children in the county of Jamtland and Sweden as a whole in 1977–1987. Acta Paediatr Scand 80:944–952
76. Williamson J, Chaplin JM (1980) Adverse drug reactions to prescribed drugs in the elderly; a multi-centre investigation. Age and Ageing 9:73–80
77. Wilson-Davis K, Mc Gavock H (2000) The Belfast Classification aggregating drugs according to the specificity of their use in general practice. In Handbook of Drug Use research Methodology. UK Drug Utilization Research Group 164–175

Gender Bias – gender research in Public Health

Ulrike Maschewsky-Schneider · Judith Fuchs

Introduction

The inclusion of gender as an essential research category in public health sciences is state of the art in the US, Canada and some other countries since 10 to 15 years. The National Institutes of Health (USA) have a gender research policy: research proposals are only accepted when men and women are included in the design (for all research problems, which are in principle relevant to men and women). Doyal (2000), Eichler (1997, 2000, 2002) and other authors showed that the exclusion of one sex – which is mostly women – leads to research biases comprising: under-representation of female diseases and conditions in research, misinterpretation of research results regarding public health policies and medical practice, and overgeneralization of results to both sexes without showing the scientific evidence for the application to both sexes. The authors' demand for systematic consideration of sex and gender in all phases of the research process and Eichler (1999, 2002) developed a comprehensive approach and a handbook of guidelines how to detect and to avoid gender bias in social sciences including public health.

While in some countries public health research was already evaluated regarding the inclusion of sex and gender in research programs (e.g. Institute of Medicine 1994) this was not ever done for Germany, though the need for women's health research and gender sensitive health sciences was claimed by scientists (Helfferich & v. Troschke 1994; Eichler 1998; Maschewsky-Schneider et al. 2001). Germany has also to comply with the European gender mainstreaming policy. This policy demands for the consideration of gender as an analytic category in all policy assessments and in all decision and implementation processes. Implications for research and research funding policies - for instance gender guidelines for application and review of research projects - in the European Community are not yet put into action. An evaluation of the European Life Science Research Program revealed an enormous lack of gender sensitivity in research, research review and funding on the European level (Klinge & Bosch 2001).

In Germany public health research and postgraduate masters programs have been established since the early 1990s at some German universities. The Federal Ministry for Education and Science initiated a public health research program to fund projects and public health research centres at German universities. More than 300 projects were conducted in five public health centres. 12 universities and several public and private research institutes are involved in the German Public Health Centres.

This paper presents results of the public health project 'Gender Bias – Gender research'[1]. The study evaluated public health research in Germany regarding the inclusion of sex and gender and the sensitivity of scientists and scientific journals for gender based analysis. The goals were: to identify gender bias and to assess to what extend gender issues are appropriately included in public health science in Germany; to give recommendations how to avoid gender bias; to ensure gender equality and equity in public health research, and to develop and publish guidelines for gender based research in Germany.

The study comprised the following research steps:

1. Analysis of the theoretical and methodological literature on gender based analysis
2. Survey of all German public health projects in the 1990ies (Fuchs & Maschewsky-Schneider 2003)
3. Review of a sample of publications in three German-language public health journals (Fuchs & Maschewsky-Schneider 2002)
4 Career-survey of public health postgraduate scientists
5. Networking between scientists from the German public health research centres and in an international context (e.g. Berlin Center of Public Health et al. 2002)
6. Advanced training of scientists and students; scientific publications; public relations
7. Research guidelines, translation and publication of Eichlers handbook (Eichler 2002; http://www.ifg-gs.tu-berlin.de/ handbuchGBA.pdf).

This paper presents selected results from the project survey [2] and the literature review [3].

Theoretical background

Theoretical framework of our study were theories and concepts of feminist social sciences and on women's health, as well as feminist methodologies to detect and avoid gender bias (e.g. Doyal 2000; Eichler 1997, 2000, 2002; Verbundprojekt 2001). Gender bias can occur when the specific conditions of men and women are analysed inappropriately, when one sex is excluded without showing evidence for the exclusion, or when theories, concepts and methods which are developed for one sex are applied to the other without proving the relevance or appropriateness for it.

The most prevalent bias was the assumption that conditions of men and women are the same and that results which were gained in male study populations can be generalized to women. A famous example comes from the research on coronary heart disease (CHD). For years scientists assumed that the risk factors for men and women were mostly the same. It was only in the 1980ies when they found out that female hormones play an important role in the causation and delay of CHD because of the protective function against coronary heart disease in women.

[1] The project was carried out at the Berliner Zentrum Public Health (BZPH) and funded by the Federal Ministry for Education and Science under funding number 01EG9821TPN11. Collaborators were: Bayrischer Forschungsverband Public Health: Dr. Hannelore Löwel, Dr. Barbara Thorand & Dr. Gabriele Bolte (GSF München); Berliner Zentrum Public Health: Dipl. Soz. wiss. Birgit Babitsch, MPH & Dr. Daphne Hahn (Institut für Gesundheitswissenschaften, Technische Universität Berlin), Prof. Dr. Kim Bloomfield (University of Southern Denmark); Norddeutscher Forschungsverbund Public Health: Dr. Ingeborg Jahn (Bremer Institut für Präventionsforschung und Sozialmedizin), Prof. Dr. Petra Kolip (Universtität Bremen), Dipl. Soz. Brigitte Stumm (Institut für Medizinische Soziologie, UKE-Eppendorf, Universität Hamburg) Nordrhein-Westfälischer Forschungsverbund Public Health: Dr. Gesinde Grande (Universität Bielefeld, Fakultät für Gesundheitswissenschaften); Sächsischer Forschungsverbund Public Health: Dr. Jutta Krappweis (TU-Dresden); Ulrike Worringen (Charité Berlin).

Eichler (2001) identifies three sources or theoretical concepts of gender bias: **Andro-centrism** is the adoption of the male perspective taking men as norm against which women are assessed. In empirical research this source of gender bias often leads to exclusion or under-representation of women and to overgeneralization of research results to both sexes. The just given example on CHD stands for this concept of gender bias. In medical and clinical research overgeneralization can be fatal when the efficacy of a new medication was positively tested in a clinical trail based on a male sample, but in clinical practice the new medication is used for men as well as for women even though it might have negative effects in women or their baby when they are pregnant.

The second source of gender bias is **gender insensitivity**. This means that sex and gender are ignored as socially or medically important variables or a false gender-neutrality is assumed (gender blindness). In scientific publications it can often be recognized that the sex of the study population is not named in the title and not given in the abstract. A specific form of gender insensitivity is householdism which often occurs in official statistics when household is the unit of analysis. The concept of household income does not allow to distinguish between the amount of money which is available for the housewife and which for the husband. De-contextualisation, another sub-form of gender insensitivity, means to deal with conditions for men and women as if they were the same (assumed gender homogeneity).

Double standard comprises evaluation, treatment or measurement of identical behaviours, traits or situations differently on the basis of sex or gender. In clinical practice symptoms and causes of symptoms of men and women are often interpreted in different ways: for men as organic malfunctions and for women as psychological disturbances - even though the underlying disease or condition might be the same. The overmedicalization of women with psychoactive drugs which could be shown in clinical practice is a fatal consequence of this form of sexual dichotomism. Another form of double standard is the reification of gender stereotypes which means the analysis or treatment of differences between men and women as if they were a necessary part of our human nature rather than a socially imposed characteristic.

With her handbook Eichler (2002) provides an instrument to detect and to avoid gender bias by asking questions regarding the three forms of gender bias on all steps of the empirical research process. Examples for diagnostic questions are:

Androcentricity

▶ Are females (males) appropriately included in all components of the research process?
▶ Are all norms comprehensive or are males taken as the norm and females compared against it?
▶ Is the study premised on an underlying notion of gender equality?

Gender insensitivity

▶ Is sex recognized as a socially relevant issue or variable?
▶ Does the analytic category or unit of analysis correspond to the level at which observations are made?
▶ Is the study contextualized in a gender sensitive manner?

Double standards

► Are the sexes dealt with differently in situations where this leads to disadvantaging females?
► Does the research treat gender stereotypes as social constructions rather than reifying them?
► Are attributes that exist in both sexes attributed to both sexes?

Design and methods

Project survey

All public health projects which were conducted between 1992 and 2001 within the German public health research centres (projects funded by the Federal Ministry for Education and Science and associated projects funded by other agencies) were included into the survey. Goal was to evaluate the gender sensitivity of public health research in Germany and the awareness of gender sensitive research among public health scientists. A questionnaire based on Eichler's concept was developed. Areas in the questionnaire for the projects were:
► Is the research subject gender-specific?
► Are gender differences taken into account in: hypotheses, design and methods, analysis of data, conclusions of the study?
► Do public health scientists in Germany demand for a high need for gender-sensitive research?

The survey was conducted as an online questionnaire; a print version was sent to researchers who demanded for it; the last call for participation also included a printed questionnaire. The online version could be filled out via internet providing each participant with his/her own login password.

A comprehensive search had to be done in the five German public health centres to retrieve a full list of all projects, names and addresses of the principal investigators and years of funding. Addresses of the scientists and/ or the institutes had to be updated by our project team. Since some of the projects had been terminated years before the survey was conducted and scientists moved to other institutes, scientific disciplines or even abroad the address-update was relatively time consuming.

Literature review

A systematic review of the three German-language public health journals was conducted to evaluate the publication practice regarding gender sensitivity or possible gender bias. The review included the following journals: Das Gesundheitswesen, Zeitschrift für Sozial- und Präventivmedizin (today: International Journal of Public Health), Zeitschrift für Gesundheitswissenschaften. The sample of publications should cover the whole period of the public health initiative in Germany and start at the beginning (1990), have a midterm sample point (1995) and a sample point at the end of the funding process (1999); the full volumes of these years were included into the sample. Selected were only original publications and reviews; excluded were letters, interviews, editorials, proceedings, etc. Based on Eichler's handbook an evaluation instrument was composed for the literature review. It covered the three main areas of scientific publications:

Formal area: language in title, abstract, text, diagrams, etc.

Substantial area: formulation of hypotheses, discussion of literature, interpretation of results, conclusions

Methodological area: sampling, description of the sample, data analysis.

No evaluation of the theoretical context, the consideration of gender aspects in the literature review, the appropriateness of methods and design, and the content of the publication itself could be made. Publications covered a whole range of different public health disciplines and topics (e.g. health economy, epidemiology, legislation, medical and physiological measurements, etc.). Only scientific experts for these disciplines would have been able to do a substantial analysis of gender bias and gender appropriateness. The public health scientists of our study who did the review had a scientific background in social sciences but no expertise in all the different fields of public health. For this reason the review could only include formal, methodological and descriptive aspects of the publications under review. The review was administered by a female and a male reviewer. The instrument was pretested by collaborating colleagues. The instrument was fully applicable for those publications only which dealt with data on individuals.

Results

Project survey

317 research projects were reported from the public health research centres. 186 scientists participated in the survey (58.4%), most of them used the online questionnaire. 170 questionnaires were filled out completely. Table 1 displays response rates by type of questionnaire and sex of project leader.

76.3% of all projects worked on issues concerning women and men, a small amount referred to women (8.6%) or men (1.1%) only; 14% worked on gender-unspecific issues like "quality assurance" or "methodology". For 8,5% of the empirical projects which included men and women the comparison between both sexes was also included into the main hypothesis, for 55.4% it was at least an auxiliary hypothesis; in 36.2% it played no role at all. 77.5% of all projects were aware of the necessity to prove the gender appropriateness of the research instruments. 23.2% did all the data analysis by sex and gender, 31% at least some of the analysis, for 16,9% it was a control variable; 14,8% applied "other"

Table 1. Response rates by type of questionnaire and sex of project leader

Response-type	Project leader		Total
	Female	Male	
Online	39 (54.9%)	110 (44.7%)	149 (47.0%)
Mail	13 (18.3%)	23 (9.3%)	36 (11.4%)
Rejection	6 (8.5%)	20 (8.1%)	26 (8.2%)
Non-response	13 (18.3%)	93 (37.8%)	106 (33.4%)
Total	71	246	317

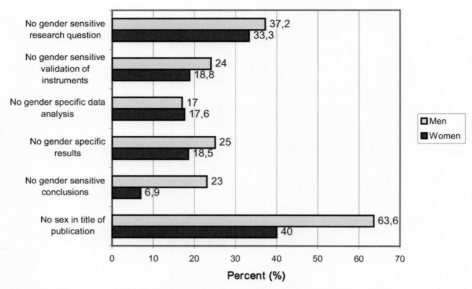

Fig. 1. Overview of the results of the public health project survey by sex of project leader

methods, and 14% did no gender-specific analysis at all. In 91 projects where quantitative analysis",7,2> on an individual level was done 76.9% found gender-specific differences. 22.2% of all projects (including either men or women or both sexes) presented specific conclusions for men and women, and an additional 36.6% did this at least regarding some aspects. Reduced to projects which included both sexes into the sample we found even higher rates: 93.1% of the female scientists and 77% of the male scientists reported that they distinguish between men and women in at least some of their conclusions.

Figure 1 gives an overview on the results of the survey for all projects which included both sexes in the study and for which the respective question was applicable (for instance when data analysis on an individual level was done). In this figure results for male and female project leaders are presented.

Literature review

517 original publications were found; they included 268 empirical or review articles which were both included into the review; 163 publications were found in "Das Gesundheitswesen, 69 in "Sozial- und Präventivmedizin" and 36 in "Zeitschrift für Gesundheitswissenschaften" (the last included articles from 1995 and 1999 only because in 1990 the journal was not yet existent). 258 publications worked on issues which are in principal relevant for men and women (excluding for instance studies on pregnancy or reproductive health problems). 210 were publications about empirical studies, 48 reviews. 88% of the publications included men and women; 5.4% (N = 14) included one sex only: 7 men- and 7 women-only studies; 6 of 7 women-only studies gave a theoretical explanation why they concentrate on one sex only, while this was true for 3 of 7 men-only studies; in 17 publications no information about the sex of the study subjects could be found. The following results include the 244 publications, which concentrate on men and women or in which no information about the sex of the study subjects was available.

Formal area: 64.3% of the publications did not mention the sex of the study subjects in the title, 25.4% used a gender-neutral formulation, 0.8% named both sexes and 9.4% had a male formulation even though the study topic applied to both sexes. In only 27.9% of the abstracts or summaries the sex of the study subjects was reported. 48.5% of the publications used a mostly gender-neutral language (e.g. human beings); in 51.1% of the articles we found mostly overgeneralization of male forms (e.g. man, participants[2], patient), and overgeneralization of female forms in 0,4%. The language used for the description of tables and figures was in 67.7% of the publications mostly gender-neutral; in 31.8% we found overgeneralization of male and in 0.5% of the publications overgeneralization of female forms.

Methodological area: Only 8% of all publications offered information on the gender-specific validity of the research instruments which were used in the study; 20.4% of the publications accounted for gender-specific differences in their theoretical concepts and research variables; 28.3% referred to the gender-specific context of at least some of the variables. Only 53.2% of all publications described the sample by sex; in these publications 41% of the data analyses were mainly done broken down by sex and gender, and 37% did at least some gender-specific analyses. In those publications where the sample was not described by sex and gender 75% of all data analyses were not broken down by sex and gender at all, 18% did some gender-specific analyses and 6% did all analyses by sex and gender.

Substantial area: To avoid gender bias in research it is very important to formulate the research questions and hypotheses in such a way that differences between men and women can be identified. This was the case in almost 50% of all publications where at least some gender-specific hypotheses were included. But there was a strong difference between the journals and the year of publication (Table 2). While "Das Gesundheitswesen" showed a significant ($p < 0.001$) decrease of publications which did not distinguish between sex and gender in the research questions this is not true for the other journals.

An improvement of gender-specific conclusions from the research results could be shown over the years. While in 1990 only 26.7% of all publications drew seperate conclusions for men and women, in 1999 this was done in 41.2% of all publications. This rate is still very low considering the practical consequences these conclusions might have for public health practice. Figure 2 shows a summary of the results of the literature review.

Table 2. Percentage of publications without distinguishing between sex and gender in research questions per journal and year of publication (%)

| | Year | | |
Journal	1990	1995	1999
Das Gesundheitswesen	73.8	64.3	39.4
Sozial- und Präventivmedizin	69.6	44.4	65.2
Zeitschrift für Gesundheitswissenschaften	–	65.2	69.2

---

[2] The German language has male and female terms like Teilnehmer (male participant) and Teilnehmerin (female participant), Patient (male patient) and Patientin (female patient) or Arbeiter (male worker) and Arbeiterin (female worker).

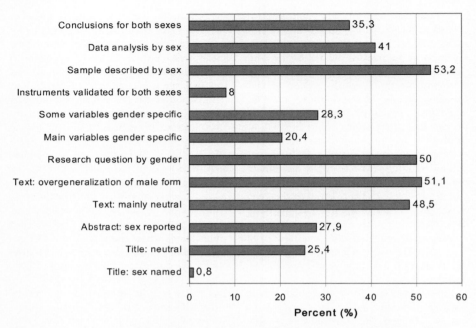

Fig. 2. Summary of the results of the literature review: percentage of gender awareness in public health publications

Conclusions

Results from the survey of German public health projects indicate a rising awareness and willingness for the inclusion of gender into public health research. Male and female researchers were both willing to carry out gender-sensitive research, but female researchers showed more sensitivity for gender issues. For all steps of the research process female researchers reported more gender-sensitive research strategies. Male and female scientists reported also a high awareness to formulate gender-specific conclusions from their research results. More than 50% of the scientists answered that they drew their conclusions separately for both sexes when results indicate those differences.

Results of the review of public health publications in Germany show that the main part of the reviewed articles included both sexes, but did not make it obvious in title or abstract. The majority of articles dealing with both sexes did not account for gender issues in the research questions, and only half of the publications accounted for the different conditions of women and men in the main variables (theoretical context). Only one third of the articles specified conclusions for men and women separately.

Survey and review results reveal quite a high awareness for gender-sensitive public health research and publications. Nothing is known about a possible response bias: more gender-sensitive scientists may have answered the questionnaire and there might also be a reporting bias. Scientists are aware of the requirement to distinguish between both sexes in research hypotheses and concepts, sampling and power calculation, and data analysis as essentials for good public health and epidemiological practice and high methodological quality. The difference between the survey (high awareness) and the review (low performance) regarding the presentation of gender-specific conclusions form the research results might be an indicator for report-bias.

Despite the rising awareness of gender issues in research our results still show remarkable gaps:

Formal level: title, abstract and text of publications/projects do not consequently reveal the sex of study subjects.

Methodologic level: research instruments have to be proved regarding gender-specific validity and the study design has to be constructed to allow for gender comparison.

Substancial level: research variables, concepts, hypothesis and especially conclusions should be systematically planned and presented under a gender perspective to avoid biases and misinterpretations in public health and clinical practice.

Eichler's concept and the results of this project can play an important role for the future of research and education not only in public health but also in medicine and other health sciences. Eichler's handbook for gender-based analysis was translated into German and is available in print (Eichler 2002) and electronic version (www.ifg-gs.tu-berlin.de/ handbuchGBA.pdf). Some scientific associations integrated gender guidelines into the research recommendations (German Epidemiologic Association: www.rki.de/GESUND/EPIDEM/ GEP_LANG.pdf), and a gender guideline was implemented into the German health report system. A discussion to implement gender guidelines in medical education and research was just started (BLK-Bildungsplanung & Forschungsförderung); even a few calls for proposals in biomedical and health research included a gender perspective.

References

Berlin Center of Public Health, European Women's Health Network, German Society for Social Medicine and Prevention (eds) (2002) Gender Based Analysis (GBA) in Public Health Research, Policy and Practice. Documentation of the International Workshop Berlin. 7–8 June 2001 (http://www.ifg-gs.tu-berlin.de)

Doyal L (2000) Gender Equity in Health: Debates and Dilemmas. Social Science & Medicine 51: 931–939

Eichler M (1997) Feminist methodology. Current Sociology 45: 9–36

Eichler M (1998) Offener und verdeckter Sexismus. Methodisch-methodologische Anmerkungen zur Gesundheitsforschung. In: Arbeitskreis Frauen und Gesundheit im Norddeutschen Forschungsverbund Public Health (Hrsg.). Frauen und Gesundheit(en) in Wissenschaft, Praxis und Politik. Huber: Bern: 4–49

Eichler M, Fuchs J, Maschewsky-Schneider U (2000) Richtlinien zur Vermeidung von Gender Bias in der Gesundheitsforschung. Zeitschrift für Gesundheitswissenschaft 8: 293–310

Eichler M (o.J.) Moving Forward: Measuring Gender Bias and More. In: Berlin Center of Public Health, European Women's Health Network, German Society for Social Medicine and Prevention (ed) Gender Based Analysis (GBA) in Public Health Research, Policy and Practice. Documentation of the International Workshop Berlin. 7–8 June 2001 (http://www.ifg-gs.tu-berlin.de)

Eichler et al. (2002) Zu mehr Gleichberechtigung zwischen den Geschlechtern: Erkennen und Vermeiden von Gender Bias in der Gesundheitsforschung. Deutsche Übersetzung und Bearbeitung von Fuchs J, Maschewsky K, Maschewsky-Schneider U. Blaue Reihe: Berliner Zentrum Public Health (http://www.ifg-gs.tu-berlin.de/ handbuchGBA.pdf)

Fuchs J, Maschewsky-Schneider U (2002) Geschlechtsangemessene Publikationspraxis in den Gesundheitswissenschaften im deutschsprachigen Raum? Ergebnisse einer Literaturreview. Das Gesundheitswesen 64: 284–291

Fuchs J, Maschewsky-Schneider U (2003) Berücksichtigung des Gender-Aspekts in der deutschen Public Health-Forschung. Ergebnisse einer Projektbefragung. International Journal of Public Health (in press)

Helfferich C, v. Troschke J (1994) Der Beitrag der Frauengesundheitsforschung zu den Gesundheitswissenschaften/Public Health in Deutschland. Schriftenreihe der Koordinierungsstelle Gesundheitswissenschaften/Public Health an der Abteilung Medizinische Soziologie der Universität Freiburg, Bd.2

Institute of Medicine, Mastroianni C, Faden R, Federmann D (eds.) (1994) Women and Health Research. Ethical and Legal Issues of Including Women in Clinical Studies. Vol. 1. National Academy Press: Washington, D.C.

Klinge I, Bosch M (2001) Gender in Research. Gender Impact Assessment of the specific programmes of the Fifth Framework Programme. Quality of Life and Living Resources. A study for the European Commission. Executive summary and recommendations. Maastricht

Maschewsky-Schneider U, Hinze L, Kolip P, Scheidig C (2001) Frauen- und geschlechtsspezifische Gesundheitsforschung in der DGSMP. Das Gesundheitswesen 63, Sonderheft 1: S89–S92

Verbundprojekt zur gesundheitlichen Situation von Frauen in Deutschland (2001) Bundesministerium für Familie, Senioren, Frauen und Jugend (ed) Untersuchung zur gesundheitlichen Situation von Frauen in Deutschland. Eine Bestandsaufnahme unter Berücksichtigung der unterschiedlichen Entwicklung in West- und Ostdeutschland. Kohlhammer: Stuttgart

Part III Health Care Services

From patient-centred medicine to citizen-oriented Health Policy-making

BERNHARD BADURA

I.

The term "patient-centred medicine" was introduced by Michael Balint and his colleagues in the late sixties of the past century. Advocates of patient-centred medicine argue that doctors and patients live in different worlds: the world of the individual patient and her or his unique experience of ill health; and the biomedical world of clinical experts.

In *the world of clinicians* a disease can be dealt with and controlled independently of the patient concerned. Diagnosis and cure of biological defects are in the centre of this model. The personal and social dimensions of an illness are perceived as irrelevant for the performance of clinical processes. Communication with patients can be neglected because high quality health care depends on the qualification of the clinician and the skilful use of medical technology alone.

In contrast, the *patient-centred model* broadens this perspective to include psychological as well as social problems. Patients are supposed to play a more active role as partners in a more egalitarian relationship. Professional dominance is replaced by shared decision-making. Since doctors and patients may have widely divergent views on the nature of the problem, on priorities, goals and treatment options shared decision-making is seen as the key to move from doctor- or illness-centred to a patient-centred care.

Shared decision-making presupposes empowerment of patients. Patients should be motivated and informed about the available evidence and potential side-effects. To put it differently: Whereas traditional medical care is technology-intensive, patient-centred care is interaction-intensive. According to the patient-centred model good clinical care includes both: a skilful use of the available knowledge as well as a skilful use of human communication.

Some advocates of patient-centred medicine emphasize an additional point as essential: a different view on the human organism as having a great capacity for self-healing. The ultimate goal of clinical care is – according to this view – to support or assist nature's capacity for self-healing instead of trying to control it.

The discussion concerning patient-centred medicine raised by Balint and his colleagues focuses on overcoming biomedical reductionism and on patient-empowerment. Looking back we might call patient-centred medicine the first important step towards the "emancipation of the patient in health care".

II.

A second important contribution to the emancipation of the patient in health care comes form the ongoing discussion on the quality of care and from a growing interest in the role of patients, their families, self-help groups and other helping networks as co-producers of care. Avedis Donabedian was among the first to stress that the effectiveness of treatment processes often depends on the co-operation and co-production of the patient and the members of her or his social network. The patient is rediscovered as part of the service production process being the third input-factor in addition to the input from the health care team and from medical technology. Especially in treating chronic illness contributions from patients, family and self-help groups are of crucial importance for the long-term success of what has been achieved by stationary and ambulatory services of the curing and caring professions. This was one main result of our own research on the effectiveness of cardiac treatment and rehabilitation.

In the scientific literature dealing with the upcoming service-economy the consumer as co-producer is a rather common issue. Donabedian first struggled with patients as co-producers of clinical care in dealing with the complex issue of "attributive validity" of clinical outcomes: that is whether or not there is a causal relationship between treatment processes and their biomedical end points. He came back to it in a later paper on "Quality assurance in health care: Consumer's role" in which he states:

"In part, the performance of patients depends on what practitioners have *permitted* them to do and how well they have *prepared* them for the task" (Donabedian 1992).

Looking at the ever-growing number of chronically ill citizens, information, advice, motivation and training of patients and their relatives become a major challenge in our move towards a better integrated, more comprehensive and indeed more citizen-oriented health care system.

III.

The discussion on patient-centred medicine is now going on for more than 30 years: Numerous papers and books try to clarify the meaning of it, how it improves patient satisfaction and medical outcomes and how to implement it efficiently. Nevertheless, we are far away from a widespread adoption of this model. It may even be the case that today the gap between the quality of health care available in Europe and the quality we could have is larger than 30 years ago. Today we should accept that the model of patient-centred medicine itself has serious limitations, which may have contributed to this situation:

The model focuses on patients without taking into account that due to cultural, socio-economic or gender differences patients enter the doctor-patient-interaction with rather different expectations and belief-systems. We need more empirical research on patient preferences and expectations depending on gender, age and on their social, educational, physical and psychological situation. High-quality clinical care from the point of view of a group of experts may not be perceived as high-quality care from the point of view of a group of patients.

▶ The model focuses on clinical medicine without sufficiently taking into account, whether it is applied in primary care, acute hospital care, rehabilitation or long-term care. It does not differentiate between different treatment situations and different treatment settings. The role of citizens or patients as co-producers is much more obvious for example in health promotion and rehabilitation than it is in intensive care.

▶ The model of patient-centred care does not take into account that today's health care is provided by numerous different highly specialized experts. Complex treatment situations need a pooling of different types of knowledge and skills from different specialists and professions. And they need a better organization and management. This raises the very serious problems of teamwork, inter-professional communication, co-ordination, and guidelines.

▶ Finally, the model focuses on medical care. And indeed, the power of modern medicine to cure and prevent diseases is undeniable. However, the reduced morbidity and mortality rates among the European population are due in large part to social, economic and psychological factors amenable to health promotion in schools, communities and work places. We public health experts agree that these factors are beyond medical care. *We need a shift of emphasis: from individual-based sickness to population based well-being.* The improvement of the doctor-patient-interaction is still an important issue. However the doctor-patient-communication is not the adequate setting to realize the urgently needed progress in health promotion, which should become a top-priority of health policy-making everywhere in Europe.

IV.

Health care systems should become better integrated, more flexible and responsive to the needs of societies and populations.

The discussion on patient-centred care concentrates on individual choices within clinical settings, on overcoming medical paternalism and a biological understanding of care. However the chances to implement patient-centred goals and processes within traditional health systems have turned out to be rather limited.

Empowerment and communication are important issues but they are not the only ones. From the public health perspective we need a fundamental redesign of goals, processes and structures of care. Health care reforms should first of all address the major health needs of populations, and they should take into account social trends and their impact on the health of populations and on the utilization of health care services. From the public health perspective major issues are: the *needs of chronically ill patients, and the expectations of a better informed, better educated and more active citizenry.* Citizens will demand more participation in clinical care. And they will demand a greater say in health care reforms and national priority setting. Citizens and patients need to know more about clinical efficacy and the quality of usual care. And they need to know more about the choices and constraints of health policy-making.

Today, a small number of chronic diseases account for the greatest share of our expenditures on curative care. Services for the chronically ill are fragmented. And they are organized around discrete episodes of care, around individual experts and institutions specialized in the application of specific skills and technologies. *This kind of organization forces excellent providers to produce low quality.* We need better integrated treatment processes, and innovations like case management and disease management.

Balint and his colleagues tried something pretty paradoxical: They tried to implement patient-centred care within the context of a provider-centred health care system. We should make a fresh start on it but with a different working-hypothesis: that the implementation of patient-centred care needs the implementation of a citizen-oriented health care system. And – whether we like the idea or not – the implementation of a citizen-oriented health care system presupposes more citizen participation in health care decision-making.

The development and continuous improvement of ways and means to achieve this goal should become a major public health issue of the 21st century.

References

Balint M (1970) The doctor, his patient and the illness – Der Arzt, sein Patient und die Krankheit.
   Fischer Bücherei, Frankfurt am Main
Donabedian A (1992) Quality assurance in health care: consumers' role. In: Quality in Health Care 1,
   pp 247–251

Influenza surveillance

PIETRO CROVARI · ROBERTO GASPARINI

Introduction

In the Middle Ages influenza epidemics were attributed to the negative influence from planets in conjunction, hence the name given to this disease.

The influenza virus was isolated only in 1933 (Smith, 1935), nevertheless the nosological picture of the disease had already been documented for a few centuries. Starting from the XVI century there are clear descriptions of epidemics in Great Britain (Thompson, 1852).

Historically, the pandemic outbreak referred to as "Spanish" is frequently mentioned. It occurred in 1918–1919 and affected 200 000 000 people, causing 20 000 000 deaths.

More recently there were two other serious pandemic outbreaks, though they were definitely less severe than the "Spanish" one. In 1957 we had the influenza known as the "Asian" outbreak and in the winter of 1968–1969 the "Hong Kong" outbreak.

The characteristics of the pathogenic agent are responsible for the recurrence of influenza epidemics. The influenza virus belongs to the *Orthomyxoviridae* family and has a particular set of genes. In fact, the genetic information is located on 8 RNA segments. This means that there is a high probability of gene rearrangement among the different strains of the virus.

What is particularly important is the presence on the surface of the virion of two glycoproteins. The first, known as haemagglutinin (H), recognises the receptor and is responsible for adhesion and fusion of the virus to the membrane of respiratory cells. The second, known as neuroaminidase (N), allows the release of newly formed viruses outside the infected cell. The peculiar epidemiological progress of the disease can be explained by variations in these two antigens.

The characteristics of the nucleoprotein enable to distinguish the 3 types of influenza viruses: A, B and C. The A viruses show greater shifts and/or minor drifts in the antigenic set. The B viruses show only minor drifts while the C viruses do not show any important variation and consequently have fairly small epidemiological relevance.

The shift in the H or N antigen represents a greater variation. When this happens the result can be widespread diffusion of the virus with very extensive epidemics.

The drifts, which are much more frequent, are instead associated with subsequent punctiform mutations in gene segments of H and N antigens, with more modest but not irrelevant consequences on the epidemiological progress of the disease.

The most authoritative hypothesis to explain the appearance of shifts is the hybridisation of human and animal viruses (birds, swine, etc.) (Scholtisseck, 1983).

At present, subtypes H3N2, H1N1 and H1N2 of the A virus circulate together, in addition to B viruses belonging to at least two genomic lineages (B/Victoria/2/87 and B/Yamagata/16/88).

The impact of the disease is particularly perceptible during pandemic outbreaks. During these circumstances, the morbidity and mortality due to influenza result in considerable social damage. Nevertheless, even during inter-pandemic periods the damage is considerable. For instance, Sullivan (1996) estimated that in the USA the disease causes an average of 17 to 50 million cases every year, from 165 to 233 million sick days, from 43 to 70 million days of limited activity or days in bed, from 4 to 24 million medical visits, 314.000 hospitalisations and 20 000 deaths. It seems that in England, every year, an average of 3000 to 5000 deaths occur, while more extensive epidemics, like the one that occurred in the winter of 1989/1990, caused 30 000 deaths. It seems that in Italy the number of influenza cases that probably occurred during the 2001/2002 winter, assessed with the method of sentinel physicians and paediatricians, was 2 610 611 during the 8 weeks of the epidemic (Crovari, Submitted for publication).

We should bear in mind that the spreading of the virus is accompanied with that of other respiratory micro-organisms, such as Respiratory Syncytial iruses, Parainfluenza viruses, Adenoviruses, Coronaviruses, Rhinoviruses, etc. Moreover, we cannot ignore other pathogens, such as *Streptococcus pneumoniae, Haemophilus Influentiae, Mycoplasma pneumoniae,* etc.

In the Northern hemisphere influenza activity occurs during winter, from October to April, whereas in the Southern hemisphere it occurs from April to October. In the tropical areas, influenza activity is always present, with recrudescence during the more cold-humid periods (Kilbourne, 1987).

Objectives and methods of influenza surveillance

The objectives of the surveillance of influenza disease are essentially two, i.e. to limit the impact of the disease (morbidity, mortality, costs, etc.) and to quickly identify the predominant viral variants.

These are the methods available. Morbidity studies through clinical/epidemiological surveillance (sentinel physicians and paediatricians), surveys on extra mortality from respiratory diseases and all other causes (Serfling, 1964; CDC, 1997), studies on extra hospitalisations (Gasparini, 1992), surveys on the use of drugs (antibiotics, antipyretics, cough remedies, etc.), surveys on absenteeism (from work, school, etc.), health economy analyses (cost-effectiveness, cost-benefits, etc.), studies on increased requests for medical house calls, etc.

Virological surveillance enables to monitor the variability of influenza viruses and answers the demand for continuous update of the composition of the vaccine.

In spite of the fact that the above-mentioned study methods provide important indications, they are individually inadequate in providing an adequate picture of the epidemiology of the disease (Nicholson, 1998).

Virological surveillance

The global virological surveillance network, created by the World Health Organisation (WHO) in 1947 (Hampson, 1996), has rapidly expanded since the Sixties and includes approximately 110 National Centres distributed in 83 countries, which collaborate very closely. They are linked to 4 WHO Centres, in Europe (London), in the USA (Atlanta), in Australia (Melbourne) and Japan (Tokyo). Their "mission" is to monitor the new variants of the influenza viruses, so as to be able to choose the most suitable ones for the production of vaccines for the following season. It is for this reason that every February experts from all over the world gather at the WHO in Geneva where the formulation for the Northern hemisphere is defined. The same thing occurs in September for the Southern hemisphere.

An attempt is currently underway to increment the exchange of information and re-agents for the typing of viral strains among the different national centres, and to ensure that all the centres be equipped with IT (Lavanchy, 1999). The FluNet Web site has been set up to provide updated data.

Since 1995 the European Influenza Surveillance Scheme (EISS) has been set up at European level. The results of participating countries, gathered in a single database, can be looked up via Internet.

In Italy, there has been for some time a virological surveillance network that includes different regions (Liguria, Lombardy, Tuscany, Emilia Romagna, Lazio, Umbria, etc.) and is linked to the National Centre in Rome. More recently, from 1st November 1999, there is an active national surveillance network (InfluNet) (Gasparini, 2001) that, through sentinel physicians and paediatricians, ensures better monitoring of the new influenza virus variants in addition to the clinical/epidemiological surveillance discussed afterwards.

Starting from the assumption that the samples coming from the population better represent the progress of virosis in the entire population (Nicholson, 1998), the Italian virological surveillance is based on the activity of free-choice general practitioners and paediatricians. The activity of the latter is extremely precious because, as is well known, children represent the prime target of the virus. It is only to identify viruses that cause more serious infections that samples coming from hospitalised patients are examined (Watson, 1995). To improve the performance of virological tests it is a good idea to examine the definition of an influenza case as specified by the WHO. In fact, influenza, at least in subjects aged >3 years, is characterised by sudden onset, high fever (often > 38–39 °C), at least one symptom of respiratory apparatus involvement (cold, pharyngitis, laryngitis, tracheitis, etc.) and at least one systemic symptom (asthenia, anorexia, muscle pains, etc.).

Laboratory diagnosis methods are different in terms of sensitivity and specificity. Today we have quick tests for diagnosis at the patient's bedside (often useful to correctly orient the treatment), isolation in embryonated chicken eggs or in cell cultures (MDCK) (Meguro, 1979), identification with the haemoagglutination inhibition test and through the polymerase amplification reaction (Polymerase Chain Reaction; PCR) (Atmar, 1996) and isolate genotyping. These last two methods allow us to focus on molecular epidemiology results, which are very useful for making forecasts. Recently, this method has enabled the Surveillance Centre at the University of Genoa to genotype a fair number of B viruses, after the identification of strains belonging to the B/Victoria/2/87 lineage, which had been absent from Europe for many years (see Fig. 1 and 2) (Ansaldi, in press).

For successful laboratory activity it is also important to take samples of the pathological material. Taking material from throat and nose seems to be the most practical way to isolate the virus (Fleming, 1995).

Clinical/epidemiological surveillance

Sentinel physicians and paediatricians carry out the clinical/epidemiological surveillance. Based on the above-mentioned definition of an influenza case, a group of healthcare professionals every day send the diagnoses of disease to a special data processing Centre. The weekly morbidity is then calculated and is reported on a special Web site, so that there is a return of information to physicians and paediatricians.

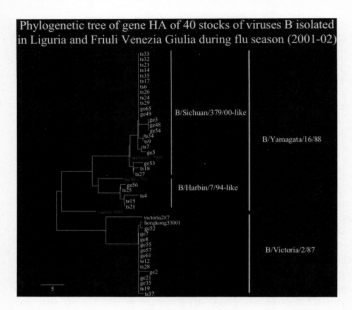

Fig. 1. Phylogenetic tree of gene HA of 40 stocks of viruses B isolated in Liguria and Friuli Venezia Giulia during flu season (2001–2002)

Aminoacidic sequence of antigenic sites A and B of 40 stocks of viruses B isolated in Liguria and Friuli Venezia Giulia during flu season (2001-02)

	Site A (145-150)	Site B (161-168)	(197-205)	
Sichuan/379/00	NATSKS	PRdDNNKT	NKTQMKNLY	
Ge49 (14 isolati)				
Ge3, Ge48, Ge54	N			B/Sichuan/379/00-like
Ge53			D	
Ge56	R	K N	.	
Ts4		K N	Y	B/Harbin/7/94-like
Ts15, Ts21, Ts25		K N		
Ge7 (10 isolati)	V_NGN	KNE	EA_AK	
Ge52, Ts37	V_NGN	KNE	TEA_AK	B/Victoria/2/87
Ge2	V_NGN	KNE	EA_AK_F	

Fig. 2. Aminoacidic sequence of antigenic sites A and B of 40 stocks of viruses B isolated in Liguria and Friuli Venezia Giulia during flu season (2001–2002)

A network of General Practitioners belonging to the English Royal College of General Practitioners exists since 1967. Through this system it has been possible to make good estimates of the onset and severity of the epidemics that occurred in England and Wales in 1989, 1993 and 1995 (Fleming, 1996).

A similar system, created in Belgium in 1985 by the Institute of Hygiene and Epidemiology (Snacken, 1996), includes approximately 50 physicians and 50 paediatricians.

In Holland, during the 1982–1992 period, the sentinel stations of physicians at the National Institute for primary care (NIVEL) were able to reduce the annual average of morbidity from influenza to 425 cases every 10000 inhabitants (Knottnerus, 1996). Even though the incidence of influenza in the community seems to be from 3 to 6 times higher

Tasso di incidenza di sindromi influenzali per settimana e per classi di età (ogni 1000 assistiti)

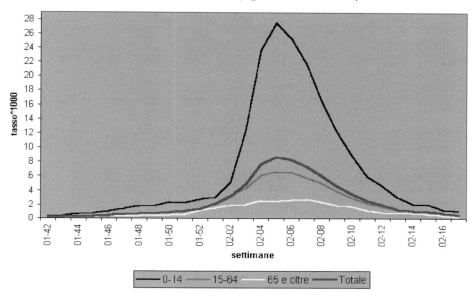

Fig. 3. Influenza morbidity (per 1000 inahabitants), in different classes of ages, in Italy during 2001/02 winter season

than that observed by physicians and paediatricians, because most of the cases do not come to the attention of physicians, the influenza activity is very well monitored by the method of sentinel healthcare professionals (Knottnerus, 1996). One of the problems to be solved has to do with the representative value of the patients monitored. They should be well distributed over the whole territory (in fact, there may be diversities in terms of age distribution, presence of conditions predisposing towards complications, vaccine coverage, etc.) and usually, given the circulation of the disease, it is estimated that at least 1% of the population should thus be monitored (Knottnerus, 1996).

The results supplied by this type of surveillance are particularly valuable in monitoring the activity trend, especially if connected with the virological data of the same population and with other clinical activity indicators (Nicholson, 1998). Another benefit is the exact identification of the start of the epidemic, through intensified virological controls and the use of specific drugs for treatment and prevention of more serious complications in subjects at risk.

At the Italian level, after local experiments implementing a detection system based on sentinel physicians, a national surveillance network is active since 1st November 1999. The gathered data are centrally processed by the Health Sciences Department at the University of Genoa and the Istituto Superiore di Sanità (Ministry of Health Institute). In addition, the results can be looked up, almost in real time, on the Web site: Cirinet.it.

The physicians who joined the Influnet system in the 2000/2001 season were 845 and the Italian population studied was an average of 1.96% of the total. The results for that season subdivided according to age groups, are shown in Figure 3. The comparison of the results of the winters 1999/00, 2000/01 and 2001/02 are shown in Figure 4.

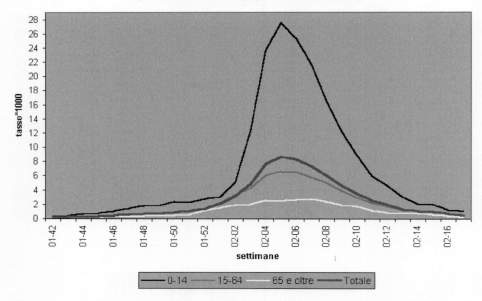

Tasso di incidenza di sindromi influenzali per settimana e per classi di età (ogni 1000 assistiti)

Fig. 4. Influenza morbidity (per 1000 inahabitants), in different classes of ages, in Italy during 2001/02 winter season

Other indicators of influenza activity

Surveillance of extra mortality and extra hospitalisations

At the time of maximum influenza virus circulation there is an increase in mortality, which is not recorded during non-epidemic periods, as can be observed from the statistical survey on all respiratory affections. This is not surprising if we consider that the influenza disease is particularly serious in elderly subjects, who pay a high toll in mortality during each epidemic occurrence.

The annual measurement of this finding (mortality due to respiratory diseases, excluding tuberculosis and tumours) is one of the most objective indices of the impact of influenza. In fact, the degree of increased mortality detected during the influenza season is a direct and reliable index of the severity of the epidemic episode that has occurred.

Farr already anticipated this surveillance system in the last century; the actual method was refined by Serfling in 1963 and has been used for 30 years by the WHO (Assaad, 1971).

The additional mortality is identified by comparing the rates of mortality from respiratory diseases with the rates one might expect (expected mortality) in the absence of influenza activity.

This methodology, not always used univocally, may be biased by, for instance, epidemics from other agents responsible for respiratory infections, etc.

Other interesting elements for the epidemiological study of influenza can be provided by the study of extra hospitalisations for influenza, pneumonias, as well as other respiratory and heart diseases. Barker in 1987 had already worked out a methodology similar to that for the study of extra mortality, which also enabled important assessments of the direct costs of the disease.

Surveillance of absenteeism from school and workplace

Very useful indications for influenza surveillance can result from surveys on absenteeism from the workplace. In Italy this is possible by examining the certificates of illness that general practitioners send to the National Institute of Social Insurance, reporting the diagnosis of the disease. Based on the cases labelled as influenza, it is possible to make reliable estimates (though probably overestimated) on its incidence. It is interesting to point out that the highest peak in absenteeism from the workplace occurs one week after that of maximum absenteeism from school. This confirms that children are the first target of the virus and represent an important link in the transmission chain.

Surveys on absenteeism from the workplace were carried out in Siena on 29 659 workers aged between 20 and 60 years (Gasparini, 2000). These surveys enabled us to extrapolate that more than 20 000 000 cases occurred among Italian workers in the 1989–1995 period.

Another parameter that enables us to assess the impact of influenza on society is school absenteeism. This indicator seems to be among the most sensitive to detect the start of an influenza epidemic. Studies on this topic (Gasparini, 1990) suggest that we are faced with an epidemic rekindling, when the daily percentage of school absenteeism is more than 10% of the pupils.

Increased demand for medical visits and use of drugs

The greatest request for medical visits for acute respiratory diseases coincides with the highest peak in influenza activity (Sullivan, 1996). Thus, this is one of the indicators that can be used for disease surveillance. This indicator has been used in two of the most important studies on the impact of influenza on the population of the USA. In the study carried out by Monto et al. (1971) in Tecumseh, the estimated number of medical calls was 26–29 visits for influenza per 1000 inhabitants per year. In the study carried out by Glezen et al. (1984) in Houston, it was 99 visits per 1000 inhabitants per year. On the basis of these results, Sullivan estimated that every year in the USA there is an average of 4 to 24 million visits for influenza.

As for the use of drugs, it is clear that the prescription of antipyretics, antibiotics and cough remedies during the periods of maximum diffusion of influenza viruses is considerably higher. It is therefore obvious that a study of increases in the use of drugs is not only useful in taking the pulse of the diffusion of the virus, but is helpful in having a better picture of the economic damage caused by this disease.

Conclusions

There are also other methods of surveillance for influenza activity, such as registration of all respiratory affections diagnosed as influenza in health clinics, emergency rooms, etc. Nevertheless, it is important to consider that some types of studies are particularly indicated to detect the initial moment of the disease (for instance the method of sentinel physicians) while others allow more accurate estimates of the actual severity of the influenza epidemic. However, it is necessary to combine several methods to have a sufficiently clear picture of the social impact of the virosis. On these bases it is then possible to carry out cost-benefit studies of vaccination or other preventive and therapeutic treatments (amantadine, zanamivir, oseltamivir, peramivir, etc.).

Based on a recently carried out survey (Crovari, submitted for publication), we were able to estimate that the cost of the influenza epidemic in the winter of 2001/2002 in Italy, during the 8 weeks of maximum diffusion, was 1 billion and 349 million Euros.

Another survey carried out in the winter of 2000/2001 (Gasparini, 2002), allowed us to estimate that the net benefit of vaccination was 110.20 Euros per elderly vaccinated subject.

It is, therefore, quite clear that surveillance of the disease is very important, also in light of the number of travels and migrations and the facility of travelling from one end of the earth to another in a few hours. This means that a viral strain that has appeared in a geographical area can be transported in every part of the world in much shorter times than in the past. This likelihood was particularly feared during the H5N1 influenza virus epidemic, which occurred in Hong Kong in 1997 (Shortridge, 1999). In that year there were serious epidemic episodes among poultry and 18 cases among the population, 6 of which deadly. It was a virus that was potentially very dangerous for man but, fortunately, the killing of 1.5 million chickens avoided the threat. This threat, however, is still present since among the many biological weapons that might be used, there is more than one utilizable influenza virus.

References

Ansaldi F, D'Agaro P, de Florentiis D, Crovari P, Gasparini R, Donatelli I, Puzzelli S, Gregory V, Bennett M, Lin Y, Hay A, Campello C: Molecular characterization of influenza B viruses circulating in Northern Italy during the 2001-2002 epidemic season. In press on J Med Virol.

Assaad F, Cockburn WC, Sundaresan TK: Use excess mortality from respiratory diseases in the study of influenza. Bull Wld Org 1973, 49:219-225.

Atmar RL, Baxter BD: Typing and subtyping clinical isolates of influenza virus using reverse transcription-polymerase chain reaction. Clin Diagn Virol 1996, 7:77-84.

Barker, WH: Excess Pneumonia and Influenza Associated Hospitalization during Influenza Epidemics in The United States. AJPH 1986, 76:761-765.

CDC: Update: Influenza activity-United States and worldwide, 1996-97 season, and composition of the 1997-98 influenza vaccine. MMWR 1997, 46:325-330.

Crovari P, Gasparini R, Lucioni C, Sticchi L, Durando P, Contos S: Costs of 2001/02 influenza epidemics in Italy. Submitted for pubblication to Pharmacoeconomics.

Fleming, DM: The Impact of Three Influenza Epidemics on Primary Care in England and Wales. PharmacoEconomics 1996, 9, Supp.3:38-45.

Fleming DM, Chakraverty P, Sadler C & Litton P: Combined clinical and virological surveillance of influenza in winters of 1992 and 1993-1994. Br Med J 1995, 311:290-291.

Gasparini R, Lucioni C, Lai P, Maggioni P, Sticchi L, Durando P, Morelli P, Comino I, Calderisi S and Crovari P: Cost-benefit evaluation of influenza vaccination in the elderly in the Italian region of Liguria. Vaccine, 2002, 20:B50-B54.

Gasparini R, Pozzi T, D'Errico A, Cellesi C, Gasparini R: Influenza in Siena (Italy): epidemiological study. Journal of Preventive Medicine and Hygiene 1990, 31:36-38.

Gasparini R, Pozzi T, Giotti M, Fatighenti D: Excess hospitalization for respiratory illnesses during the influenza epidemics in Siena between 1987 and 1990. Journal of Preventive Medicine and Hygiene 1992, 33:107-110.

Gasparini R, Pozzi T, Bonanni P, Fragapane E, Montomoli E: Valutazione dei costi di un'epidemia influenzale nella popolazione lavorativa di Siena. Giornale Italiano di Farmacoeconomia, 4:3-9, 2000.

Gasparini R., Lucioni C, Lai P, De Luca S, Durando P, Sticchi L, Garbarino E, Bacilieri S, Crovari P: Influenza surveillance in the Italian region of Liguria in the winter of 1999-2000 by general practitioners and paediatricians: socio-economics implications. Journal of Preventive Medicine and Hygiene, 2001; 42:83–86

Glezen WP, Six HR, Perrotta DM: Epidemics and their causative viruses community experience. In Stuart-Harris C, Potter CW, editors. The molecular virology and epidemiology of influenza. New York, Academic Press, 1984.

Hampson AW, Cox NJ: Global surveillance for pandemic influenza: are we prepared? In Brown LE, Hampson AW & Wbster RG (eds) Options for the Control of Influenza, Vol 3. Elsevier, Amsterdam, 1996.

Kilbourne ED: Influenza. Plenum, New York, 1987.

Knottmerus: Influenza in The Netherlands. PharmacoEconomics 1996, 9, Supp. 3:46–49.

Lavanchy D: The importance of global surveillance of influenza. Vaccine 1999, 17:S24–S25.

Meguro H, Bryant JD, Torrence AE, Wright PE: Canine kidney cell line for isolation of respiratory viruses. J Clin microbiol 1979, 9:175–179.

Monto AS, Napier JA, Metzner HL: Tecumseh study of respiratory illness: I. Plan of study and observation on syndromes of acute respiratory disease. Am J Epidemiol 1971, 94:269–279.

Nicholson KG, Webster RG, Hay AJ: Textbook of Influenza. Blackwell Science Editor, Oxford, 1998.

Scholtisseck C, Burger H, Bachman PA, Hannun C: Genetic relatedness of haemagglutinins of the HI subtype of influenza A viruses isolated from swine and birds. Virology 1983, 129:521–523.

Serfling RE: Methods for current statistical analysis of excess pneumonia-influenza deaths. Publ Hlth Rep 1963, 78:494–499.

Shortridge KF: Poultry and the influenza H5N1 outbreak in Hong Kong, 1997: abridged chronology and virus isolation. Vaccine, 1999, 17:S26–S29.

Smith W: Cultivation of the virus of influenza. Br J Exp Pathol 1935, 16:508–512.

Snacken R: Weekly Monitoring of Influenza Impact in Belgium (1993–1995). PharmacoEconomics 1996, 9, Supp. 3:34–37.

Sullivan KM: Health Impact of Influenza in The United States. PharmacoEconomics 1996, 9, Supp. 3:26–33

Thompson T: Anonymous Annals of Influenza in Great Britain 1510–1837. Sydenham Society, London 1852.

Watson JM, Dedma D, Joseph C, Zambon M & Timbury MC: Influenza Types and patient population (letter), Lancet 1995, 346:515–516.

The mental health care system on its way to integration in general health care

Heinz Häfner

"Today, some 450 million people suffer from a mental or behavioural disorder...mental health and mental disorders are not regarded with anything like the same importance as physical health. Instead they have been largely ignored or neglected" (WHO 2001, p. 3). The neglect of the mentally ill with simultaneous violation of their human and civil rights culminated in the killing of some 200000 of these people between 1939 and 1945 by the National Socialist regime in Germany. But in other countries and at other times, too, mentally ill people have been left behind in terms of social privileges and resources, as shown by the death rates for selected German mental hospitals (Table 1) and a British county mental hospital during World War I (Table 2).

Social stigma and discrimination are the main reasons why lack of knowledge of mental disorders and their treatment continues to be widespread even in modern European societies (Angermeyer & Matschinger 1997). Consequently, persons falling mentally ill are frequently unable to recognize or accept what they are suffering from and to seek help without delay. Even in high-income countries with well-developed health care systems merely some 40% of persons with severe mental disorders receive treatment in the first year fol-

Table 1. Deaths – as a percentage of total of patients (old and new stays) – in selected German mental hospitals during World War I

State/Hospital	1914 [%]	1915 [%]	1916 [%]	1917 [%]	1918 [%]
Prussia [1]	6.6	8.8	11.2	19.3	15.5
Eichberg [2]	5.6	8.7	16.3	24.3	17.9
Weilmünster [3]	7.2	10.0	17.0	36.5	30.0

[1] Based on statistic yearbooks for the state of Prussia, vol. 16 (1920) and 18 (1922), Berlin
[2] Calculated on the basis of male and female rates
[3] Based on "Verhandlungen des 50. bis 54. Kommunallandtages", Wiesbaden 1916–1920
Source: Faulstich 1999, modified

Table 2. Deaths (mean number and % per year) due to malnutrition among some 600 inmates of the Buckinghamshire County Asylum (GB) during World War I

Year	1910–1914	1915	1916	1917	1918
∅	67	81	110	129	257
%	~ 11	13.5	18.3	21.5	43.0

Source: Based on Crammer 1990

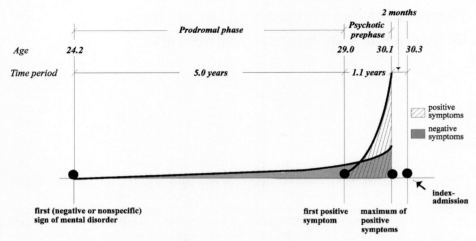

Fig. 1. The prephases of schizophrenia from first sign of mental disorder to first admission – N = 232 (108 males, 124 females) – for both sexes together. Source: Häfner et al. 1995

lowing illness onset (WHO International Consortium in Psychiatric Epidemiology 2000). On average, treatment is initiated several years after illness onset and delays of more than 10 years are common, as demonstrated by Olfson et al. (1998) for example for anxiety disorder. Figure 1, based on results from our population-based ABC sample of first illness episodes, demonstrates this for schizophrenia, a disorder of immense public health relevance. On average, five years elapse from illness onset to the first psychotic symptom and another 1.3 years to appropriate treatment (Häfner et al. 1995). And it is in this early illness phase, and thus, before treatment beginning that most of the social consequences emerge, causing social stagnation in early-onset and social decline in late-onset cases (Häfner et al. 1999).

Mentally ill persons often unable to look after their interests rely on a humanitarian health policy and a strict observation of ethical principles within the health care system. The three main principles, as formulated in the United Nations Resolution 46/119 of December 17, 1991 entitled "Principles of the protection of persons with mental illness and for the improvement of mental health care", are:

1. All persons have their right to the best available mental health care, which shall be part of the health and social care system.
2. All persons with mental illness or who are being treated as such persons shall be treated with humanity and respect for the inherent dignity of the human person.
3. There shall be no discrimination on the grounds of mental illness.

Similar principles have also been adopted by the Council of Europe, most recently in the White Paper of January 3, 2000.

For centuries concern about premature death used to govern the outlook on illnesses both in medicine and among people in general. It has helped to combat common serious diseases associated with high mortality rates. The targets were first epidemics such as cholera, the plague, typhus and smallpox and later coronary heart disease, stroke, cancer and diabetes. In this way physical medicine has succeeded in reducing most of the causes for premature death. It has essentially contributed to a large increase in the life expectancy of elderly people since the 19th century and it has reduced, though not eliminated, the years

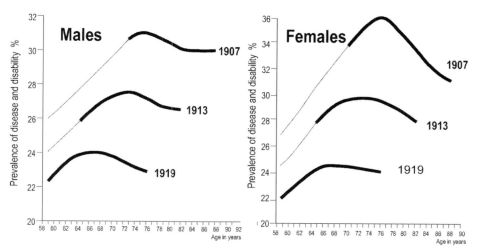

Fig. 2. Age-related prevalence of disease and disability from age 60 years on for males and females born in 1907, 1913 and 1919 in Germany. Source: Dinkel 1999, modified

elderly people have to live with illness and disability. This is illustrated by a comparative analysis of three successive birth cohorts from 1907 to 1919 from Germany (Dinkel 1999) (Fig. 2). It shows significantly decreasing prevalence rates for disease and disability in old age, especially from 1970 to 1980 for men and from 1980 to 1990 for females.

With the enormous decrease in mortality life years that people have to live in illness and disability have become the main cause for concern. Disability constitutes a burden not only to the persons affected and their families, but also to the health care system and the national economy. "With this shift in perspective," the Director-General of the WHO writes, "mental illness...suddenly bulks very large indeed. It may not in itself be fatal, but it causes extensive disability..." (Brundtland 2000).

With a considerable delay a wide range of therapeutic instruments has become available for most mental disorders since the mid 20th century. As a consequence, revolutionary changes have occurred in mental-health care systems. Year-long stays on closed wards of remote mental hospitals have given way to effective treatment and care provided by open services in the patients' own community. As a consequence, lengths of stay, illustrated for Germany from 1970 to 1997 in Figure 3, and numbers of occupied beds at mental hospitals have declined drastically. In many cases patient's living conditions and the therapies they receive have improved decisively. At the same time the responsibility for caring for the seriously disabled has been shifted from mental hospitals to the families or the community. Along with the immaterial costs mostly also the financial burden has been shifted away from the public sector to the families and the community.

The size of the problem

It was not until the disease burden caused by disability and premature mortality was combined into a single measure "disability-adjusted life years" (DALY) in 1993 (World Bank 1993, Murray & Lopez 1996) that disability was generally recognized as a public-health problem. In the original estimates calculated for 1990 mental and neurological disorders:

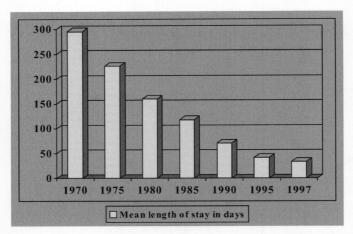

Fig. 3. Mean length of stay in mental hospitals and units in Germany. Based on data from the statistics yearbooks 1979 to 1997

depression, anxiety, substance-abuse disorder, schizophrenia, dementia and epilepsy accounted for 10.5% of the total DALYs globally. The estimate for 2000 is 12.3% and for 2020 15% (Murray & Lopez 1996).

Only "years of life lived with disability" (YLDs) in the most active period in human life (age 18–45) considered, mental disorders rank among the 10 leading causes because of their mostly early age of onset and low mortality. At 43% the YLD rate is highest for Europe, compared with 31% worldwide.

But are governments, health-care systems and people adequately responding to this huge need for mental health care and preventive action?

Basic aspects of mental health care systems

The concern for mental health

Society and the government have the duty to keep economic and social disadvantage caused by illness and disability to a minimum. This quality criterion, called fairness, is defined as a basic value of a health care system. In European countries with their social and humanitarian orientation it should be taken very seriously.

The quality criterion has two implications

1. All citizens must have access to mental health care free of any economic and social barriers.
2. All ill and disabled individuals no longer capable of earning their living must be given the financial, social and, if necessary, institutional support they need.

Because of the high risk of disability involved, the major mental disorders pose serious social and economic problems. These have been markedly compounded by the large-scale mental hospitals programmes. In countries with large low-income populations, for example in the former communist countries, many families do not have the resources for caring for their mentally disabled members. In rich countries such as Germany patients requiring long-term residential care are often placed in remote homes hardly distinguishable from the old mental hospitals. Serious deficits in the social care of the seriously mentally ill may lead to destitution, as shown for example by Fuller Torrey in 1988 for the USA.

Affected by social inequality are also the families caring for their mentally ill or disabled members. The caregivers are restricted in their personal, social and in part also economic activities, and they are themselves at risk for mental-health problems. For this reason society should provide for these people ample support to reduce their burden as well the stigma and discrimination involved. Self-help groups play an important role in this context.

The mental health care system is undergoing sweeping changes. I have tried to outline the humanitarian, economic and social dimensions of this process. An urgent target of this reform process is fully integrating mental health care in the general health care system without giving up its close ties to the system of social care.

In the World Health Report 2001 Gro Harlem Brundtland (2001a) points out the inseparableness of the aetiological factors underlying both mental and physical diseases and stresses the necessity for an overarching medical competence. And the same holds for diagnosing and therapy. Having realized this most European countries have included in their health care programmes the objective of reintegrating mental health care in general health services at all levels, from primary to hospital care. But the countries show great differences in their progress towards this goal.

Cooperation of the health and the social care system and coordination at the political, the organizational level and in individual cases are organized very differently from country to country. And the best solutions have not always been chosen. In well-developed national economies it is not a good solution to confer social care on health services or medical care on social services. The reason is the limited competence of both sides for fulfilling one another's tasks and different professional orientations of the two disciplines. A purely social orientation neglects chances for a possible therapy and a purely medical orientation the need of the mentally disabled for social support and reintegration. Combined, the two orientations provide the most favourable basis for optimally caring for the seriously mentally ill.

Secondary prevention and early treatment

Because of the delayed initiation of treatment and early occurrence of social consequences in serious mental illness their early recognition and early treatment are urgently needed. The preconditions are 1) knowledge of these disorders, their early symptoms and possible therapies, 2) early recognition or diagnosis and availability of appropriate treatment, and 3) adequate help-seeking behaviour and therapy acceptance. In the last decade comprehensive early-intervention programmes have been developed especially for psychosis. First successes have been reported from controlled randomised studies of interventions administered at the prodromal stage of psychotic illness (McGorry et al. 2002, Morrison et al. 2002, McGlashan et al. 2002). But we are still far from an optimal solution. Deficits still abound concerning treatment acceptance and awareness among at-risk populations as well as potent instruments of early recognition and filters in the services provided.

Primary prevention and improving mental health education

The gap to physical medicine is widest in the field of primary prevention. One reason certainly is a shortage of large-scale prospective, epidemiological studies in psychiatry. Another is a lack of knowledge and health education in the population concerning mental disorders. In most European countries elementary schools provide good basic information about physical diseases and their risk factors. This means that health education starts at an age ensuring long-term benefits. In addition, there are supranational (WHO), national and local programmes educating and encouraging people to change their habits and lifestyles in a way to reduce health risks.

To improve the prevention of major mental disorders, a Europe-wide programme is required to spread knowledge at schools and among adult populations. Provided awareness of mental-health risks is increased and unfavourable stereotyped attitudes are combated, the preconditions can be created for treating mental disorders earlier, for markedly improving their primary prevention as research advances and, finally, for closing the gap to physical medicine.

To finish by quoting WHO's Director-General: "There is no development without health and no health without mental health" (Brundtland 2001 b).

References

Angermeyer MC, Matschinger H (1997). Social distance towards the mentally ill: results of representative surveys in the Federal Republic of Germany. Psychol Med 27, 131–141.

Brundtland GH (2000). Mental health in the 21st century. Bulletin of the World Health Organization 78 (4), 411.

Brundtland GH (2001a). Message from the Director-General. In: The World Health Report 2001. Mental health: new understanding, new hope. WHO, Geneva, pp. ix-x.

Brundtland GH (2001b). Introduction. In: Mental health – a call for action by world health ministries. WHO, Geneva.

Crammer J (1990). Asylum history. Gaskell, Royal College of Psychiatrists, London.

Dinkel RH (1999). Demographische Entwicklung und Gesundheitszustand. Eine empirische Kalkulation der Healthy Life Expectancy für die Bundesrepublik auf der Basis von Kohortendaten. In: Häfner H (ed) Gesundheit – unser höchstes Gut? Springer, Berlin Heidelberg New York, pp. 61–83.

Faulstich H (1999) Der Eichberg im Ersten Weltkrieg. In: Vanja C, Haas S, Deutschle G, Eirund W, Sandner P (eds) Wissen und irren. Psychiatriegeschichte aus zwei Jahrhunderten – Eberbach und Eichberg. Historische Schriftenreihe des Landeswohlfahrtsverbandes Hessen (vol. 6), Kassel, pp 129–141.

Häfner H, Maurer K, Löffler W, Bustamante S, an der Heiden W, Riecher-Rössler A, Nowotny B (1995). Onset and early course of schizophrenia. In: Häfner H, Gattaz WF (Hrsg.) Search for the causes of schizophrenia III. Springer: Berlin Heidelberg, pp 43–66.

Häfner H, Maurer K, Löffler W, an der Heiden W, Könnecke R, Hambrecht M (1999). Onset and prodromal phase as determinants of the course. In: Gattaz WF, Häfner H (eds.) Search for the causes of schizophrenia, vol. IV: Balance of the century. Steinkopff-Verlag, Darmstadt, Springer, Berlin, pp. 1–24.

McGlashan TH, Zipursky RB, Perkins DO, Addington J, Miller TH, Woods SW, Marquez E, David SM, Tohen M, Breier A (2002). A prodromal trial of olanzapine vs. placebo: baseline results (Abstract). Acta Psychiatr Scand 106:42

McGorry PD, Yung AR, Phillips LJ, Yuen HP, Francey S, Cosgrave EM, Germano D, Bravin J, Adlard S, McDonald T, Blair A, Jackson H (2002). Can first episode psychosis be delayed or prevented? A randomized controlled trial of interventions during the prepsychotic phase of schizophrenia and related psychoses. Arch Gen Psychiatry (in press).

Morrison T, Bentall R, French P, Kilcommons A, Green J, Lewis S (2002). Early detection and intervention for psychosis in primary care. (Abstract) Acta Psychiatr Scand 106 (Suppl. 413), 44.

Murray CJL, Lopez AD (1996). The global burden of disease. Harvard School of Public Health on behalf of World Health Organization and World Bank. Distributed by Harvard University Press, Cambridge, MA.

Olfson M, Kessler RC, Berglund PA, Lin E (1998). Psychiatric disorder onset and first treatment contact in the United States and Ontario. Am J Psychiatry 155:1415–1422.

Torrey EF (1988). Nowhere to go. The tragic odyssey of the homeless mentally ill. Harper & Row, New York.

WHO International Consortium in Psychiatric Epidemiology (2000). Cross-national comparisons of the prevalences and correlates of mental disorders. Bulletin of the World Health Organization 78, 413–426.

WHO (2001). The world health report 2001. Mental health: new understanding, new hope. WHO, Geneva.

World Bank (1993). World development report 1993: Investing in health. Oxford University Press for the World Bank, New York.

The role of acute day hospital treatment for mental health care: Research context and practical problems of carrying out the international multi-centre EDEN-study

Thomas Kallert · Stefan Priebe · Matthias Schützwohl · Jane Briscoe
Matthias Glöckner · and the EDEN-study group

The role of acute psychiatric day hospital evaluation in the European context

In many European countries dramatic changes in mental health care are an ongoing process [5, 15, 18, 38, 43]. The realisation of community-oriented psychiatric care principles differs significantly between the individual countries. Although needs-orientation, increasing professional quality of care in spite of cost-containment, individualisation, social integration and improvement of patients' quality of life are generally accepted principles of mental health care, their transformation to the practice of care and health services is highly heterogeneous [4, 24]. Care- or service-planning- and treatment-standards in various sectors of mental health service systems are not established in a cross-nationally homogeneous way.

Contrasting to these differences, it is one of the major health political goals of the European Commission to harmonize the conditions and chances for the treatment of mentally ill persons, simultaneously aiming towards strengthening their rights and autonomy as well as decreasing their reservations related to psychiatric treatment settings and approaches [11, 16, 21].

Due to the search for alternatives to cost-intensive psychiatric inpatient treatment health policy plans, defined particularly for several countries to be associated to the European Union attribute to day hospitals that they can be one cost-effective alternative [5, 51]. Furthermore, mostly as a reflection of the European process of decreasing the number of hospital beds and deinstitutionalisation especially in the last 5 years these clinical institutions themselves increasingly change their program functions to the conceptualisation of providing acute psychiatric treatment [22, 26, 34, 45]. With regard to the scientific state of the art, it still has to be stated that the number of empirical studies especially studies respecting the outlined change of program functions is yet limited, with randomised controlled trials only being conducted in few centres in the Netherlands, in UK and the USA [12–14, 19, 30, 31, 39, 46, 49, 50, 52, 53], i.e. countries with different approaches to acute day hospital treatment. Thus, several requirements for further research have been established, giving top priority to a multi-centre randomised controlled trial (RCT), using a common set of outcome measures and carefully describing the applied methods as well as untoward events [34].

Therefore, the European Commission also defined a high public health policy priority for evaluating this treatment approach and funded the European Day Hospital Evaluation (EDEN)-study (for more information on current European mental health services research projects see chapter Becker et al. in this book). This study realizes the outlined main requirement for future research in this field and is the first RCT in this configuration of mental health services spanning former western and eastern block countries.

But, this project also contributes to the social goals of the European Union as follows:
► According to the studies available to date, patients' quality of life outcomes are more positive when the community-psychiatry approach to mental health care is applied rather than psychiatric care in an inpatient setting [20, 26, 33].
► Based on its direct connection to the social environment of the individual psychiatric patient, the propagation of such a setting also seems suitable for reducing the stigma attached to mental disorders and for lowering the threshold to taking advantage of psychiatric therapy.
► Furthermore, treatment in a day hospital setting implies for the patients their independent and completely voluntary consultation regarding this treatment approach and strengthens the position of the psychiatric patient in terms of an active and responsible co-formation of therapy [11, 16, 42].

This chapter focuses on some important aspects of this international mental health services research project. Firstly, the rationale for scientifically ambitious, but expensive randomised controlled trials in this field of research is explained. Secondly, general objectives, some characteristics of the sites, and important details of the study design are presented. Thirdly, practical problems of carrying out the project are outlined. And finally, based on a few preliminary results the so far achieved public health impact of the project is demonstrated.

Why conduct randomised controlled trials in mental health services research?

Several important fields of psychiatric treatment still lack an evidence-based choice of alternatives for allocating patients. This statement applies to long-established traditional (conventional) treatment approaches for individuals as demonstrated by the Cochrane review [44] on seclusion and restraint for people with serious mental illnesses as well as to more recently established approaches focusing on mental health services as demonstrated in reviewing clinical case management [9].

This clinical uncertainty leads to the ethical requirement to design and execute randomised controlled trials (RCTs) focusing on clinically important research questions aiming to help in deciding upon which interventions to use [23]. Because of the above-mentioned lack of satisfactory empirical work – contrasting to four decades of international establishment of day hospitals with dramatically increasing capacity of these treatment settings within the last years – this requirement also applies to the current situation of day hospital evaluation.

There is increasing criticism surrounding the definition of RCTs as kind of a gold standard for mental health services research. Firstly, there are practical objections (mainly focusing on costs and logistical challenges) for assessing rare but important outcomes such as suicide and violence committed by mentally ill persons as well as for evaluating long-term outcomes [23]. Secondly, there are methodological concerns that contributions to the evidence-base using other well-established methodologies in the field of social sciences are neglected [48]. This could lead to narrowed and skewed clinical recommendations strengthening the (strictly medical/biological) position of pharmacotherapy and decreasing the importance of psychological and social interventions also established on the basis of evidence. Thirdly, especially in RCTs assessing clinical as well as cost-effectiveness there can be an ethical dilemma because studies that attempt to address economic questions should be powered on economic variables. But then they would almost certainly be overpowered with respect to the clinical outcomes [7, 17, 37]. Some might argue that it would be inappropriate to continue a trial beyond a point at which clinical superiority has been determined beyond reasonable doubt. Others might argue that failure to recruit enough patients to give unequivocal treatment and health policy/cost recommendations could be seen as unethical. Fourthly, statisticians demonstrated that several popular theoretical arguments in favour of randomisation are either incorrect or imprecise [1]: 1. Randomisation is not sufficient for comparability: in fact, randomisation only implies the equality of the distributions of variables measurable at the time of randomisation. It leads to the statistical control of imbalance in the baseline variables and permits probability statements on differences between the groups regarding these variables. It has no influence on what happens between randomisation and the assessment of the outcome. 2. Randomisation is not the basis for statistical significance tests. 3. Randomisation is only one of many criteria that can be used for judging causal relations, it is not the basis for causal inferences on treatment effects. 4. Randomisation is not a sufficient condition for blinding.

Abel and Koch [1] conclude that the true achievements of randomisation are on a pragmatic rather than epistemological level. Six arguments for supporting the summarizing statement that randomisation should not be avoided without compelling need can be outlined: 1. The most important argument is the eminent importance of balancing prognostic variables for evaluating treatment effects. 2. Randomised studies belong to a larger class of high-quality studies, namely, prospective parallel comparisons with a written protocol specifying important aspects of patient enrolment, treatment, observation, analyses etc. [2, 35, 36]. 3. Investigators who randomise are more credible. 4. Randomisation makes a fundamental difference in defending positive study results against criticism. 5. Randomised studies have a much better reputation than non-randomised studies. 6. The conduct of randomised trials has a positive educational effect on the participating clinicians and clinical units.

Especially the outlined "meta-scientific" arguments contain some major advantages/achievements that need to be protected for the field of mental health services research in which randomised studies are still an exception.

To make this methodological approach really relevant it is imperative that RCTs are carried out under usual service conditions and that an atmosphere of collaboration between clinicians and researchers in designing and executing pragmatic RCTs is created [23]. Furthermore, for implementing this study design into the clinical routine of mental health services it is essential to solve clinical and organisational/ethical problems affiliated with the practise of randomisation. The following paragraphs outline in detail how the EDEN-study dealt (successfully) with these problems.

General objectives, design and participants of the EDEN-study

Main objectives and design of the EDEN-study

The EDEN-study (duration of funding: December 2000–June 2003) aims to evaluate the effectiveness of acute psychiatric treatment in a day hospital setting in five European centres: Dresden (D), London (UK), Wroclaw (PL), Michalovce (SK) and Prague (CZ).

The main objectives of the study are as follows: a) to evaluate the viability and effectiveness of day hospitals for acute psychiatric treatment; b) to identify subgroups of patients with a more or less favourable outcome so that the treatment setting might be specifically applied; and c) to ascertain the cost-effectiveness of day hospital treatment compared to conventional inpatient treatment.

Patients receiving psychiatric/psychotherapeutic treatment in either a day hospital or a completely inpatient setting at the 5 centres are studied in a temporally parallelised randomised experimental pre-post design (see Table 1). Each centre already has reached sufficiently large sample sizes (N > 200 patients included in the study in each centre) with regard to basic features of comparable patient populations in both of the settings. The obser-

Table 1. The Eden-study design

Questionnaire	t_1 admission	t_2 1 week after admission	t_3 4 week after admission	t_4 discharge	t_5 3 months after discharge	t_6 12 months after discharge
Client Sociodemographic and Clinical History (CSCHI)[1]	+	−	−	ask for changes	ask for changes	ask for changes
Schedules for Clinical Assessment in Neuropsychiatry (SCAN 2.1)[2]	+	−	−	add clinical diagnosis	−	optional
Brief Psychiatric Rating Scale (BPRS)[3]	+	+	+	+ only if t_3–t_4 > 1 week	+	+
Groningen Social Disabilities Schedule (GSDS)[4]	+	−	−	+ only if t_1–t_4 is at least 6 weeks	+	+
Berliner Bedürfnisinventar (Berlin Needs for Care Inventory), Questionnaire for Clients[5]	+	−	−	−	+	+
Berliner Bedürfnisinventar (Berlin Needs for Care Inventory), Questionnaire for Carer[6]	+ within 5 days	−	−	−	+	+
The Manchester Short Assessment of Quality of Life (MANSA)[7]	+	−	−	+	+	+
Clients' Scale for Assessment of Treatment (CAT)[8]	+ 3rd day after admission	+	+	+	−	−
The Helping Alliance Scale (HAS)[9]	−	−	−	−	+	+
Client Service Receipt Inventory (CSRI)[10]	+	−	−	+	+	+
Involvement Evaluation Questionnaire (IEQ, incl. GHQ-28)[11]	+ within 1 week	−	+	−	+	+

[1] Standardized documentation sheet (adapted to the special national conditions in a comparable way) of the individual patient's sociodemographic data and psychiatric history (regarding the development and course of the mental disorders as well as previous treatments); [2] standardized clinical interview for establishing ICD-10 diagnoses of mental disorders (developed under the auspices of the World Health Organisation); [3] assessment of psychopathological symptoms; [4] assessment of social disabilities in 8 major social roles; [5] evaluation of the care needs on the part of the patient and; [6] the need for care from the vantage point of professional carers, as well as the respective degree of coverage in 16 areas of need; [7] assessment of (area-specific) subjective quality of life; [8] assessment of the patient's satisfaction with the treatment; [9] assessment of the quality of the therapeutic relationship; [10] assessment of the individual patient's direct and indirect health care costs (including a detailed recording of the specific characteristics of the index-treatment using a documentation system developed for the purposes of this study); [11] assessment of the (psychological, social and financial) burden on the patient's closest reference person(s)

vation period has been chosen so that the persistent effects of the therapy in either setting can be evaluated prospectively over a 12-month period in terms of a multilevel observation, independent of when semi-, respectively completely inpatient treatment is concluded. Outcome criteria assessed at defined time-intervals during and after the period of acute treatment (Table 1) are psychopathology (SCAN 2.1, BPRS), social disabilities (Groningen Social Disabilities Schedules), quality of life (Manchester Short Assessment of Quality of Life), satisfaction with care (Client's Scale for Assessment of Treatment), needs for care (Berlin Needs Assessment), the psychological/financial burden of the relatives (Involvement Evaluation Questionnaire), and costs for treatment (Client Service Receipt Inventory). The health economic part of the study is based upon the compilation of direct and indirect costs of care; assessment of costs is independent of the treatment settings used over the course [for more details see 28].

Sample recruitment and randomisation

All patients admitted to acute psychiatric services who do not meet the exclusion criteria and fulfil the inclusion criteria are eligible to take part in the study. The exclusion criteria are as follows: under 18 or over 65 years of age; admission to the psychiatric hospital without consent of the patient (according to the legal regulations of the respective countries); degree of severity of the disorder requires measures restrictive of the patient's freedom on the day of admission, or a 1:1 supervision, or deems such probable; acute intoxication; presence of a somatic disorder requiring complete inpatient care; direct transfer from a different hospital; homelessness; one-way journey to hospital longer than 60 minutes; requires constant pick-up and delivery service to manage the journey to and from the hospital (for example due to limited mobility); inability to give informed consent; admission for diagnostic reasons only (e.g. PET).

After application of the exclusion criteria, the following inclusion criteria must be fulfilled: presence of a mental disorder with current symptoms whose degree of severity is sufficient to provoke a moderate disturbance in role performance in more than one area of daily living or which endangers the residential or financial status of the patient, or whose degree of severity implies a danger to the patient himself or to others [3]; available external (non-inpatient) treatment was not sufficiently effective (or if not attempted – is assessed as unsuitable for the current mental state of the patient) to prevent a deterioration of the mental state; no hospital treatment other than at the participating hospital is available to the patient.

Patients who did not meet the exclusion criteria while at the same time fulfilling the inclusion criteria received an explanation of the study; those who consented to participate were randomly assigned to the day hospital or to in-patient services. The allocation sequence was computer generated and concealed in sequentially numbered, opaque, sealed envelopes (2). The assignment happened prior to admission or shortly thereafter.

Random allocation was independent of availability of space in the treatment setting. A change in allocation was made, however, if no corresponding treatment place could be found within 24 hours. If no treatment place was available within this treatment setting either, the patient was then switched to a treatment setting in which a space is available, regardless of the random distribution.

Brief description of the EDEN-study catchment areas

The city of Dresden (470 000 inhabitants) is the capital of the Free State of Saxony, one of the five new German federal states that have been re-established after German reunification in 1990. Dresden's economic growth over the last years is based on science (6 universities with ca. 40 000 students), technologies, and public services.

The East London borough of Newham is the third most deprived and culturally the most diverse borough in the UK. Over half of the population (220 000 inhabitants) have an Afro Caribbean or Asian ethnic origin. There are more than 30 ethnic minorities in the borough. The birth rate is the highest in London. According to an Annual Residents Survey, rising crime, lack of jobs and quality of the health service constitute the three main problems in the area.

Wroclaw is one of the largest cities in Poland (637 000 inhabitants) and has been formed by many cultures. The city is situated in the Southwest of the country and constitutes the economical, cultural and intellectual (16 universities and academies with ca. 70 000 students) capital of the Lower Silesian Region, an area productive in agriculture and mining.

The town of Michalovce is situated in Eastern Slovakia and constitutes the economic and cultural centre of the lower-Zemplin region (320 000 inhabitants). The lower-Zemplin region possesses rural, agricultural character and is economically less developed.

As today's capital of the Czech Republic, Prague (1 200 000 inhabitants) is a centre of engineering, electronics and chemical industry. Besides Charles University the city has several other academies and research institutes.

The participating centres

The Clinic and Policlinic for Psychiatry and Psychotherapy at the University Hospital of the Dresden University of Technology has offered treatment at the day hospital for over 30 years and is thus one of the oldest in the entire German-speaking area. The clinic has 58 full inpatient treatment places, the day hospital offers 25 places in separate facilities.

The Unit for Social and Community Psychiatry is part of the Department of Psychiatry at St. Bartholomew's and the Royal London School of Medicine and Dentistry (Queen Mary and Westfield College), University of London. It was established in 1997. In 1999, a new acute day hospital with 20 places was opened, initially intended to be an alternative to acute in-patient care.

The Department of Psychiatry at Wroclaw Medical University is an educational and scientific institution sited in the Mental Health Care Centre with inpatient wards (55 beds) and 2-day hospitals (70 places).

The Psychiatric Hospital in Michalovce (SK) was opened in 1990. It has 260 inpatient-beds and 25 places at the day hospital, which was opened in 1993. As a model-institution, the Hospital is organised according to the community-oriented intentions of the Slovakian psychiatry-reform.

The Psychiatric Clinic of the General Faculty Hospital in Prague is the oldest psychiatric hospital in the Czech Republic. There are 5 inpatient wards with a total capacity of 119 beds and an unfixed number of integrated day hospital treatment places; a new day care centre for adolescent patients (15 places) was opened in 2000.

The institution in Prague contributes its model of integrated day hospital treatment (i.e. day hospital treatment on a ward that also provides complete inpatient care to patients), while the other centres work with day hospital treatment models that are institutions completely separate from the fully inpatient care wards of the hospital but which are nonetheless affiliated with them.

The differentiated listing of the clinical staff (Table 2) firstly reflects the distribution of clinical tasks in the hospitals, e. g. assigning the highest number of nurses and physicians to the most acute (closed) wards (P-1 in Dresden, P-W in London, IW-I in Wroclaw, SUPS in Michalovce, W-6 in Prague) where patients need a high level of supervision, psycho-pharmacological interventions and general health care. Secondly, this listing shows the current standard of general multidisciplinarity of the therapeutic teams in all clinical units, but also demonstrates significant variation in the employment of therapists not uniformly accepted as the "core clinical professions" in psychiatric hospitals. Thirdly, not only concerning the personnel structure, but especially related to the mean staff hours per week available per treatment place the situation in 4 EDEN-day hospitals is quite similar (the respective (lower) figures in DH-II in Wroclaw can be attributed to the fact that this is a brand-new clinical department). While the distribution of the clinical professions working in the day hospital in Michalovce can be more or less compared to the other centres, the available staff hours per treatment place only reach 55–60% of the input which can be provided in the other sites. (Note: Because the amount of personnel input could not be separately calculated for integrated day hospital treatment in Prague it can be supposed that the statement characterizing the situation in the Michalovce DH also applies to this treatment approach in the Czech EDEN-centre.) This calculation, fourthly, as an example points to the fact that the general level of staffing in the psychiatric hospitals in Michalovce and Prague is 30–50% beneath the level in the other EDEN-hospitals.

The specific personnel and organisational structure as well as the program functions of the participating day hospital and inpatient settings cannot be analysed according to established international standards. Only in Germany, since 1990 the Psychiatrie-Personalverordnung (Psych-PV) provided a directive for staff levels in in-patient psychiatric services (at a federal level, i. e. for the whole country) and has given new impetus to improving quality of care in in-patient services (32). The directive applies to general adult, substance misuse and child and adolescent psychiatric in-patient services. It provides a matrix of care classes or groups, and it allocates minutes of staff time per professional group (e. g., psychologist, nursing staff) and week on the basis of these categories.

Oriented to this standard which is fulfilled in the German centre, all EDEN day hospitals, except Michalovce (which is the only EDEN-centre where the academic staff is not resourced by the status of a university department), have a quite similar multidisciplinary personnel structure as demonstrated by the available weekly treatment time per place. Contrasting to this, the level of staffing in the Eastern European inpatient settings is significantly lower than in the Western European study centres. None of the other EDEN centres fulfils the high German standard of staffing inpatient services.

In general, these staff differences do not affect the level of diagnostic measures which can be provided in the hospitals (Table 3). Especially the accessibility to specific somatic diagnostic measures and to those examinations using technical equipment depends on the integration of the psychiatric hospital into a general (university) hospital which is given in the Dresden, Wroclaw and Prague site. The provision of neurological examinations in the psychiatric departments depends on the professional qualifications of the employed physicians as well as on the establishment of an on-site neurological consultancy service, which again requires the integration of the psychiatric hospitals into general hospitals.

Table 2. Personnel structure[1] in the EDEN-day hospital (i.e. DH) and inpatient settings (i.e. other acronyms)

	Dresden				London				Wroclaw				Michalovce					Prague					
	DH	P-1[d]	P-2	P-3	DH	P-W	E-W	R-W	DH-I	DH-II	IW-I	IW-II	DH	PSS	SUPS	Admission	Quiet	ADC	W-1	W-2	W-3[E]	W-5	W-6[d]
Form of organisation[1]	1				2				4	5			1					3					
Fixed number of treatment places	25	14	24	20	20	25	25	25	35	35	29	26	30	25	10	34	34	15	15*	18*	24*	30*	32*
Physicians	3 / 120	3 / 120	3.5 / 140	3 / 120	0.5 / 21	1.85 / 74	2.1 / 84	2.15 / 86	3 / 120	2 / 80	6.12 / 245	3 / 120	1.5 / 63.8	2 / 85	1 / 42.5	2 / 85	1 / 42.5	2 / 80	2.5 / 100	2 / 80	3 / 120	3 / 120	3.5 / 140
Nurses	2.7 / 108	16 / 640	13 / 520	12 / 480	3 / 111	15 / 562.5	11 / 412.5	7 / 262.5	3 / 120	2 / 80	12 / 480	9 / 360	3 / 127.5	4 / 159.5	9 / 360	9 / 360	5 / 200	1 / 40	11 / 440	4 / 160	6 / 240	11 / 440	11 / 440
Psychologists	0.8 / 32	0.2 / 8	1 / 40	0.5 / 20	0.4 / 14				1 / 40	1 / 40	0.36 / 14.4	1 / 40	0.8 / 35.5	0.07 / 3		0.05 / 2	0.05 / 2	0.7 / 28	0.7 / 28	0.7 / 28	0.7 / 28	0.7 / 28	0.7 / 28
Psycho-therapists									1 / 40		0.36 / 14.4								0.2 / 8	0.2 / 8	0.2 / 8	0.2 / 8	0.2 / 8
Occupational therapists	1 / 40	1 / 40	1 / 40	1 / 40	2 / 72	1 / 37.5	0.8 / 30	1 / 37.5	1 / 40	1 / 40	1 / 40		0.63 / 27	0.78 / 33.3		0.78 / 33.3	0.78 / 33.3	0.15 / 6	0.15 / 6	0.15 / 6	0.15 / 6	0.15 / 6	0.15 / 6
Music therapists	0.8 / 32	0.1 / 4	0.1 / 4	0.1 / 4						0.33 / 13.2	0.5 / 20	0.33 / 13.2	0.01 / 0.5	0.02 / 1		0.02 / 1	0.02 / 1						
Dance therapists													0.1 / 4.5	0.05 / 2			0.14 / 6						
Sport therapists							0.05 / 2				2 / 80	0.5 / 20											
Art therapists					0.2 / 7				1 / 40	1 / 40	2.5 / 100	0.25 / 10	0.035 / 1.5	0.08 / 3.5		0.19 / 8	0.19 / 8	0.2 / 8					
Physio-therapists	0.25 / 10	0.25 / 10	0.25 / 10	0.25 / 10									0.09 / 4	0.12 / 5		0.09 / 4	0.19 / 8	0.57 / 23	0.57 / 23	0.57 / 23	0.57 / 23	0.57 / 23	0.57 / 23
Social worker	0.8 / 32	0.3 / 13.3	0.3 / 13.3	0.3 / 13.3					1 / 40	0.25 / 10	1 / 40	0.25 / 10	0.08 / 3.5	0.08 / 3.5	0.3 / 13	0.4 / 18	0.19 / 8	0.43 / 17	0.43 / 17	0.43 / 17	0.43 / 17	0.43 / 17	0.43 / 17

Table 2 (continued)

	Dresden				London				Wroclaw				Michalovce					Prague					
	DH	P-1^d	P-2	P-3	DH	P-W	E-W	R-W	DH-I	DH-II	IW-I	IW-II	DH	PSS	SUPS	Admission	Quiet	ADC	W-1	W-2	W-3^E	W-5	W-6^d
Secretary	0.5 / 20	0.5 / 20	0.5 / 20	0.5 / 20	2 / 72	0.5 / 18	0.5 / 18	1 / 35	1 / 40	1 / 40	5 / 200	4 / 160		0.14 / 6	0.14 / 6	0.14 / 6	0.14 / 6	0.43 / 17	0.43 / 17	0.43 / 17	0.43 / 17	0.43 / 17	0.43 / 17
Other	3 / 120		2.1 / 84	2.5 / 100	0.1 / 4	8.5 / 318.7	8 / 300	1 / 37.5						0.2 / 8.5									
Sum	9.85 / 394	24.3 / 971	21.8 / 871	20.2 / 807	8.2 / 301	26.8 / 1010.7	22.4 / 846.5	12.2 / 458.5	14 / 560	7.58 / 303	30.8 / 1234	18.8 / 723	6.165 / 264.3	7.54 / 310.3	10.44 / 421.5	12.67 / 517.3	7.84 / 314.8	5.48 / 219	15.98 / 639	8.48 / 339	11.48 / 459	16.48 / 659	16.98 / 679
Mean staff hours per week available per treatment place	15.76	69.35	36.3	40.35	15.05	40.4	33.9	18.34	16	10.1	42.55	27.8	8.81	12.4	42.15	15.2	9.26	14.6	42.6	18.83	19.12	21.96	21.2

Cl: closed ward; E: special unit for treatment of eating disorders; *The number shows the fixed number of beds. However, as an integrated day hospital, an unfixed number of further patients may be assigned to the ward, but treated as day hospital patients. ^{1}The first line gives the number of staff positions and the second line gives the number of available weekly working hours. ^{2}Form of organization (cf. Schene, 2001): 1. Not freestanding, but organizationally independent and equipped with own units; 2. Freestanding on the terrain of a psychiatric hospital and organizationally independent; 3. Integrated on a psychiatric unit with few own units; 4. Organizationally independent and freestanding with the administration of the Psychiatric Clinic located in the same building; 5. Freestanding in another district but organizationally dependent

Table 3. Available diagnostic measures in the EDEN-day-hospital (i.e. DH) and inpatient settings (i.e. other acronyms)

	Dresden				London				Wroclaw				Michalovce				Prague						
	DH	P-1[cl]	P-2	P-3	DH	P-W	E-W	R-W	DH-I	DH-II	IW-I	IW-II	DH	PSS	SUPS	Admission	Quiet	ADC	W-1	W-2	W-3[E]	W-5	W-6[cl]
Psychological tests	++	++	++	++	++	++	++	++	++	++	++	++	++	++	++	++	++	++	++	++	++	++	++
Blood tests	++	++	++	++	++	++	++	++	++	++	++	++	++	++	++	++	++	++	++	++	++	++	++
Urine tests	++	++	++	++	++	++	++	++	++	++	++	++	++	++	++	++	++	++	++	++	++	++	++
EEG	++	++	++	++	+	+	+	+	++	++	++	++	+	+	+	+	++	++	++	++	++	++	++
CT	++	++	++	++	+	+	+	+	+	+	+	+	+	+	+	+	++	+	+	+	+	+	+
X-rays	++	++	++	++	+	+	+	+	++	++	++	++	+	+	+	+	+	+	+	+	+	+	+
Other diagnostic procedures of somatic specialities	++	++	++	++	-	-	-	-	+	+	+	+	+	+	+	+	+	+	+	+	+	+	+
Physical examination	++	++	++	++	+	++	++	++	++	++	++	++	++	++	++	++	++	++	++	++	++	++	++
Nurological exmination	++	++	++	++	-	++	++	++	++	++	++	++	+	+	+	+	+	+	+	+	+	+	+
Interviews of relatives	++	++	++	++	+	++	++	++	++	++	++	++	++	++	++	++	+	++	++	++	++	++	++
Others	++	++	++	++	-	-	-	-	+	+	+	+	+	+	+	+	+	+	+	+	+	+	+

Cl: closed ward; E: special unit for treatment of eating disorders; ++: measures regularly used in the clinical unit/psychiatric hospital; +: measured used off-site at another hospital; -: measures not available

Some practical problems of implementing the randomised controlled EDEN-study protocol and respective quality assurance measures

Should randomisation and allocation to treatment setting be disconnected?

In clinical routine patients approach a treatment setting not only with specific expectations concerning helpful treatment elements, but also – in the case that this is not their first contact – with pre-existing experiences in definite treatment settings. Especially concerning day hospital treatment clinical studies [26, 42] demonstrate that patients with former admission to this setting have a more favourable attitude towards this setting than patients without prior day hospital admissions. Furthermore, the patients' initial global satisfaction with this setting is identified as a major predictor for the treatment course related to the improvement of psychopathological symptoms.

Therefore, discussion in the EDEN-group on the practise of clinical implementation of the randomisation process in the participating institutions (note: as demonstrated above these are not at all "Rolls Royce" services, see the criticism concerning external validity of Hotopf et al. [23]) had to weigh the ethical argument of ignoring patients' preferences for a special treatment setting [6, 10] associated with a more favourable clinical outcome and the scientific argument to decrease herewith immanent bias effects. Because the finding that there is a correlation between initial satisfaction and psychopathological improvement is currently established only for schizophrenic patients, but if replicated and examined for other mental disorders could have high clinical relevance and because of the possibility to deal with this research question in the first multi-site study following a strict randomised controlled study design (approved by 5 national ethical committees) comparing day-hospital and inpatient psychiatric treatment the decision was that there has to be an indissoluble connection during the explanation session(s) and in the respective written materials for the patients (and their relatives) between participating in the randomisation procedure to the treatment setting and in the defined clinical assessments. In order to assess one main limitation of RCTs' external validity and without disclosing the following definition to the clinicians responsible for the treatment the EDEN-study group agreed on the following procedure: To form a special subgroup of those patients absolutely not willing to be randomised (and therefore allocated to their preferred treatment setting) but approving to be clinically assessed over a 1-year-period and also to perform their clinical assessments defined in the study protocol for the first half of the whole randomisation period. Within the first eight months of the study 6 patients (total number of randomised patients in the 5 centres within this period: 583) constituted this special subgroup.

The preliminary conclusion from an ongoing study for RCTs' in other psychiatric treatment settings could be that randomisation and allocation to the setting should be an integrated procedure to be communicated (orally and using written material) to possible study participants. The resulting limitation of the study's external validity is a minor problem.

Are randomisation rates independent of the level of clinical experience of the professional responsible for enrolling participants?

While there is no doubt in general (see item 10 of the CONSORT-statement, [2]) that failure to separate creation of the allocation sequence from assignment to study group (40) may introduce bias up to now there is no statement based on empirical data how the level of clinical qualifications of those responsible for the enrolment of participants into a trial influences the result of the randomisation. Concerning studies in psychiatric treatment settings and the needed clinical assessment of the defined eligibility criteria – e.g. suicidal risk or risk for others – this is of eminent importance to guarantee a high safety-standard for possible participants and also to minimize resistance of those responsible for the treatment in the settings patients are randomly assigned to.

The differences concerning the refusal rates of patients fulfilling the inclusion criteria in the centres of the EDEN-study – although this variable is also influenced by cultural differences, experience of the centre with mental health services research, number of the involved clinicians and wards to be covered for recruitment etc. – indicate to a certain extent that low refusal rates are associated with the clinical experience of those responsible for formal enrolment. In one centre where research assistants (young psychiatrists) fulfil this task the refusal rate for the first eight months of the study is 31% (decreasing from 44% (1st month) to 14% (5th month) to 21% (6th month)), in another centre where a senior clinician (15 years of clinical experience) is in charge of this project task the refusal rate is only 11%.

For the moment, the conclusion is that randomisation to clinical settings requires profound clinical experience and should be done by experienced psychiatrists ranking higher in the hierarchy of the participating institutions. At least the qualification of those in charge for this process has to be reported that possible bias effects resulting from these differences (decreasing especially external validity) can be judged.

Is a standardized procedure for involving the clinical institution needed?

Platt et al. [41] reported on a randomised trial to evaluate day hospital care as an alternative to inpatient treatment in the acute phase of psychiatric illness which was abandoned when too few patients were admitted to the trial to enable any valid generalization to be made concerning the total at-risk population. In accounting for the failure of the experimental design, the authors draw special attention to the inability of the research team to influence the organization of the unit. Although the design was modified, allowing the medical staff to exclude randomised patients from the trial aiming to modify the prevailing ideology and decision-making process (i.e., "Who goes there") there was no change in the rate of entry into the trial which floundered ultimately on this lack of administrative control.

To minimize this problem, the EDEN-study team established the following quality assurance measures: 1. Every centre sends a monthly report concerning the ongoing process of randomisation – according to the elements of the CONSORT-diagram [2, 36] to the project co-ordinator who can compare and comment or clarify possible difficulties. 2. Each local research team analyses the monthly rates of randomised and excluded patients, discusses continuously the definitions of the exclusion criteria with the responsible clinicians and tries to reduce "clinical (and not definitely defined) reasons for exclusion", e.g. suicidality or degree of severity of the disorder. 3. Every 3 months the whole EDEN-team discusses problems of randomisation in each centre during the regular project meetings and puts possible solutions down in the project's research logbook.

There are various conceptualisations of psychiatric day hospitals, ranging from social rehabilitation after inpatient treatment to crisis intervention and psychotherapy of personality disorders [26, 45]. Furthermore, in contrast to the situation with inpatient treatment on open wards, organizational structures and number of staff are not established in a way that one institution can be compared with another. For a research study focusing on acute day hospital treatment as an alternative to inpatient treatment [22, 34] there is a need to reorganize clinical procedures and provision of treatment elements [25] and to communicate clinical guidelines for this task to the involved staff in the participating institutions. To compound matters, these explanations and request for involving clinical units into a specific research task face a different level of staff's clinical experience and attitudes of the distinctive, not alternative functions of the treatment settings. This holds true for senior staff with a distinct experience concerning the conceptualisation of a clinical unit as well as for junior staff who e.g. didn't have a contact with a day hospital (also due to lacking regulations from the respective educational bodies concerning the professional training). To influence the prevailing beliefs about patients not being suitable for day hospitalisation (see 41) is a constant task for those responsible for the research approach.

The EDEN-group used the following strategies to control these influences: 1. Prior to the official start date there was a conference for the whole staff of each hospital explaining the main objectives and work plan of the project. Every staff member received a short information sheet (3 pages) summarizing the presentation. 2. Also prior to the official start date there was a special conference for the staff of each day hospital with a more detailed oral presentation concerning the main objectives. Each staff member of the day hospital received a detailed information pack (20 pages) outlining the essentials of the proposal and literature on the situation of day hospitals in other countries. 3. Regular meetings for questions of the staff concerning consequences for the daily clinical routine/professional tasks for the staff in the day hospital were established as well as constant informal discussions (e.g. associated to clinical rounds). 4. Special conferences for the nurses and for the senior physicians of the participating hospitals were held for reporting the progress of the project. 5. The principal investigator and director of the department in every centre prepared – before the start of the project – written material with clear definitions how to handle admission procedures (e.g. during weekends) for all physicians/head-nurses of the hospital.

Conclusion: The aims of the study have to be communicated intensely to all colleagues involved in the admission process. Their attitudes concerning the advantages/disadvantages of a specific treatment setting should be changed using a defined dissemination strategy.

Implementing the randomisation before or directly into the process of admission?

Concerning randomisation into different mental health treatment settings up to now there is no clear definition when this should exactly take place during the admission process [2]. But, e.g. dealing with admissions at the weekends is one of the difficult and practically important issues of the implementation of a research design. There are several arguments for integrating randomisation as early as possible into the clinical admission procedure and finish this process before placement into a clinical setting has been decided: If the study aims to compare effectiveness of the treatment in a specific setting this should not be influenced by a short prior treatment in a different clinical setting. This may also have some impact on the stability of conducting the treatment in the setting patients are randomised, if e.g. acute psychopathological symptoms improved using a high dose of medication e.g. for 2 days at an acute ward before the patient changes e.g. to the day hospital, and is against the setting-specific intention-to-treat approach. Previously cited empirical studies (see above) furthermore demonstrate that building a high degree of satisfaction with the treatment setting within the first days after admission is highly predictive for the treatment success of the whole admission period. In practise it is also quite understandable and normal that patients make themselves familiar with their surroundings, staff and treatment conditions what influences their willingness to take the risk for changing the setting after 2 or 3 days. Within this period also attitudes of the responsible clinicians concerning adequateness and effectiveness of the current clinical setting will have been communicated to the patient.

Conclusion: Besides the necessity and standard clinical practice to assess exclusion criteria as well as the patient's capacity to give informed consent as early as possible in the admission process the arguments outlined above should lead to practical definitions in a research design to finish the randomisation process before the definite allocation into a treatment setting has happened. This will also improve the position of those responsible for this process to discuss or modify preferences and attitudes towards treatment settings which are held by the patient, the relatives and by the clinicians (e.g. in private practice or in outpatient departments) initiating the assignment (e.g. to an inpatient or a day hospital setting).

Preliminary results from the EDEN-study

Because data collection for all time-points of assessment as well as the establishment of the final corrected database is not yet finished while writing this chapter, only some preliminary results are presented in this paragraph.

Randomisation rates range from 24.1% to 43.5% in the participating centres, thus confirming results from single site RCTs that the given percentage of acute general psychiatric patients admitted to a hospital can be successfully treated in a day hospital setting. No major untoward events were reported for the index-treatment episodes [27].

With caution, results on effectiveness (based on analyses of the total sample recruited in the first year of the study (December 2000–November 2001)) of the index-treatment episode can be summarized as follows: Improvements of psychopathological symptoms in day hospital settings are equal to the improvements in inpatient settings in all centres [29]. – Concerning the improvement of social disabilities advantages of the day hospital settings in all EDEN-centres could be demonstrated. – No significant difference was found between the two treatment settings on subjective evaluation criteria (quality of life, needs, satisfaction with treatment). However, there was a significant centre setting effect on the subjective evaluation criteria [8]. – The burden for caregiving relatives is significantly decreased both by day hospital treatment and inpatient treatment, whereas, in general, day hospital and inpatient treatment do not significantly differ with respect to the extent of relief provided during the first four weeks of treatment. But, as concerns the strained interpersonal atmosphere between patient and caregiver and the caregivers' task of supervising the patients' medicine intake, sleep and dangerous behaviour, the effect size was generally greater for the inpatient setting compared to the day hospital treatment. However, the development of burden related to caregivers is not consistent in all centres and seems to be affected by cultural factors [47].

Public health – related achievements of carrying out the project

Participating in this multi-centre EC-funded trial with a high scientific standard had a significant impact on the ranking of the participating centres in their countries (especially for the Eastern European centres) and for the mental health services research approach in general. The most important examples to underline this statement are as follows: 1. The Dresden and London study centres significantly increased their involvement in multinational research projects and designed (as co-ordinator or as principal contractor) and started new mental health service research projects funded by the European Commission (for details see chapter Becker et al. in this book). 2. Because of the high reputation associated with participating in an EC-funded multinational project the Polish EDEN-centre received a special grant from its National Committee of Scientific Affairs to restructure the respective department's scientific activities and the technical and housing equipment needed for this purpose. 3. All Eastern European study centres wrote successful grant applications to national ministries in the respective countries for financial support of the EDEN-study. 4. The Slovakian EDEN-study centre recently started an internationally funded transformation project aiming to reorganize the mental health service system of the whole respective catchment area towards establishing a community-oriented care approach. 5. The Czech EDEN-study centre established a research centre for social psychiatry at the psychiatric department; young researchers are now allowed to write theses for academic graduation on social psychiatry research issues.

The translation of instruments – representing not only international research standard but also comprising a range of outcome variables (objective as well as subjective ones, including social disabilities, health care costs and burden on relatives) – can be viewed as a major achievement especially for the Eastern centres (besides BPRS all instruments were not used in these countries before the start of the project). All centres not only gained and some already used the opportunity to publish their translations and spread the instruments in their countries. They can also implement these into further research projects and can use the established contacts to the original authors and to WHO to participate in further developments in this field. Together with the successful implementation of the ambitious scientific design in the clinical reality of the participating institutions, it can be stated that the study created a reliable research basis of current and adequate international standard especially in the participating Eastern centres for mental health services research in general.

Furthermore, the study caused major improvements for the participating day hospitals and increased interest for this treatment approach/setting at a professional, health political and financial level. The following examples of respective achievements try to illustrate this process: The day hospitals in three study centres moved to more comfortable facilities. One study centre opened a new day hospital. In 2002, all study centres organized special symposia on "Treatment in Day Hospitals", mostly attached to the national conferences of the Psychiatric Associations, but also aiming towards audiences interested in health politics and financing. Furthermore, the study group was accepted to organize special symposia on the EDEN-project at all major international scientific conferences worldwide. Especially due to carrying out national day hospital surveys in the participating countries, and due to widely distributing a special project newsletter interest for the project's results, but also for the day hospital setting in general increased among professional colleagues, health politicians (e.g. all German state ministries of health and social affairs announced their interest) and national financial carriers of mental health care.

So far, two direct health political implications of the project can be reported. In Southwestern Poland the project initiated a governmental audit of the situation in day hospitals which caused a significant improvement of staff levels and of the standard of clinical procedures in these services. The Slovakian centre could significantly influence a new directive of the national Ministry of Health defining that each Slovak psychiatric hospital has to establish a day hospital.

Conclusions

The study closes a gap in the European region with regard to scientific work and usable health policy data.

Detailed definitions of the randomisation procedure do not guarantee high performance quality and randomisation rates. Continuous precise assessment of the implementation into the clinical routines of every study centre, adaptation according to specific conditions and personal discussions with all participants are obligatory to establish and keep a high quality of this important research procedure.

Any standardization of randomisation procedures will be a compromise and not suit each site in the same way. The heterogeneously successful implementation of the EDEN-study design seems to be dependent on the different structure of the participating hospitals' clientele, ethnic factors, the current structure of the regional mental health service systems, as well as on specific traditions and specializations of each hospital. These differences have to be taken into account while conducting international multi-centre mental health services research projects.

Should the effectiveness of treatment in a day hospital setting be corroborated in the final analyses, this could well result in a reinforced consideration and acceptance of this therapy setting at the expert and health policy level and increase the safety of therapy for the individual patient.

Although these results are not yet established, this project could already increase professional and health political interest in this treatment setting, and influence health policy decisions aiming towards further establishment of acute day hospitals as well as towards improving the standard of care provided in these services.

Summary

Recent reviews of the effectiveness of acute psychiatric day hospitals – increasingly important for mental health systems which restructure their treatment approaches giving top priority to the reduction of expensive inpatient treatment capacity – suggest that there is a lack of methodologically sound empirical work in this area. Implications for further research prioritise the need for a multi-centre randomised controlled trial, using the most common sets of outcome measures and describing the results according to the CONSORT-standard.

The European Day Hospital Evaluation (EDEN) study, conducted in 5 European centres in 5 European countries (Czech Republic, Germany, Poland, Slovak Republic, UK), realizes this scientific recommendation and is the first randomised controlled trial in mental health service configuration spanning former western and eastern block countries.

This chapter focuses on some important aspects of this international mental health services research project. Firstly, the rationale for randomised controlled trials in this field of research is explained. Secondly, general objectives, some characteristics of the sites, and important details of the study design are presented. Thirdly, practical problems of carrying out the project are outlined. And finally, based on a few preliminary results the so far achieved public health impact of the project is demonstrated.

Acknowledgement

The multi-site research project (Acronym: EDEN-study; website: www.edenstudy.com) "Psychiatric day hospital treatment: An alternative to inpatient treatment, being cost-effective and minimising post-treatment needs for care? An evaluative study in European countries with different care systems" is funded by the European Commission (Quality of Life and Management of Living Resources Programme, contract no. QLG4-CT-2000-01700). Additional national grants supporting the project have been provided by Roland-Ernst-Stiftung für Gesundheitswesen and the Faculty of Medicine at the Dresden University of Technology (for the German centre), the National Health Service Executive Organisation and Management Programme (for the London centre), the Polish National Committee of Scientific Affairs (for the Wroclaw centre), and the Slovak Ministry of Education (for the Michalovce centre). Pfizer Pharmaceutical Company supported travel and accommodation for the EDEN project meetings.

References

1. Abel U, Koch A (1999) The role of randomisation in clinical studies: Myths and beliefs. J Clin Epidemiol 52:487–497
2. Altman DG, Schulz KF, Moher D, Egger M, Davidoff F, Elbourna D, Gotzsche PC, Lang T (2001) The revised CONSORT statement for reporting randomized trials: Explanation and elaboration. Ann Intern Med 134:663–694
3. American Academy of Child & Adolescent Psychiatry, American Psychiatric Association (1996) Criteria for short-term treatment of acute psychiatric illness. American Academy of Child & Adolescent Psychiatry
4. Becker T (1998) Gemeindepsychiatrie. Entwicklungsstand in England und Implikationen für Deutschland. Thieme, Stuttgart New York
5. Becker T, Vázquez-Barquero JL (2001) The European perspective of psychiatric reform. Acta Psychiatr Scand 104 (Suppl. 410):8–14
6. Brewin CR, Bradley C (1989) Patient preferences and randomised clinical trials. BMJ 299:313–315
7. Briggs A (2000) Economic evaluation and clinical trials: size matters. BMJ 321:1362–1363
8. Briscoe J (2002) Cultural differences and subjective evaluation criteria: findings from a European multi-centre study. Eur J Public Health 12:p 43
9. Burns T, Fioritti A, Holloway F, Malm U, Rössler W (2001) Case management and assertive community treatment in Europe. Psychiat Serv 52:631–636
10. Charles C, Gafni A, Whelan T (2000) How to improve communication between doctors and patients. BMJ 320:1220–1221
11. Corrigan PW, Jakus MR (1993) The patient satisfaction interview for partial hospitalization programs. Psychol Rep 72:387–390
12. Creed F, Black D, Anthony P, Osborn M, Thomas P, Tomenson B (1990) Randomised controlled trial of day patient versus in-patient psychiatric treatment. BMJ 300:1033–1037
13. Creed F, Mbaya P, Lancashire S, Tomenson B, Williams B, Holme S (1997) Cost effectiveness of day and inpatient psychiatric treatment: results of a randomised controlled trial. BMJ 14:1381–1385
14. Dick P, Cameron L, Cohen D, Barlow M, Ince A (1985) Day and full time psychiatric treatment: A controlled comparison. Brit J Psychiatry 147:246–250
15. Goldberg D (1999) The future pattern of psychiatric provision in England. Eur Arch Psychiatry Clin Neurosci 249:123–127
16. Goldstein JM, Cohen P, Lewis SA, Struening EL (1988) Community treatment environments. Patient vs. staff evaluations. J Nerv Ment Dis 176:227–233
17. Gray AM, Marshall M, Lockwood A, Morris J (1997) Problems in conducting economic evaluations alongside clinical trials. Brit J Psychiatry 170:47–52
18. Haug HJ, Rössler W (1999) Deinstitutionalization of psychiatric patients in central Europe. Eur Arch Psychiatry Clin Neurosci 249:115–122

19. Herz MI, Endicott J, Spitzer RL, Mesnikoff A (1971) Day versus in-patient hospitalization: a controlled study. Am J Psychiatry 10:1371–1382
20. Hoffmann K, Kaiser W, Isermann M, Priebe S (1998) Wie verändert sich die Lebensqualität langzeithospitalisierter psychiatrischer Patienten nach ihrer Entlassung in die Gemeinde? Gesundheitswesen 60:232–238
21. Hoge MA, Farrell SP, Munchel ME, Strauss JS (1988) Therapeutic factors in partial hospitalization. Psychiatry 51:199–210
22. Horvitz-Lennon M, Normand SLT, Gaccione P, Frank RG (2001) Partial versus full hospitalization for adults in psychiatric distress: A systematic review of the published literature. Am J Psychiatry 158:676–685
23. Hotopf M, Churchill R, Lewis G (1999) Pragmatic randomised controlled trials in psychiatry. Brit J Psychiatry 175:217–223
24. Kallert TW, Leiße M, Bach O (1999) Community-oriented psychiatric care for schizophrenic patients in the Dresden area. In: Manz R, Kirch W (eds) Public Health Research and Practice: Report of the Public Health Research Association Saxony 1993–1998, Vol. I. Roderer, Regensburg, p 159–178
25. Kallert TW, Schützwohl M (2002) Wirkfaktoren der Behandlung in psychiatrischen Tageskliniken aus Patientensicht. Überlegungen zu daraus abzuleitenden Behandlungsmodalitäten. Krankenhauspsychiatrie 13:46–53
26. Kallert TW, Schützwohl M (2002) Clientele, assessment and efficacy of psychiatric day hospital treatment: implications resulting from existing research findings (in German). Schwz Arch Neurol Psychiatr 153:144–152
27. Kallert TW, Priebe S, Kiejna A, Nawka P, Raboch J (2002) The relevance of acute day hospital treatment for restructuring European mental health care systems. Eur J Public Health 12:p 29
28. Kallert TW, Schützwohl M, Kiejna A, Nawka P, Priebe S, Raboch J (2002) Efficacy of psychiatric day hospital treatment: Review of research findings and design of a European multi-centre study. Arch Psychiatry Psychother 2:55–71
29. Kiejna A, Raboch J, Nawka P, Priebe S, Kallert TW (2002) Is acute psychiatric day hospital treatment as effective as inpatient treatment? Eur J Public Health 12:p 29/30
30. Kluiter H, Giel R, Nienhuis FJ, Rüphan M, Wiersma D (1992) Predicting feasibility of day treatment for unselected patients referred for inpatient psychiatric treatment: Results from a randomized trial. Am J Psychiatry 149:1199–1205
31. Kris EB (1965) Day hospitals. Curr Ther Res 7:320–323
32. Kunze H, Kaltenbach L (1996) Psychiatrie-Personalverordnung. 3. erweiterte Auflage. Kohlhammer, Stuttgart Berlin Köln
33. Levitt AJ, Hogan TP, Bucosky CM (1990) Quality of life in chronically mentally ill patients. Psychol Med 20:703–710
34. Marshall M, Crowther R, Almarez-Serrano A et al (2001) Systematic reviews of effectiveness of day care for people with severe mental disorders. (1) Acute day hospital versus admission; (2) Vocational rehabilitation; (3) Day hospital versus outpatient care. Health Technol Assess 5 [21]
35. Moher D, Jones A, Lepage L (2001) Use of the CONSORT Statement and quality of reports of randomized trials. JAMA 285:1992–1995
36. Moher D, Schulz KF, Altman DG for the CONSORT Group (2001) The CONSORT statement: Revised recommendations for improving the quality of reports of parallelgroup randomized trials. Lancet 357:1191–1194
37. Mulward S, Gotzsche PC (1996) Sample size of randomized double-blind trials 1976–1991. Dan Med Bull 43:96–98
38. Munk-Jørgensen P (1999) Has deinstitutionalization gone too far? Eur Arch Psychiatry Clin Neurosci 249:136–143
39. Nienhuis FJ, Giel R, Kluiter H, Rüphan M, Wiersma D (1994) Efficacy of psychiatric day treatment. Course and outcome of psychiatric disorders in a randomised trial. Eur Arch Psychiatry Clin Neurosci 244:73–80
40. Ogundipe LO, Boardman AP, Masterson A (1999) Randomisation in clinical trials. Brit J Psychiatry 175:581–584
41. Platt SD, Knights AC, Hirsch SR (1980) Caution and conservatism in the use of a psychiatric day hospital: Evidence from a research project that failed. Psychiat Res 32:123–132
42. Priebe S, Gruyters T (1994) Patients' and caregivers' initial assessments of day-hospital treatment and course of symptoms. Compr Psychiatry 35:234–238
43. Rössler W, Salize HJ, Biechele U, Riecher-Rössler A (1994) Stand und Entwicklung der psychiatrischen Versorgung. Ein europäischer Vergleich. Nervenarzt 65:427–437

44. Sailas E, Fenton M (2001) Seclusion and restraint for people with serious mental illnesses. Cochrane Library: Cochrane Collaboration
45. Schene AH (2001) Partial hospitalization. In: Thornicroft G, Szmukler G (eds.) Textbook of community psychiatry. Oxford University Press, Oxford, p 283–289
46. Schene AH, van Wijngaarden B, Poelijoe NW, Gersons BPR (1993) The Utrecht comparative study on psychiatric day treatment and in-patient treatment. Acta Psychiatr Scand 87:427–436
47. Schützwohl M, Matthes C, Kallert TW (2002) Acute day hospital treatment and its burden on relatives. Eur J Public Health 12:p 30
48. Slade M, Priebe S (2001) Are randomised controlled trials the only gold that glitters? Brit J Psychiatry 179:286–287
49. Sledge WH, Tebes J, Rakfeldt J, Davidson L, Lyons L, Druss B (1996) Day hospital/crisis respite care versus inpatient care, Part I: Clinical outcomes. Am J Psychiatry 153:1065–1073
50. Sledge WH, Tebes J, Wolff N, Helminiak TW (1996) Day hospital/crisis respite care versus in-patient care, Part II: Service utilization and costs. Am J Psychiatry 153:1074–1083
51. Tomov T (2001) Mental health reforms in Eastern Europe. Acta Psychiatr Scand 104 (Suppl. 410):21–26
52. Wiersma D, Kluiter H, Nienhuis FJ, Ruphan M, Giel R (1995) Costs and benefits of hospital and day treatment with community care of affective and schizophrenic disorders. Brit J Psychiatry 166 (Suppl. 27):52–59
53. Zwerling J, Wilder JF (1964) An evaluation of the applicability of the day hospital in the treatment of acutely disturbed patients. Isr Ann Psychiatry Rel Disciplines 2:162–185

Evidence-based mental health services research. The contribution of some recent EU-funded projects

Thomas Becker · Lorenza Magliano · Stefan Priebe · Hans-Joachim Salize
Matthias Schützwohl · Thomas Kallert

Introduction

Thornicroft and Tansella [1] have addressed the issue of how community-based and hospi-tal-based mental health care can be balanced. In looking at the prerequisites they empha-sise (a) needs assessment at the country/regional level, the local level and the individual level, (b) strengthening the evidence base on treatment effectiveness, and (c) the task of looking at various interfaces between (i) the various components of the mental health ser-vice, (ii) those within the health service, i.e. between mental health and other health ser-vices, and (iii) those between health and other public services, including social services and housing departments.

Reform processes of mental health care are still ongoing in Europe [2]. Although public and political interest increased during the last decade, and although several European gov-ernments established ambitious health policy plans for the future development of this area, the evidence base in European mental health services research to guide such important de-cisions is still slender. Especially, there is a scarcity of methodologically sound multi-centre studies aiming to establish more uniform standards of care across Europe.

Most recently, and particularly within the framework of their "Quality of Life and Man-agement of Living Resources" – Program [3] the European Commission defined a priority for such studies covering issues of major public health impact (see also Kallert et al. in this book). This chapter introduces five of these multi-centre studies (Table 1) to the sci-entific audience. These studies cover the following topics:

▶ The improvement of community care for persons with chronic psychotic disorders (**MECCA** Study);
▶ The problems encountered in implementing behavioural family treatment for people with schizophrenia into routine practice across Europe, such interventions having been proven to be as effective as psychopharmacological treatment regarding the frequency of relapse and re-hospitalisation, but not currently available in clinical practice (**Psy-choedutraining** Study);
▶ The identification of factors leading to treatment- and non-treatment seeking in people suffering from posttraumatic stress disorders following war and migration in the Bal-kans (**STOP** Study);
▶ The variations of the legal framework for involuntary admissions/coercive measures in Europe; and
▶ The evaluation of variations of coercive psychiatric treatment in 12 European coun-tries - entailing infringements of patients' rights – and the development of European guidelines on best clinical practice of coercive treatment in psychiatry (**EUNOMIA** Study).

Table 1. Five European mental health service research studies: Public health relevance

Study/ Acronym	Theme	Aims/Hypotheses	N European centres	Design	N	Intervention	Duration of follow-up	Outcome(s)	Focus on process	Treatment fidelity addressed?	Focus on training	Public health relevance	Policy implications
MECCA	Individual outcome management (OM) in SMI	OM will improve outcome in CMH care	6	Cluster RCT	480	Feedback of key outcome domains to patient	1 year	Quality of life, psychopathology, service satisfaction, compliance with treatment, needs, empowerment, therapeutic relationship, activities and costs	Yes, CMH care	Yes	Yes	Yes	Yes
PSYCHO-EDUTRAIN-ING	Dissemination of psycho-education in SMI	Improving psycho-education availability will improve patient and carer out-come	6	RCT	48 families (1 member with schizophrenia)	2 approaches of staff training in behavioural family therapy	1.5 years	Clinical state, coping, social network and function, carer burden	Yes, relevant to treatment process	Yes	Yes	Yes	Yes
STOP	PTSD in Balkan civil war victims	Provide empirical basis for care programmes for PTSD sufferers	6	1: health service use, coping (exploratory, cross-sectional), 2: investiga-tion of treat-ment programmes	1. 150 in 4 centres; 2. 110 in 4 centres		1 year	PT stress, psychological problems, psychopathology, QoL, health service utilisation and cost	Yes, focus on treatment components	–	–	Yes	Yes

Table 1 (continued)

Study/ Acronym	Theme	Aims/Hypotheses	N European centres	Design	N	Intervention	Duration of follow-up	Outcome(s)	Focus on process	Treatment fidelity addressed?	Focus on training	Public health relevance	Policy implications
EUNOMIA	Variation in coercive psychiatric treatment, its influencing factors and outcomes	Establish European guideline for best practice of coercive treatment	12	Naturalistic mental health services research approach	320 per centre	–	3 months	Perceived coercion, satisfaction and compliance with treatment, psychopathology, severity of illness, service use, social integration	Yes, focus on patients' experiences and rights	–	–	Yes	Yes
INVOLUNTARY ADMISSION/ COERCION	Mental health legislation, involuntary treatment practice	Standardised description, systematic analysis of legislation on involuntary treatment	All EU-member states	Basic documentation, narrative	–	–	–	–	Yes	–	Yes	Yes	Yes

CMH – community mental health; PT – post-traumatic; PTSD – post-traumatic stress disorder; QoL – quality of life; RCT – randomised controlled trial; SMI – severe mental illness

The idea of this contribution is not to report the results of these projects but to outline their core themes, study design and methods, and to discuss their public mental health implications.

Five EU-funded mental health services research projects

The impact of routine outcome measurement on treatment processes in community mental health care (MECCA study)

Three issues characterise the background to the MECCA study: A) throughout Europe, most patients with severe forms of psychotic disorders are cared for in the community. The challenge now is to make processes in community mental health care more effective. B) There are widespread calls to implement regular outcome measurement in routine settings. This, however, is more likely to happen, if it provides a direct benefit to clinicians and patients. C) Whilst user involvement is relatively easy to achieve on a political level, new mechanisms may have to be established to make the views of patients feed into individual treatment decisions.

Although widely called for, outcome management has not been widely implemented [4]. Recently, there have been initiatives to implement outcome measurement in routine settings in various countries. Outcome management on a service or regional level – in different ways – is likely to develop in many European places rather soon. For example, the National Health Service is planning to implement some of the techniques of outcome management in secondary mental health care services for all adult patients. Pilot studies to test feasibility and identify practical problems are underway. Although the precise assessment measures have not yet been decided upon, there is the expectation that every patient should have their morbidity, quality of life and treatment satisfaction regularly assessed in all mental health services throughout the country. However, routine assessment alone is likely to be perceived as just another piece of time consuming paperwork and will only happen if there is some benefit for patients and clinicians. If, however, clinicians and patients can use the information that is routinely collected in a meaningful way in the therapeutic process, they are more likely to comply with the requirements of data collection, and routine outcome management is more likely to happen. Outcome management on a service or regional level may have to be combined with some form of outcome management in the individual therapeutic process in the direct clinician-patient-interaction.

The MECCA study is a cluster randomised controlled trial following the same protocol in community mental health teams in six European countries (participating centres: University of London, United Kingdom; Central Institute for Mental Health Mannheim, Germany; University of Lund, Sweden; University of Zurich, Switzerland; University of Granada, Spain; University of Groningen, Netherlands). In the experimental group, patients' subjective quality of life, treatment satisfaction and wishes for different or additional help are assessed in key worker-patient meetings every two months and intended to inform the therapeutic dialogue and treatment decisions.

The trial tests the hypothesis that the intervention – as compared to current best standard practice – will lead to a better outcome in terms of quality of life and other criteria in patients with psychotic disorders over a one year period. Moreover, the study will hopefully reveal new insights into how therapeutic processes in community mental health care work and how they can be optimised. Changes in psychopathology are not hypothesised to differ between the two groups. Concerning treatment costs in the two groups, the study is exploratory. One might expect higher as well as lower costs in the experimental group.

Higher costs could occur due to additional input as a result of patients' wishes and joint decisions. The intervention could be associated with lower costs when it helps to prevent costly hospital admissions or emergency interventions. If the one year outcome will indeed be more favourable in the intervention group, we further hypothesise that the positive outcome will be mediated through more appropriate therapeutic interventions as decided by the clinician and patient or a better therapeutic relationship in line with a partnership model of care or both.

Assessing the patient's perspective on their quality of life, treatment satisfaction and needs for care will be at the heart of a concurrent outcomes management intervention to be tested in the MECCA study. It involves the key worker regularly assessing outcome and feeding the results back to the patient during their routine meetings. The key worker asks patients about their subjective quality of life, i.e. satisfaction with mental and physical health, accommodation, job situation, leisure activities, friendships, relationship with family/partner, personal safety, and treatment satisfaction, i.e. satisfaction with practical help, psychological help and medication. Ratings are given for each question on a simple 1 to 7 rating scale. Each satisfaction question is followed by a question as to whether the patient wishes additional or different help. If the patient expresses such a need there should be some information as to what kind of additional or different help is desired. Thus, there are only 11 regular questions, each with the complementary question on wishes for change. The assessment is completed by the key worker and patient every two months.

All responses from the patient will be entered by the key worker onto a hand held computer, with the results being available immediately. The quality of life and satisfaction scores, along with needs for additional care, rated in the current and the previous assessment are presented in a graphical colour display. This feedback highlights change over time, dissatisfaction with life domains and aspects of treatment, and needs for additional or different help.

It is expected that the results will feed directly into the therapeutic dialogue and be discussed by the patient and key worker together. The discussion is intended to address, in particular, all areas where the patients expressed dissatisfaction or ratings that have changed since the previous assessment.

Inclusion criteria for key workers are a professional qualification in mental health and/or a minimum of one-year professional experience in an outpatient setting. Key workers are randomised to either the experimental or the control condition. Out of the caseload of each key worker, patients are randomly selected who fulfil the following criteria: living in the community and treated as outpatients by community mental health teams; a history of at least 3 months of continuous care in the current service; fulfilling DSM IV criteria for 295, i.e. schizophrenia and other psychotic disorders; aged between 18 and 65 years of age; having at least one contact with their key worker every two months; capable of giving informed consent; and sufficient knowledge of the language of the host country.

Exclusion criteria are: living in 24 hour supported hostel type of accommodation; organic psychiatric illness or primary substance abuse; expectation to discharge the patient from the service within the next 12 months.

At baseline and 12 month follow up, all outcome criteria are assessed by a researcher in both groups. The outcome criteria assessed in pre-post evaluation include quality of life, psychopathology, service satisfaction, compliance with treatment, needs, empowerment, therapeutic relationship and activities and costs.

In brief, MECCA is a European multi-centred RCT investigating the effects of routine assessment and review of subjective outcome criteria on the individual treatment level. The study aims to explore therapeutic processes in community mental health care whilst trying to find measures to shift therapeutic relationships towards a more effective partnership model of care.

Impact of two alternative staff training programmes on the implementation and effectiveness of a psychoeducational intervention for families of patients with schizophrenia (PSYCHOEDUTRAINING Study)

In spite of their proven efficacy psychoeducational interventions for relatives of patients with schizophrenia are not being routinely offered in mental health services of the European Community. One of the main limiting factors is the availability and content of training courses for the staff. The aim of this study is to assess, in six European countries, the impact of two alternative staff training programmes on the implementation and effectiveness of a well-known psychoeducational intervention (i. e. behavioural family therapy) for relatives of patients with schizophrenia [5]. In each country, the leading centre will select four mental health services whose staff will be trained, and in which the psychoeducational intervention will be applied for 1.5 years in families of patients with schizophrenia. The impact of the two programmes is evaluated by assessing: (a) the families who received the intervention; (b) the adherence of trained staff to the intervention protocol; (c) the treated families' burden, coping strategies, and social network at 1 and 1.5 years after the start of the intervention; (d) the patients' clinical status and social functioning at 1 and 1.5 years after the start of the intervention; and (e) patients' relapses and time spent in hospital during the follow-up period.

Family intervention (FI), compared with routine case management has been shown to significantly reduce patient relapse rates (fourfold at one-year, and twofold at two-year follow up). FI improves patient compliance to antipsychotic drug treatment, and they have been shown to reduce the overall cost of care. However, FI is not routinely available to patients across Europe. Proportions of families having ever received FI varied from none to 15%. The application of FI in clinical settings depends critically on the availability of training courses. This study addresses the questions of (1) whether it is possible to increase the availability of FI to families in routine clinical settings, (2) what training should be offered to staff, (3) differences in FI outcome in different contexts, and (4) to differentiate specific and non-specific effects of the intervention on patients and families. Project participants/ centres include Naples, Birmingham, Dresden, Athens, Lisbon, and Granada (Italy, United Kingdom, Germany, Greece, Portugal, Spain).

The study comprises four phases: (1) development, and (2) implementation of training materials (including training guidelines, videos, audiocassettes, information and training materials on family engagement, the assessment of family relationships and relatives' needs, schizophrenia and its treatment, communication skills, and problem solving techniques) and programmes, (3) providing the psychoeducational intervention, and (4) the evaluation of the impact of training on the effectiveness of FI at 1 and 1.5 years after its start. It compares two FI training programmes both of which include a basic course on a psychoeducational FI, regular supervision meetings, whereas the augmented training programme, as an add-on, includes training sessions and supervision meetings on the implementation of FI in routine settings, and practice sessions on the use of the FI techniques in routine clinical work during the core training phase. Training materials include: guidelines and exercises on coping with conflicts and organisational problems, a guide for staff training in FI, assessment instruments, i. e. the family intervention schedule (FIS), the staff adherence to the psychoeducational intervention schedule (SAPIS), and guides for staff training in psychoeducational interventions and in the use of assessment procedures. In phase 2, a random 10% sample of all public mental health services in each country was contacted by mail and asked for study participation of which four services were randomised into one of the alternative training programmes. Two professionals in each service entering the study were trained in FI and involved in its implementation, and one professional was trained in the administration of outcome assessment instruments. In phase 3 the staff were trained in the psychoeducational intervention by means of either a five-day intensive basic course and regular supervision meetings or the augmented training programme. Interviewers were trained in the use of the assessment instruments. Each of the six national lead centres has one trainer and one researcher, and 24 mental health services across the sites each have two professionals to be trained in the psychoeducational intervention and one trained in the use of assessment instruments. The intervention is then administered by trained professionals to at least four families of patients with a DSM-IV diagnosis of schizophrenia with relatives living with the patient or having spent at least fifteen hours per week at face to face contact with the patient during the last three months. The impact of the two programmes implementing FI is then assessed. At 1 year and 1.5 year follow-up carer burden, coping strategies, and social network as well as patients' clinical status, relapses and social functioning are assessed.

In late 2002, a guide on training professionals in FI had been developed in six European languages, and assessment instruments for the trainees' difficulties in the provision of the psychoeducational intervention and their competence in the use of psychoeducational techniques were also available in the various languages. 48 mental health service staff had been trained in FI, and 24 had been trained in the use of assessment instruments. Supervision meetings are still ongoing. Each trained professional is working with at least two families of patients with schizophrenia. Preliminary data suggest that it is possible to increase the number of families of patients with schizophrenia receiving psychoeducational interventions through a short training package.

Treatment seeking and treatment outcomes in people suffering from posttraumatic stress following war and migration in the Balkans (STOP Study)

War and migration in the Balkans caused traumatic experiences in great parts of the population. About four million victims living in former Yugoslavia as well as about 100 000 refugees living in different European countries are estimated to suffer from on-going and severe psychological symptoms of post-traumatic stress, and many of these people, although in need of treatment, do not seek treatment. Given the fact that, if untreated, post-traumatic stress reactions tend to persist for many years, often resulting in impairment and disability secondary to the symptom complex, offering appropriate care is a special challenge to health services.

With regard to this context, the multi-centre STOP study includes partners from the UK (London) and Germany (Dresden) as EU member states, and from Bosnia (Sarajevo) and Herzegovina (Rijeka), Croatia (Zagreb), and Serbia (Belgrade) as the biggest countries in the area of former Yugoslavia. The study aims to provide an empirical basis for designing care programmes for people suffering from post-traumatic stress following war and migration in the Balkans who currently do not seek treatment, and to improve the cost-effectiveness of treatment programmes for those patients who are cared for in specialised treatment centres.

The civil war in Yugoslavia caused traumatic experiences in great parts of the population, including combat, loss of relatives, persecution through ethnic cleansing, rape, being shot and wounded, and forced migration. Millions of people fled their homes and took refuge either in other parts of Yugoslavia or in Western European countries, the USA, Australia, and New Zealand. Germany, for example, gave temporary protection to about 350 000 Bosnian refugees, about half of all Bosnians who sought protection in Western European countries during the Bosnian war. Such traumatic war experiences can lead to serious and long-lasting psychological distress. The prominent posttraumatic stress disorder is characterized by unwanted recollections, nightmares, emotional numbing and signs of hyperarousal, such as sleeplessness and irritability. It is associated with impaired social functioning and often accompanied by marital, occupational, and other health problems. Studies on Yugoslavian refugees living in the USA or the Netherlands, for example, as well as studies on civilians still living in Yugoslavia show that a high number of participants suffer from high levels of posttraumatic stress, with war experiences often resulting in a complex and difficult to treat form of PTSD [6–8]. In terms of symptom reduction, RCTs showed the effectiveness of different forms of pharmacological and psychotherapeutic treatment, such as CBT or EMDR [9]. The generalizability of the existing well-controlled studies, however, is limited, given that most studies evaluated well-defined treatments in well-selected participants. Patients suffering from the mentioned complex PTSD often need combinations of different treatment interventions. Thus, little is known about treatment outcomes and predictors of treatment outcomes in this population.

Another problem is that patients suffering from posttraumatic stress often do not receive specialised treatment for their mental health difficulties. Studies on health service utilization of traumatized patients showed that most victims seek medical treatment, and PTSD is deemed to be associated with nearly the highest rate of service use, and the highest per capita cost of any mental illness [10]. But only a minority seeks or receives, respectively, mental health treatment, which means that only a minority seeks or receives specialised treatment that holds the promise of shortening the duration of symptoms and impairment. Knowledge on the barriers to specialised mental health treatment is rather limited. Several studies showed that mental health treatment seekers suffer from a higher level of symptoms, particularly the PTSD symptoms of intrusion and hyperarousal. In a study on survivors of disaster it has been found that traumatized victims were reluctant to use mental health services because of the fear that painful memories would be aroused. And another study on rape victims found that medical treatment was considered as a less stigmatising form of treatment than mental health treatment, and this was suggested as being an important reason why the rape victims were more likely to seek medical treatment.

And finally: It has to be mentioned that most published research on refugees is on refugees who emigrated to countries with an appropriate infrastructure. To what extent results gained in refugee groups apply to people who stayed in the post-war area, is still unclear.

Given this background, the workplan of the STOP study has been divided into two parts, one of which is on health service utilization of people suffering from posttraumatic stress, the other of which is on the investigation of treatment programmes offered in specialised centres in the mentioned Ex-Yugoslavian countries.

A first part which is the part on health service utilization covers three main research questions:

▶ What are the barriers to specialised treatment in people suffering from post-traumatic stress who have not received specialised treatment?

▶ What are the coping strategies of people suffering from posttraumatic stress who have not received specialised treatment?

▶ Are characteristics and coping strategies of people suffering from post-traumatic stress and having not received specialised treatment in refugee populations different from those who stayed in the post-war area?

To answer these questions, participants will be recruited in four centres, namely in Dresden and London, and in Belgrade and Zagreb. We defined the following inclusion criteria: (i) Balkan origin; (ii) age between 18 and 65 years; (iii) experience of war and/or forced migration in the Balkans; (iv) no severe mental impairment due to organic causes and no severe physical disability; and (v) capability of giving written informed consent.

In a next step, seven screening questions on symptoms of post-traumatic stress since war/migration will be asked. Participants reporting two or more symptoms will be asked to complete the full interview which comprises the CAPS and the IES-R for the assessment of posttraumatic stress, the SCL-90-R for the assessment of psychological problems and symptoms of psychopathology, and the MANSA for the assessment of quality of life. Costs of health service utilization and other support will be assessed using the CSRI. Barriers to treatment, coping strategies and social support will be assessed using open questions, with in depth interviews being conducted with approximately 30 participants per centre. Altogether, about N = 150 participants will be recruited in each centre. Thus, the design clearly shows that this part of the study is a cross-sectional, mainly exploratory and partly qualitative study. It will reveal results on the barriers to treatment, on coping strategies and it will allow the comparison of non-treatment receivers in Germany and the UK with non-treatment receivers in Croatia and Serbia.

A second part of STOP aims at the investigation of treatment programmes offered in specialised centres in the mentioned Ex-Yugoslavian countries. Again, three research questions could be specified:

▶ What outcomes in changes of symptoms, treatment satisfaction and quality of life are to be expected for different sub-groups of patients in specialised treatment centres?
▶ What baseline characteristics and treatment components are consistently associated with a more favourable outcome across treatment centres?
▶ What are the treatment and support costs for patients suffering from posttraumatic stress and how are costs linked to outcome?

Participants will be recruited in specialised treatment centres in Belgrade, Rijeka, Sarajevo, and Zagreb. The inclusion criteria have been defined as in Part A, which is Balkan origin, aged between 18 and 65 and so on. Furthermore, to be included into the study, the potential participants must suffer from posttraumatic stress and be accepted for treatment by the respective centre.

Patients will be interviewed at baseline which is a pre-treatment assessment, after three months and after 12 months. About N = 110 patients will be recruited at baseline in each centre, so that about N = 75 patients will be interviewed after 12 months. The set of instruments is largely identical to that used in Part A of the study. Again, the CAPS and the IES-R will be used for the assessment of posttraumatic stress, the SCL-90-R for the assessment of psychological problems and symptoms of psychopathology, the MANSA will allow the assessment of the patients' subjective quality of life, and the CSRI will allow the assessment of costs of health service utilization. Open question will be asked on coping strategies, social support, expectations concerning treatment and, later on, on the experiences with the given treatment. All components of the received treatment, i.e. pharmacological interventions, psycho-education, behavioural techniques and so on will be continuously recorded. Using symptom change and treatment adherence as main outcome predictors, this part of the study will allow answering the research questions by calculating analyses using baseline variables and treatment components as predictors.

European evaluation of coercion in psychiatry and harmonization of best clinical practice (EUNOMIA Study)

In all European countries reforms in mental health care focused on the reduction of hospital beds, the diagnosis-specific differentiation of inpatient treatment, the de-institutionalisation of people with chronic mental illness [11], the establishment of community mental health care structures and treatment approaches [12]. In general, guiding principles of this process were: strengthening the autonomy of the patient, individual needs- or consumer-orientation, flexibility of the treatment approaches in mental health services and the normalisation of the living conditions of those affected [13–15]. In sharp contrast to these fundamental principles, there is a lack of research into inpatient psychiatric treatment of the acutely mentally ill, especially those involuntarily admitted to hospital, and this is particularly the case at the European level. No national or European guidelines or standards of best practice have been established, and this applies both to the legal aspects and the issues of clinical practice.

On the other hand, most European countries report current increasing rates of involuntarily admitted psychiatric patients or currently are planning to revise existing legal regulations. These are processes which lack an adequate empirical basis. This scarcity of evidence is underlined by the wide variability across Europe with different legal regulations. The literature reports a factor of nearly 20 between different parts of Europe [16, 17]. All this collides with one of the most important general goals of the European Union: approximation of health care opportunities and living conditions of the citizens in the individual member countries. Furthermore, especially the past decade has seen an increasing focus on the consumer of mental health services and on the question whether psychiatric treatment can be considered successful if the recipients of such services are dissatisfied. A frequent and serious cause of negative feelings toward psychiatric treatment is being treated involuntarily. It is often difficult to correlate patients' legal status of admission and numbers of involuntary admissions with patient variables or varying legal situations. There is some pressure to abolish involuntary hospitalisation or to narrow the criteria by which people qualify for involuntary hospitalisation. Mental health professionals and family groups have lobbied with equal fervour that civil commitment be maintained, often with broadened criteria. These discussions, inconsistent findings and controversies add to a growing concern that coercive measures in psychiatry may entail unnecessary infringements of patients' rights [18]. Furthermore, it is unknown in which ways involuntary admissions and coercive measures can be meaningfully compared between nations, because they might constitute quite different procedures in different countries.

The major goal of this project is to analyse existing variation in coercive psychiatric treatment (i.e. forced admission to a psychiatric hospital, involuntary detention after voluntary admission, seclusion/isolation in a room that the patient is not allowed to leave, restraint/fixation by holding and/or mechanical devices, forced medication), its influencing factors and outcomes. This requires to combine a wide range of different European countries and regions, and to use a naturalistic methodological mental health services research approach. The detailed research objectives are:

► to systematically describe and compare patients admitted both on a legally voluntary and on a legally involuntary basis with regard to variables associated with coercive treatment measures or to patients' subjective perception of being treated coercively;
► to explore the connection between coercion during treatment, treatment outcome and future treatment seeking;
► to identify conditions of coercion and to link them to outcome criteria on a European cross-cultural basis;
► to identify views of staff, users and family members on coercive measures on a European cross-cultural basis;
► to understand better which factors influence staff to select coercive treatment measures in favour of non-coercive alternatives.

In designing the project regions of comparable size from all parts of Europe were included in order to cover as much of the existing variation as possible. The regions included are: Dresden, Germany; Sofia, Bulgaria; Prague, Czech Republic; Thessaloniki, Greece; Tel-Aviv, Israel; Naples, Italy; Vilnius, Lithuania; WrocÅaw, Poland; Michalovce, Slovakia; Granada,

Spain; Ārebro, Sweden; East-London, United Kingdom. Systematic description and comparison of the socio-demographic characteristics and mental health services of these regions was achieved by using the following standardized instruments: European Socio-Demographic Schedule (ESDS) and Area Socio-demographic Sheet to collect information on the socio-demographic profile of a catchment area; information on multi-ethnicity and criminality rates in the respective catchment areas is covered by neither of the mentioned instruments, but will be established as well; European Service Mapping Schedule (ESMS) for standardized assessment of the established mental health services in the catchment areas; International Classification of Mental Health Care (ICMHC) for a standardised description of the level of specialization of inpatient clinical units for acute treatment participating in EUNOMIA. This instrument classifies activities aimed directly at the users of these services.

The main part of the study is the 21-month phase of data collection. During this phase the study will include two sub-samples of patients: an "involuntarily admitted" group and a "voluntarily admitted" group. Both groups (N = 320 in each centre) will be assessed at three time points (within the first week after hospital admission, 4 weeks and 3 months after admission), at each using identical instruments for both groups. To separate both groups, legal status of admission based on a court's decision cannot be used. The national law or mental health act used to justify the actual procedure of admission, will be used to separate both groups. This is because of the different possible definitions of coercion and because of the legally permissible practise of patients being admitted against their will, but changing their legal status to voluntary shortly after admission. The inclusion of a group of voluntarily admitted patients in this study is necessary because patients' legal status can be changed to "involuntary" some time after admission and in some countries it is possible to administer coercive treatment to legally voluntary patients. Furthermore, as mentioned above, the correlation between observable coercive treatment and perceived coercion is at best moderate. The instruments (MacArthur Admission Experience Survey; Cantril Ladder of perceived coercion, Client's Assessment of Treatment, Compliance-rating with treatment, Modified Over Aggression Scale, Clinical Global Impression Scale, Brief Psychiatric Rating Scale, items rating perceived coercion and pressures concerning stay in hospital, items assessing social outcome variables and use of services) which will be implemented in a specially designed computerised documentation system acting as central assessment tool have been chosen so that they will provide a valid and reliable assessment of the constructs of interest, while accommodating the limited mental capacity of the participating patients and the fact that some instruments will have to be integrated into clinical routine (for more details please visit: www.eunomiastudy.net). In a standardized way staff will have to record details of each coercive measure applied in the first 4 weeks after index admission, and will also rate the patient's perceived coercion.

In order to assess staff's and relatives' attitudes towards coercive measures, self-compiled interviews using open questions will be conducted on subjective definitions of violence and coercion, their subjective criteria for the use of coercive measures as well as their attitudes toward violence and coercion.

Further objectives of the project include, (a) to provide information on the legal basis for coercive measures in the participating countries and on current practice; and (b) to establish a critical mass for influencing future research in this area as well as legal and political decisions in order to harmonise the clinical practise of coercive measures in psychiatry on both a national and a European level. To realize these objectives the project will establish (i) local focus groups comprising all relevant institutions and groups involved. Their task will be to discuss procedural issues of involuntary admissions and treatments, to discuss results from the empirical part of the project, and to establish local or national guidelines for good clinical practice; it will (ii) establish a special legal counselling group, involving one expert from each country; it will (iii) organise a European board of advisors, involving relevant health institutions, professional associations, ethical experts and a representative of European patient organisations.

Project targets include: the development and implementation of a standardised computerised system for basic documentation and documentation of coercive measures in psychiatry, thereby facilitating continuous quality assurance, clinical and legal certainty, and the preparation of public health reports; the collection of data in naturalistic settings on both objective characteristics of coercive measures used during psychiatric treatment and on subjective views of patients, clinicians and family with regard to coerced psychiatric treatment; the description of the clinical practice of coercive treatment in each of these regions; the description of variation between regions in the variables studied; the identification of the best clinical practice of coercive treatment in psychiatry on the basis of the observed variation; the development of a European guideline ("patient charter") for the best practice of coercive measures in psychiatry, and the dissemination of the results of this study to professional, user and legal organisations in order to advocate the harmonisation of best practise across Europe.

Compulsory admission and involuntary treatment of mentally ill patients-legislation and practice in EU-Member States

The involuntary placement and involuntary treatment of mentally ill patients are central issues in mental health care. Their massive impact upon the liberty and freedom of the persons concerned have made them a topic of controversial legal and ethical debates for more than 100 years. These debates evolve from the necessity to apply coercive measures in certain circumstances, a fact which singularly distinguishes psychiatry from most other medical disciplines. Thus, during the 19th and 20th centuries different approaches to regulating the application of coercive measures were developed across Europe and all over the world that depend on a variety of cultural or legal traditions, as well as on different concepts and structures of mental health care delivery.

The legal frameworks for the involuntary placement or treatment of the mentally ill, or the application of coercive measures still differ widely. Overviews of national approaches are scarce. Moreover, there is a lack of methodologically sound studies. Statistics on compulsory admission from official sources are rarely published internationally. When such comparisons are available, they usually include only selected nations. Consequently, the Assembly of the Council of Europe criticised the lack of comparative European studies in the field [19]. Against the background of the rapid European integration process, a standardised description or systematic analysis of commitment laws or other legal instruments for regulating involuntary placements across the European Union Member States seems to be overdue. The study "Compulsory admission and involuntary treatment of mentally ill patients-legislation and practice in EU-Member States", funded by the Health and Consumer Protection Directorate-General of the European Commission, attempts to bridge this gap. The study aimed at gathering, describing and analysing information on the differences or similarities of legal frameworks for involuntary placement or treatment of mentally ill patients across the European Union Member States. Involuntary placement or treatment in this context did not include the treatment of mentally ill offenders or any other aspect of forensic psychiatry, which was seen as another topic, requiring a different scientific approach. For the first time, this study describes legal frameworks and routine procedures of compulsory admission and involuntary treatment in European Union member states in a comprehensive, systematic and standardised manner. Furthermore, epidemiological data from official national sources are provided, detailing the compulsory admission rates for most of the Member States for the last decade.

The study lasted from October 2000 to January 2002. A network of experts and collaborators from each Member State was set up. The experts filled in a questionnaire for gathering structured information about the current situation and practice concerning legislation for compulsory admissions and involuntary treatment of mentally ill patients in each member state. The experts also contributed a chapter describing specific characteristics of their respective member states (e.g., regional differences, historical changes). Numbers and rates of admission per 100 000 population for the most recent available year were assessed in all 15 European member states. Time series for the last decade which are scarce but available for some countries were also looked at. General trends are described and correlations between compulsory admission rates, their change over time and the respective legislation in member states are analysed and discussed.

Based on the detailed national information the study's co-ordinating centre (in Mannheim, Germany) compiled a synopsis of the current situation in the EU. One of the major results of the study was that legal regulations as well as routine procedures for detaining the mentally ill differ considerably across the European Union, whether or not they are regulated by a separate mental health act. National legal traditions, structures or standards of quality with regard to the provision of general health care, as well as national approaches or philosophies regarding mental health care, most strongly determine the legal frameworks or the practice of involuntary placement or treatment of mentally ill patients. Thus, the most significant characteristic of the European Union member states' legal frameworks regarding involuntary placement or treatment of mentally ill is their variety. Although common patterns among member states were identified in comparing crucial legislative or procedural details, these patterns were far from being consistent across all analysed items or approaches. Although compulsory admission is seen as an intervention of last resort across the European Union, only to be applied in an acute crisis or state of emergency, even the most basic legal criteria qualifying a person for involuntary placement in a psychiatric facility differ widely. For a global overview, these criteria can be categorised into three groups, providing probably the most significant distinction for characterising a member state's legal approach towards involuntary placement or treatment of mentally ill persons: a serious threat of harm to the person himself and/or to others ("dangerousness criterion"), an ultimate need for psychiatric treatment ("need-for-treatment criterion"), and a combination of both. The global inconsistency in legal frameworks and practices constitutes a major obstacle to any mutual European actions or policies. However, ongoing activities in the member states to reform or adapt their mental health legislation might offer opportunities for harmonising legal instruments across the European Union. One major problem, however, for increasing the harmony of national laws, acts or procedures according to the policies or experiences in other countries is the shortage of evidence that could guide best practice (the EUNOMIA study aims to fill this research gap). Currently, even within some member states, there might be several legal instruments, each with a different regional scope or pertaining to selected patient groups, in effect simultaneously. The most significant example is Germany, with one nationwide guardianship law and sixteen state commitment laws (according to the sixteen German Federal States) currently in effect that differ remarkably with regard to crucial details. Separate mental health acts are also in effect for large parts of the United Kingdom (Scotland and Northern Ireland), Denmark (Greenland) or other Member States.

The final report of the study [20] provides numerous further information or data, describing and analysing the legal frameworks or national approaches by detailing the crucial aspects of the topic (e.g. acts, criteria, practice, rights of persons concerned, procedures, epidemiology). This information is essential to any discussion of this issue on a European level.

Discussion

The studies described in this chapter differ widely in themes, hypotheses, design, the instruments used, types of data and other material collected, and also in the approach to the data collected. However, there are a few elements they have in common.

▶ Firstly, the studies bear witness to the fact that mental health service researchers concentrate on the detail of the care process. MECCA aims at establishing whether a feedback to service users on some outcome domains may strengthen the therapeutic relationship, improve symptoms, medication and overall self-management by patients, and whether there are effects on patient outcome. PSYCHOEDUTRAINING looks more closely at different ways of improving both staff training in and the availability of psychoeducational family interventions. STOP examines the effects of PTSD interventions that are suited to the social, economic and general ecological situation in the Balkan region, and it does not uncritically infer from therapy studies on the disorder performed elsewhere. Finally, EUNOMIA and the Involuntary Admission/Coercion Study both attempt to elucidate current practice to define the basis for research into a key element of debates around mental health care. Thus, there is some groundbreaking work here which lays the foundation for multidimensional service evaluation with an eye to practice and routine implementation.

▶ Secondly, several of these studies (MECCA, PSYCHOEDUTRAINING, STOP) address the important step in health care research and planning which separates efficacy and effectiveness research in that they explicitly address practice transfer and staff training.

▶ Thirdly, the studies bear witness to the ethical issues involved in mental health care. Szmukler [21], in addressing "ethics in community psychiatry", discusses the following ethical dilemmas: privacy (relevant to the debate on assertive community treatment), confidentiality, coercion, and conflicts of duty to patient versus others including the issue of harm to others and informal carers. In approaching the ethical problems he suggests ways of helping clinicians to resolve the ethical dilemmas such as: increasing patient involvement in their care; addressing the issue of paternalism; and facing conflicts of duty. MECCA is pertinent in this respect, and the two studies on coercion reflect the importance of this ethical issue for the future of psychiatric services in Europe.

Conclusions

In conclusion, studies of this kind could help to inform and stimulate future practice. Some European studies have opened the field by developing methodology and instruments, adapting them for cross-national use and describing mental health care structure, process, service use and cost [22–24]. The studies presented above document that progress is being made in this field of mental health services research, that study aims, methodology and scope are evolving towards more complex issues on the one hand and towards an increasing focus on the issues of implementation and routine care on the other hand.

Acknowledgements: Projects are/were funded by the European Commision: MECCA (QLG5-CT-2002-01938), PSYCHOEDUTRAINING (QLG4-CT-2000-01554), STOP (ICA2-CT-2002-10002), EUNOMIA (QLG4-CT-2002-01036), compulsory admission and involuntary treatment of mentally ill (SI2.254882[2000CVF3-407]).

References

1. Thornicroft G, Tansella M (2002) Balancing community-based and hospital-based mental health care. World Psychiatry 1:84–90
2. Becker T, Vázquez-Barquero JL (2001) The European perspective of psychiatric reform. Acta Psychiatr Scand 104 (Suppl. 410):8–14
3. European Commission (2002) Improving the Quality of life. An overview of Public Health Research projects 1994-2002. (websites: http://biosociety.cordis.lu or www.cordis.lu/life or http://europa.eu.int/comm/research/rtdinfo)
4. Slade M (2002) Editorial: Routine outcome assessment in mental health services. Psychol Med 32:1339–1343
5. Falloon I, Mueser K, Gingerich S, Rappaport S, McGill C, Graham-Hole V (1996) Behavioural family therapy. Workbook. Second edition. Buckingham, UK
6. Bauer M, Priebe S, Häring B, Adamczak K (1993) Long-term mental sequelae of political imprisonment in East Germany. J Nerv Ment Dis 181:257–262
7. Kozaric-Kovacic D, Marusic A, Ljubin T (1999) Combat-experienced soldiers and tortured prisoners of war differ in the clinical presentation of posttraumatic stress disorder. Nordisk Psykiatrist Tidsskrift (Nordic Journal of Psychiatry) 53:11–15
8. Ebbinghaus R, Bauer M, Priebe S (1996) Behandlung der posttraumatischen Belastungsstörung. Eine Übersicht. Fortschr Neurol Psychiat, 64:433–443
9. Arbor A (1998) Comparative efficacy of treatments for posttraumatic stress disorder: a meta-analysis. Clin Psychology Psychotherapy 5:126–144
10. Bramsen I, Van der Ploeg HM (1999) Use of medical and mental health care by World War II survivors in the Netherlands. J Traumatic Stress 12:243–261
11. Munk-Jorgensen P (1999) Has deinstitutionalization gone too far? Eur Arch Psychiat Clin Neurosci 249:136–143
12. Thornicroft G, Szmukler G (eds) Textbook of Community Psychiatry. Oxford University Press, Oxford 2000
13. Priebe S, Gruyters T (1995) Patients' assessment of treatment predicting outcome. Schizophr Bull 21:87–94
14. Ruggeri M (1994) Patients' and relatives' satisfaction with psychiatric services: the state of the art of its measurement. Soc Psychiatry Psychiatr Epidemiol 29:265–276
15. Kallert TW, Leiße M (2001) Schizophrenic patients' normative needs for community-based psychiatric care – Evaluative study throughout the year post hospital release in the Dresden region –. Soc Psychiatry Psychiat Epidemiol 36:1–12
16. de Girolamo G (2001) Der gegenwärtige Stand der psychiatrischen Versorgung in Italien. Nervenarzt 72:511–514
17. Nenonen M, Pelanteri S, Rasilainen J (2000) Mielenterveyden häiöiden hoito Suomessa 1978–1998 – Treatment of mental disorder in Finland 1978–1998. National Research and Development Centre for Welfare and Health, Statistical report 3/2000 (available from the author)
18. Nilstun T, Syse A (2000) The right to accept and the right to refuse. Acta Psychiatr Scand (Suppl.) 101:31–34
19. Assembly of the Council of Europe (1994) – Recommendation 1235 in psychiatry and human rights.
20. Salize HJ, Dressing H, Peitz M (2002) Compulsory admission and involuntary treatment of mentally ill patients - legislation and practice in EU-Member States. European Commission – Health & Consumer Protection Directorate-General. Final report.
21. Szmukler G (1999) Ethics in community psychiatry. In: Bloch S, Chodoff P, Green SA (eds) Psychiatric Ethics, 3rd edition, Oxford University Press, Oxford: 363–381
22. Becker T, Knapp M, Knudsen HC, Schene A, Tansella M, Thornicroft G, Vázquez-Barquero JL, and the EPSILON Study Group (1999) The EPSILON study of schizophrenia in five European countries: Design and methodology for standardising outcome measures and comparing patterns of care and service costs. Brit J Psychiatry 175:514–521
23. Beecham J, Munizza C (2002) Assessing mental health in Europe. Acta Psychiatr Scand 102, suppl 405
24. Knapp M, Chisholm D, Leese M, Amaddeo F, Tansella M, Schene A, Thornicroft G, Vázquez-Barquero JL, Knudsen HC, Becker T, and the EPSILON Study Group (2002) Comparing patterns and costs of schizophrenia care in five European countries: The EPSILON Study. Acta Psychiatr Scand 105:42–54

Cost-effectiveness of mental health service systems in the European comparison

MATTHIAS C. ANGERMEYER · CHRISTIANE ROICK · THOMAS BECKER
REINHOLD KILIAN

Introduction

As other sectors of medical care, mental health care has to struggle with the problems of raising health care costs and the limitations of financial resources (Häfner et al. 1991; Knapp et al. 1990; Salize et al. 1996). And as in somatic medicine, most mental health experts agree that the current financial problems should not be solved by reducing the standard of care but by improving the efficiency of existing and by developing more efficient treatment methods (John et al. 2001; Wasem et al. 2001). Most experts further agree that health economic methods such as cost-outcome analysis are important tools for the assessment of treatment efficiency and for the forecasting of the possible economic consequences of innovative treatment strategies (Knapp 2000).

Usually four approaches of cost-outcome analysis are distinguished:

(I)   Cost-efficiency studies are conducted when the outcomes of all possible treatment alternatives are equal and the goal of the analysis is to find the most inexpensive treatment alternative. The problem of cost-efficiency analysis is that conclusive evidence for the equal effectiveness of treatment alternatives is hardly to find in psychiatric treatment.

(II) Cost-benefit analysis is a rarely used method in health economy because it requires that both costs and outcomes are calculated in monetary units, which is regarded as impossible for most medical outcomes.

(III) In cost-effectiveness analysis only the costs have to be calculated in monetary units and the outcome may be calculated in units which are more appropriate to the particular kind of outcome. Limitations of this approach result from the fact that most health interventions have multiple outcomes which cannot be measured with a common metric. Therefore, it is difficult to integrate the different outcomes to assess overall effectiveness.

(IV) Cost-utility analysis is an extension of cost-effectiveness analysis by using utility measures which combine numeric preference weights of several outcome indicators yielding a single utility value as outcome. The quality adjusted life year (QALY) is an example of an utility measure which is widely used in health economic studies. The advantage of cost-utility analysis is the comparability of different interventions with different outcomes. The disadvantage is the difficulty of obtaining reasonable preference values. Particularly in psychiatry, utility assessment is not well developed and therefore cost-utility analysis is only rarely used.

At present, cost-effectiveness analysis is the method of cost-outcome analysis which is most frequently used for the evaluation of psychiatric treatment. However, most of the existing studies are focused on the comparison of the cost-effectiveness of treatment alternatives in controlled clinical settings (Chan et al. 2000; Clark et al. 1998; Creed et al. 1997; Dixon et al. 2002; Essock et al. 2000; Ford et al. 1997; Knapp et al. 1998; Lave et al. 1998; Reinharz et al. 2000; Rosenheck et al. 1998; Seshamani 2002; UK700 Group 2000). By contrast to somatic medicine, the particular nature of mental disorders and, as a consequence, the particular nature of psychiatric treatment makes it difficult to apply existing methods of health economic assessment. Difficulties of comprehensive cost-assessment result from the great variety of services and from the variety of financing systems (Salize et al. 1996). Difficulties of outcome assessment also result from the variety of outcome dimensions and the lack of methods to combine several outcome parameters to a single value. A further difficulty results from the fact that most psychiatric patients are not in an acute but in a chronic state of the illness. In an acute state of mental illness the reduction of symptoms is the primary task of treatment and the change of symptom severity can be used as a reasonable indicator of treatment effectiveness. However, in a chronic state of a severe mental illness such as schizophrenia, the primary goal of psychiatric treatment is keeping the condition of the patient stable and preventing psychotic relapse and inpatient episodes. This means that the system may work most effectively when nothing changes. However, this does not mean that stability of clinical outcome parameters is a sufficient criterion of effectiveness since clinical stability can be reached at a low level of subjective quality of life. Therefore, clinical as well as non-clinical outcome parameter are needed which reflect the effectiveness of the mental health care system for patients in acute as well as in chronic states. Most of these problems are multiplied when it comes to international comparisons due to the great variety of systems for the provision and the financing of mental health care (Chisholm et al. 2000; Knapp et al. 2002).

Since the 1970s psychiatric services in most European countries have fundamentally changed from mainly hospital based to community based health care systems. During this process the number of beds in mental hospitals has been more or less drastically reduced and the capacities of outpatient and complementary services have been significantly increased. However, although the goals of the reform process were quite similar in all Western European countries, the current systems of mental health care still show a number of considerable differences which reflect distinct traditions in health care as well as diverse financing systems (Becker et al. 2001).

The comparison of basic figures of the mental health care systems in six selected European countries shows a large variation of the number of psychiatric beds. While in the Netherlands 187 beds per 100 000 population are provided, followed by Denmark with 151 per 100 000, there are only 17 per 10 000 in Italy. There is also a large variation as concerns the various groups of mental health professionals. Most psychiatrists and psychologists are found in Denmark, fewest in Spain. The number of psychiatric nurses is highest in UK and in the Netherlands, and again lowest in Spain. Social workers appear to be most pre-

Table 1. Psychiatric services in six European countries (Number per 100 000 population)

	N	DK	UK	E	I	D
Psychiatric beds	187	151	58	44	17	76
Psychiatrists	9	16	11	3,6	9	7,3
Neurologists	3,7	3	1	2,5	?	2,5
Psychologists	28	85	9	1,9	3	?
Psychiatric nurses	99	59	104	4,2	26	52
Social workers	176	7	58	?	2,7	?

Source: Department of Mental Health and Substance Dependence, WHO, Geneva 2002

Table 2. Financing of psychiatric services in six European countries (Figures indicate the primary sources of mental health financing in descending order)

	N	DK	UK	E	I	D
Social Insurance	1		3			1
Tax based		1	1	1	1	3
Private Insurance	3		2	3	3	2
Out of Pocket	2		4	2	2	4

Source: Department of Mental Health and Substance Dependence, WHO, Geneva 2002

valent in the Netherlands, representing the most important professional group in the mental health field in this country. The density of all mental health professionals taken together is highest in the Netherlands, followed by Denmark and UK, and lowest in Spain.

As concerns the financing of mental health care, in Germany and in the Netherlands social insurances are the primary source of money while all other countries finance their mental health care systems mainly by taxes. Modes of financing show the greatest variety in Germany and the UK, while in Denmark mental health care is exclusively financed by taxes.

It must be assumed that these differences in the provision and financing of mental health care have consequences for the quality and the costs of psychiatric treatment. However, currently only few studies have addressed this question. Recently some publications from the project "European Psychiatric Services: Inputs Linked to Outcome Domains and Needs" (EPSILON) provided comparisons of needs, costs and outcomes of schizophrenia treatment in five European countries (Becker et al. 1999; Gaite et al. 2002; Knapp et al. 2002; McCrone et al. 2001). In cooperation with the EPSILON study the project "Cost-Effectiveness Analysis of Psychiatric Health Care Systems in the European Comparison" has been carried out in Leipzig. In this paper the results from both projects will be used to address the following questions:

▶ To what extent are the differences between European mental health care systems reflected by the costs and the outcome of schizophrenia treatment?

▶ To what extent are the differences of clinical and non-clinical outcome parameters between schizophrenia patients from different European countries reflected by differences of service costs?

▶ To what extent are the costs of schizophrenia treatment in different European countries related to service needs and to the severity of illness?

▶ To what extent is the relationship between costs and outcomes of schizophrenia treatment stable over time?

Methods

The EPSILON study has been carried out in Amsterdam (N), Copenhagen (DK), London (UK), Santander (E) and Verona (I). Aims of the study were the development of European wide standardized instruments for the assessment of costs and outcomes of schizophrenia treatment and the application of these instruments in a comparative study to obtain basic data on the quality and the costs of schizophrenia treatment in Europe (Becker et al. 1999). The following instruments have been developed by the EPSILON study: The Camberwell Assessment of Need (CAN-EU) for the assessment of mental health service needs

(McCrone et al. 2001); the Client Sociodemographic Service Receipt Inventory (CSSRI-EU) for the assessment of mental health service use and the estimation of costs (Knapp et al. 2002); the Involvement Evaluation Questionnaire (IEQ-EU) for the assessment of caregiver burden (van Wijingaarden et al. 2000); the Lancashire Quality of Life Profile (LQoLP-EU) for the assessment of quality of life (Gaite et al. 2002); and the Verona Service Satisfaction Scale (VSSS-EU) for the assessment of service satisfaction (Ruggeri et al. 2000). For the comparative assessment of costs and outcomes of schizophrenia treatment these instruments were applied to samples of patients with schizophrenia (n = 404) in each of the study sites (Becker et al. 1999). To get data which are comparable to those of the EPSILON study the instruments developed by the EPSILON study were adapted for the use in German speaking countries (Bernert et al. 2001; Kilian et al. 2001a; Kilian et al. 2001b; Mory et al. 2001; Roick et al. 2001). The study sample recruited in Leipzig consists of 307 patients with the diagnosis of schizophrenia (ICD-10 F 20.0), age of 18–64 years, who were treated by psychiatric services in the city of Leipzig. Since in Germany no psychiatric case register exists the number of patients who are using psychiatric services is widely unknown. Therefore it was necessary to assess how many patients were treated for schizophrenia during the three months before the study onset by means of a survey including all psychiatric service institutions and all office based psychiatrists in the city. On the basis of this information the study participants where recruited from all outpatient clinics, all community mental health centres, all office based psychiatrists and from the psychiatric hospitals and the psychiatric day hospitals in the city of Leipzig. Participants from each type of service were consecutively recruited until the stratification of patients across services in the sample was equivalent to the stratification of the population of persons with schizophrenia who were treated in Leipzig in the three month period before the study onset. Resulting from this sampling procedure 10.75 percent of the study participants were recruited during an inpatient stay, 79.15 percent from outpatient facilities and 10.10 percent from residential homes. These figures were found to be very similar to those which were reported from a national study on the stratification of patients across services in Germany (Besthehorn et al. 1999). Participants were asked to sign a written consent before they were included in the sample.

In addition to the instruments developed in the EPSILON study, all study sites used the Brief Psychiatric Rating Scale (BPRS) for the assessment of psychopathological symptoms (Ventura et al. 1993) and the General Assessment of Functioning (GAF) for the assessment of functional disability (American Psychiatric Association 1987). Furthermore all centers used the European Service Mapping Schedule (ESMS) for a structured compilation of mental health services for adults with severe mental illness which are provided by the health services, social services, voluntary sector and private sector providers within a catchment area. The ESMS allows comparisons between catchment areas regarding the structure, range and level of provision of services (Johnson et al. 2000).

Results

The provision of mental health services

The provision of psychiatric services in the six study sites is presented in Table 3. In Copenhagen, most hospital beds are provided for people with severe mental illness, almost twice as many as in Leipzig which ranks second. Fewest beds exist in Verona and London. It is also in Copenhagen where most residential places are found, 250 per 100000 population, which is in sharp contrast to Santander where this type of setting is almost not exist-

Table 3. Provision of mental health services for people with severe mental illness in 6 European study sites (Assessed by means of the European Service Mapping Schedule ESMS)

Services	Amst.[1]	Cop.[1]	Lon.[1]	Sant.[1]	Ver.[1]	Lei.[2]
Inpatient[3]	117	279	63	89	53	147
Residential[4]	78	250	44	4	52	29
Day & Structured activity[5]	221	375	426	–	90	717
Out-patient & Community[6]	736	1259	1105	2716	558	997

[1] Becker et al. 2002; [2] Leipzig study; [3] Number of beds per 100 000 population; [4] Number of places per 100 000 population; [5] Number of users per 100 000 population per working day; [6] Number of contacts/users per 100 000 population per month

ing. Thus, there is no inverse relationship between the two, hospital beds and residential places, as one might have expected.

Most day care/structured activity providing facilities exist in Leipzig, none in Santander. By contrast, in Santander, there are by far most outpatient and community based services, more than twice as many as in Copenhagen which ranks second. The fewest exist in Verona. As regards the ratio between the rates of users of outpatient and community services and beds/places in inpatient/residential services, Santander ranks first (29.2), London second (14.3), Leipzig third (9.7), Verona fourth (6.2), Amsterdam fifth (4.4) and Copenhagen sixth (3.1).

Patient characteristics and needs for mental health services

The main characteristics of the patient samples in the different study sites are presented in Table 4.

Table 4. Characteristics of schizophrenia patient samples in six European study sites

	Amst.[1]	Cop.[1]	Lon.[1]	Sant.[1]	Ver.[1]	Lei.[2]
Age μ	39.9	39.4	43.8	39.9	43.0	43.7
95% CI	37.4–42.4	36.7–42.1	41.1–46.5	38.1–41.7	40.6–45.4	42.5–44.9
% male	67	60	58	59	49	50
% working	13	35	8	14	30	15
% living alone	49.2	65.4	41.7	7.0	15.0	39.9
Admissions μ	3.8	5.1	5.7	2.4	3.9	4.8
95% CI	2.7–4.9	3.4–6.8	4.5–6.7	1.9–2.9	2.9–4.9	4.2–5.4
Years Ill μ	14	13	17	13	13	16
95% CI	11.7–16.3	10.5–15.5	14.4–19.6	11.4–14.6	11.1–14.9	14.8–17.1
GAF μ	56.5	53.6	58.7	59.0	56.6	54.6
95% CI	53.5–59.5	49.6–57.6	56.3–61.1	55.3–62.7	53.4–59.8	52.8–56.4
BPRS μ	1.6	1.7	1.5	1.6	1.5	1.4
95% CI	1.5–1.7	1.6–1.8	1.4–1.6	1.5–1.7	1.4–1.6	1.36–1.43
N	61	52	84	100	107	306

[1] McCrone et al. 2001; [2] Kilian et al. 2001

Table 5. Needs for psychiatric services of patients with schizophrenia in six European study sites

	Amst.[1]	Cop.[1]	Lon.[1]	Sant.[1]	Ver.[1]	Lei.[2]
Number of met needs	3.8	3.6	3.9	3.2	3.6	2.9
95% CI	(3.2–4.4)	(3.0–4.2)	(3.3–4.5)	(2.8–3.6)	(3.2–4.0)	(2.7–3.0)
Number of unmet needs	2.4	0.8	2.3	1.7	1.6	1.0
95% CI	(2.0–2.8)	(0.4–1.2)	(1.9–2.7)	(1.3–2.1)	(1.2–2.0)	(0.9–1.1)
Number of total needs	6.2	4.4	6.2	4.9	5.3	3.8
95% CI	(5.6–6.8)	(3.6–5.2)	(5.6–6.8)	(4.5–5.3)	(4.7–5.9)	(3.7–4.0)
Met needs/total needs	0.61	0.82	0.63	0.65	0.68	0.76
N	61	52	84	100	107	306

[1] McCrone et al. 2001; [2] Kilian et al. 2001

The similarities between patient samples prevail. Most notable differences with regard to socio-demographic characteristics concern the living situation, with significantly fewer patients living alone in Santander and Verona, and the working situation, with the highest percentage of those having a job in Copenhagen and the lowest in London. There were no significant differences with regard to general functioning. Patients from Leipzig did show slightly fewer symptoms than those from Santander, Amsterdam and Copenhagen.

According to McCrone et al. needs are to be defined as "the requirements of individuals to enable them to achieve, maintain or restore an acceptable level of social independence or quality of life" (McCrone et al. 2001). Needs were assessed by interviewing the patient as well the case manager or another mental health expert familiar with the situation of the patient, using the CAN. Resulting from this procedure the number of needs that are met by mental health services, the number of needs that are not met by the service system and the total number of needs was assessed for each patient.

Table 5 shows the comparison of met, unmet and total service needs and the relation of met to total service needs between the six European study sites. Number of met service needs is highest in the London and lowest in Leipzig, where they are significantly lower than in Amsterdam, London and Verona. Unmet service needs are lowest in Copenhagen and highest in Amsterdam. Differences between Copenhagen and Leipzig on the one side and the other sites are significant at the five percent level. Ratios between met and unmet service needs are presented in the third row. With 0.82, they are highest in Leipzig and Copenhagen, indicating that 82% of the total needs for services are met by the existing service system. The lowest ratios of 0.61 and 0.63 are found in Amsterdam and London, which indicates that only 61% or 63%, respectively of the total service needs are met in these two study sites.

Quality of life

Table 6 shows the comparison of the specific and overall subjective quality of life between the six study sites.

General quality of life is highest in Copenhagen and lowest in London. The comparison of the confidence intervals shows that the differences between London and other sites with the exception of Verona are significant at the five percent level. Quality of life with regard to the work situation is highest in Copenhagen and lowest in Verona, which is astonishing

Table 6. Quality of life of patients with schizophrenia in six European study sites

	Amst.[1]	Cop.[1]	Lon.[1]	Sant.[1]	Ver.[1]	Lei.[2]
Average	4.80	5.11	4.35	4.73	4.63	4.79
95% CI	(4.6–5.0)	(4.8–5.3)	(4.1–4.5)	(4.6–4.9)	(4.4–4.8)	(4.7–4.9)
Work	4.32	5.29	4.25	4.07	3.73	4.85
95% CI	(3.9–4.7)	(4.8–5.7)	(3.8–4.6)	(3.7–4.3)	(3.4–4.0)	(4.5–5.2)
Leisure	4.95	5.06	4.50	4.56	4.50	4.71
95% CI	(4.6–5.2)	(4.7–5.3)	(4.2–4.7)	(4.3–4.8)	(4.3–4.7)	(4.6–4.8)
Finances	4.57	5.23	3.94	4.08	4.13	4.11
95% CI	(4.1–5.0)	(4.7–5.7)	(3.5–4.3)	(3.7–4.4)	(3.7–4.5)	(4.0–4.2)
Social	4.77	4.92	4.47	4.86	4.57	4.86
95% CI	(4.4–5.1)	(4.5–5.3)	(4.2–4.8)	(4.6–5.1)	(4.3–4.8)	(4.8–5.0)
Health	5.05	4.83	4.10	4.60	4.77	4.72
95% CI	(4.7–5.4)	(4.5–5.2)	(3.8–4.4)	(4.4–4.9)	(4.5–5.0)	(4.6–4.8)
N	61	52	84	100	107	306

[1] Gaite et al. 2002; [2] Kilian et al. 2001

since, as shown in Table 6, the patients from the Italian study site had the second highest percentage of employment. Differences between Copenhagen and the other sites, with the exception of Leipzig, are significant at the five percent level. Satisfaction with leisure activities is again highest in Copenhagen and lowest in London and in Verona. However, the differences are small and not significant. Satisfaction with the financial resources is also highest in Copenhagen and lowest in London. The same picture emerges for satisfaction with social relationships which is highest in Copenhagen and lowest in London without any of the differences being significant. Satisfaction with health is highest in Amsterdam and lowest in London. With the exception of Santander, all differences between London and the other countries are significant. Taken together, the Danish mental health care system seems to be most successful in keeping the quality of life of patients with schizophrenia at a high level while Leipzig is located in the middle field and London at the lower end of the six countries.

The costs of schizophrenia treatment

The comparison of mental health service costs in Table 7 shows that total costs are highest in Copenhagen ($\mu = 7460$ £; 95% CI = 2542 £ – 12857 £) and lowest in Santander ($\mu = 1444$ £; 95% CI = 279 £ – 2878 £). The comparison of the confidence intervals indicates that only the difference between Santander and the other sites is significant at the five percent level. With the exception of Amsterdam, the greatest proportion of money is spent in all countries for inpatient treatment. Expenditures for the several types of outpatient care (outpatient, community and day care) are highest in Amsterdam and lowest in Santander, while London and Verona build the upper and Copenhagen and Leipzig the lower part of the middle field. Significant differences occur particularly between Santander and the other countries but also between Leipzig and London for outpatient treatment, between Copenhagen and the other countries for community care, and between Amsterdam, Copenhagen and London on the one side and Santander, Verona and Leipzig on the other side for day care.

Table 7. Costs of schizophrenia treatment in six European study sites

	Amst.[1]	Cop.[1]	Lon.[1]	Sant.[1]	Ver.[1]	Lei.[2]
Inpatient care	320	5772	3659	1456	2705	1894
95% CI	(0-2614)	(1442-10588)	(1217-6753)	(129-2861)	(933-5268)	(1309-2479)
Hospital outpatient care	236	376	139	0	627	232
95% CI	(107-383)	(0-1020)	(29-177)	(0-37)	(481-771)	(218-246)
Day care	2293	774	1091	–	1650	255
95% CI	(1443-3068)	(402-1432)	(415-1879)	90	(738-2589)	(118-392)
Community based care	551	241	1086	(0-195)	459	959
95% CI	(211-947)	(1-478)	(722-1520)	–	(130-876)	(800-1118)
Residential care	764	130	749	1444	298	1158
95% CI	(510-1092)	(0-446)	(372-1276)	(279-2878)	(30-642)	(677-1639)
Total	4112	7460	6771	1456	5730	4489
95% CI	(2063-6452)	(2542-12857)	(4231-10155)	(129-2861)	(3703-8160)	(3667-5330)
N	61	5772	84	100	107	306

[1] Knapp et al. 2002; [2] Kilian et al. 2001

Cost-effectiveness of schizophrenia treatment

As stated above, the main criterion of the effectiveness of mental health services for people in a chronic state of illness is clinical stability at a high level of quality of life. As a necessary precondition mental health service provision must be primarily oriented on the needs of the patients. Therefore, the relationship of met to unmet needs is a further main indicator of service effectiveness. Since stability cannot be assessed in a cross-sectional comparison only quality of life and the relation between met and unmet needs are considered in the following. To take socio-demographic or clinical status differences of patients into account means of costs, quality of life and service needs will be adjusted for age, gender, living situation, job status, number of admissions, psychopathology (BPRS), general functioning (GAF), and alcohol abuse.

In order to get cost-effectiveness ratios the summed rank of the mean quality of life score and of the met needs to total needs ratio were divided by the rank of the total costs. Putting the information of the comparison of effectiveness and costs together into a relation of the ranks of effectiveness and the ranks of costs, it can be seen in Table 8 that the best cost-effectiveness rank ratio of 6 is found for Santander, followed by Amsterdam and Leipzig with a ratio of 3, Copenhagen with a ratio of 2, Verona with a ratio of 1.5 and London with a ratio of 0.6.

Table 8. Ratio between ranks of effectiveness and rank of costs of schizophrenia treatment for six European study sites

	Amst.	Cop.	Lon.	Sant.	Ver.	Lei.
Met needs/total needs	1	6	2	3	4	5
Quality of life	5	6	1	3	2	4
Total costs	2	6	5	1	4	3
1+2/3	3	2	0.6	6	1.5	3

Beyond the comparison of costs and outcomes the relations between costs, clinical parameters and service needs is regarded as a further indicator of cost-effectiveness because "...*the relationship between service needs and costs is an indication of the responsiveness of care resources and agencies to the health and social welfare needs of clients*" (Knapp et al. 1990). So it will be expected from an effective service system that service costs are positively related to severity of illness and met service needs, and negatively or not related to unmet service needs.

For the comparison of the relations between service needs and costs linear regression models with total service costs as dependent variable were computed for each study site. Due to the highly skewed distribution of total service costs the dependent variable must either be transformed or non-parametric standard errors must be computed which are robust against non-normality and heteroscedasticity of the residuals. Since regression coefficients are easier to interpret and in order to permit cost predictions in the original metric we decided to compute a linear model with the untransformed cost variable and to assess standard errors and 95% confidence intervals by bootstrapping with 2000 replications. A comparison of the regression parameters in Table 9 shows only few significant effects and not all of them are in the expected direction. Only in Spain and in Germany, the number of previous hospital admissions, which serves as a criterion of severity of illness, is positively related to total service costs. The other criterion of severity, symptoms measured by the BPRS, is positively related to costs only in Amsterdam and in Leipzig. Met service need are positively related to costs in London and Leipzig. In Santander and Verona unmet service costs are positively related to costs which indicates that costs increase with the number of unmet needs. A comparison of the adjusted R^2 values indicates that the propor-

Table 9. Linear regression models for the impact of clinical and social variables on the costs of schizophrenia care in six European study sites (unstandardized regression coefficients, bold figures are significant at $p < 0.05$)

	Amst.[1]	Cop.[1]	Lon.[1]	Sant.[1]	Ver.[1]	Lei.[2]
Age (years)	−150	503	66	−169	−12	−70
Education (years)	−9.5	596	−390	−144	−574	23
Gender (1 = male)	−2248	−21948	2993	828	1972	−855
Marital Status (1 = married/other)	−1420	182	−2026	1604	−4043	−1817
Ethnicity (1 = not European national)	−3431	−2204	584	–	–	–
Language (1 = non-national)	1383	24509	−6446	–	–	–
Living situation (1 = with others)	1692	15940	9595	1130	−7649	2271
Employment (1 = not employed)	4642	3635	2579	−1207	−263	−164
Admissions (n)	123	−445	115	880	201	533
GAF	89	−514	−118	−3.9	97	43
BPRS	7339	−4702	−1775	39	−2244	5927
CAN-EU met	−237	616	2488	−467	917	997
CAN-EU unmet	−1004	−1395	−604	914	2037	337
LQoLP-EU	−1167	4974	−5178	807	603	123
VSSS-EU	−2199	−14826	−4077	−2385	−745	−585
Const.	8182	55723	35731	11622	9336	7007
Adj. R2	0.167	0.101	0.342	0.179	0.125	0.380
N	57	43	80	100	93	220

[1] Knapp et al. 2002, [2] Kilian et al. 2001

tion of explained cost variance is highest in Leipzig ($R^2 = 0.38$) and in London ($R^2 = 0.34$) and lowest in Copenhagen ($R^2 = 0.10$).

The longitudinal analysis of mental health service costs

For the assessment of the stability of the relationships between costs and service needs a random-effect regression model for three points of measurement covering a 1.5 year period has been computed. The random effect-model provides estimations of the combined within and between effects taking into account the incompleteness of the panel data. Within effects are the effects of the intra-personal transitory changes of the independent variables on the intra-personal transitory changes of the dependent variable. Between effects are the effects of the time invariant inter-personal differences of the independent variables on the time-invariant interpersonal differences of the dependent variable. The random effect model provides the proportion of variance explained by the transitory changes (R^2 within) and the proportion of variance explained by the time-invariant interpersonal differences (R^2 between) and the proportion of variance explained by both effects (R^2 overall).

Due to the skewness of the distribution of the dependent variable standard errors and 95% confidence intervals of the regression coefficients were assessed by means of bootstrapping with 2000 replications. The results of the random-effect model are presented in Table 10. The regression coefficients indicate that the 1.5 year total costs of mental health care are positively related to symptoms, to met service needs, and to the number of previous hospital admissions. Furthermore costs are higher for patients who live with others

Table 10. Random effect regression model for the longitudinal analysis of the impact of clinical and social variables on the costs of schizophrenia care in Leipzig

	b	se[1]	95% CI[1]	
Age (years)	−92.68	36.22	−141.44	3.44
Education (years)	−209.85	232.39	−652.54	270.70
Gender (1 = male)	190.18	673.76	−1137.39	1557.20
Marital status (1 = married/other)	−3122.30	1024.51	−5719.72	−1569.27
Living situation (1 = with others)	2697.03	1171.63	865.58	5266.19
Employment (1 = not employed)	−1622.50	1184.25	−3698.19	971.26
Admissions (n)	303.23	113.44	22.91	454.83
GAF	−39.76	44.76	−114.29	61.75
BPRS	5623.50	1768.59	1576.01	7894.31
CAN-EU met	666.42	223.73	575.43	976.09
CAN-EU unmet	−16.88	317.78	−628.61	626.96
LQoLP-EU	130.25	274.86	−401.17	659.15
VSSS-EU	−848.35	635.05	−2364.77	142.21
Constant	4932.51	5092.33	−5048.27	14913.29

R^2 within = 0.039
R^2 between = 0.311
R^2 overall = 0.223
N = 268

[1] se and 95% CI estimated by nonparametric bootstrapping with 2000 replications

in comparison to patients who live alone, and married patients cause lower costs than singles.

The parameters for the model fit show that four percent (R^2 within = 0.039) of the intra-personal cost variance over time is explained by intra-personal transitory changes but 31 percent (R^2 between = 0.311) of the interpersonal time invariant cost variance is explained by time-invariant differences between the patients. The proportion of the total (intra- and inter-personal) cost variance explained by the independent variables is 22 percent (R^2 overall = 0.223).

Discussion

What does the comparison of outcome and costs mean with regard to cost-effectiveness? Due to the limitations of the study and the complexity of the subject the answer must be preliminary. At the one hand patients at the Danish study site seem to receive the most effective mental health service at the highest costs. On the other hand at the Spanish study site expenditures are very low but patients show a medium level relation between met and unmet needs and a medium level of quality of life. By contrast at the UK study site service expenditures are nearly as high as in Denmark but patients show the worst relation between met and unmet needs and the lowest level of quality of life on four out of six domains. Germany shows a high level relation of met to unmet needs and a mean level of quality of life while the treatment expenditures are at a mean level. Italy shows a mean level met to unmet needs relation, a mean level of quality of life, and costs are also at a mean level. The Netherlands show a low met to unmet needs relation, but the second best profile of quality of life values while expenditures are at the second lowest. Taking together the ranks of effectiveness and the ranks of costs, the best relation is found in Spain and the worst in the UK. Germany is located in the middle between these two extremes.

Looking at the relations between service needs and costs it becomes obvious that the expected positive relations between symptoms and costs was found only in Germany and in the Netherlands and the expected positive relation between met needs and costs was found only in Germany and the UK. On the other hand, positive relation between unmet service needs and costs were found in Spain and in Italy. While positive effects of met service needs and symptoms on costs indicate that the allocation of resources is responsive to the needs of the patients the positive effect of unmet needs on costs signalizes that the resource allocation is not need oriented. For Leipzig the need orientation of the resource allocation was found to be stable over time.

Conclusion

Currently, the empirical basis for comparative cost-effectiveness analysis of mental health services in the European context is small. The presented results of existing studies are in great part preliminary and explorative. Further studies with adequate case numbers and longitudinal study designs are necessary to make cost-effectiveness analysis useful for the estimation of the economic consequences of different service options.

References

American Psychiatric Association (1987) Diagnostic and statistical manual of mental disorders (DSM-III-R). 3 edn, APA, Washington DC.

Becker T, Vázques-Barquero JL (2001) The European perspective of psychiatric reform. Acta Psychiatr Scand 104 (suppl. 410):8–14.

Becker T, Knapp M, Knudsen HC, Schene A, Tansella M, Thornicroft G, Vázquez-Barquero JL (1999) The EPSILON study of schizophrenia in five European countries. Design and methodology for standardising outcome measures and comparing patterns of care and service costs. Br J Psychiatry 175:514–521.

Bernert S, Kilian R, Matschinger H, Mory C, Roick C, Angermeyer MC (2001) Die Erfassung der Belastung der Angehörigen psychisch erkrankter Menschen: Die deutsche Version des Involvement Evaluation Questionnaire (IEQ-EU). (The assessment of burden on relatives of mentally ill people.) Psychiat Prax 28 (Sonderheft 2):S97–S101.

Besthehorn M, Tischer B, Glaser P, Mast O, Schmidt D (1999) Representative study on the distribution of schizophrenia patients to medical health care institutions in Germany. Fortschr Neurol Psychiatr 67:487–492.

Chan S, Mackenzie A, Jacobs P (2000) Cost-effectiveness analysis of case management versus a routine community care organization for patients with chronic schizophrenia. Arch Psychiatr Nur 2000:98–104.

Chisholm D, Knapp M, Knudsen HC, Amaddeo F, Gaite L, van Wijngaarden B, and the EPSILON Study Group (2000) Client Sociodemographic and Service Receipt Inventory-European Version. Br J Psychiatry 177 (suppl. 39):S28–S33.

Clark RE, Teague GB, Ricketts SK, Bush PW, Xie H, McGuire T, Drake RE, McHugo GJ, Keller AM, Zubkoff M (1998) Cost-effectiveness of assertive community treatment versus standard case management for persons with co-occuring severe mental illness and substance use disorder. Health Serv Res 33:1285–1308.

Creed F, Mbaya P, Lancashire S, Tomenson B, Williams B, Holme S (1997) Cost-effectiveness of day and inpatient psychiatric treatment: Results of a randomised controlled trial. Br Med J 314.

Dixon L, Hoch JS, Clark R, Bebout R, Drake R, McHugo G, Becker D (2002) Cost-effectiveness of two vocational rehabilitation programs for persons with severe mental illness. Psychiatr Serv 53:1118–1124.

Essock SM, Frisman LK, Covell NH, Hargreaves WA (2000) Cost-effectiveness of clozapine compared with conventional antipsychotic medication for patients in state hospitals. Arch Gen Psychiatr 57:987–994.

Ford R, Raftery J, Ryan P, Beadsmoore A, Craig T, Muijen M (1997) Intensive case management for people with serious mental illness – Site 2: Cost-effectiveness. J Ment Health 6:191–199.

Gaite L, Vázques-Barquero JL, Borra C, Ballesteros J, Schene A, Welcher B, Thornicroft G, Becker T, Ruggeri M, Herrán A, the EPSILON Study Group (2002) Quality of life in patients with schizophrenia in five European countries: the EPSILON study. Acta Psychiatr Scand 105:283–292.

Häfner H, an der Heiden W (1991) Evaluating effectiveness and cost of community care for schizophrenic patients. Schizophr Bull 17:441–451.

John J, Wismar M, Geraedts M (2001) Aktuelle Forschungsperspektiven von Gesundheitssystemforschung und Gesundheitsökonomie in Deutschland. (Current research perspectives of health systems research and health economics in Germany.) Gesundheitswesen 63 (Sonderheft 1):S73–S78.

Johnson S, Kuhlman R (2000) The European Service Mapping Schedule (ESMS): Development of an instrument for the description and classification of mental health services. Acta Psychiatr Scand s405:s14–s23.

Kilian R, Bernert S, Matschinger H, Mory C, Angermeyer MC (2001a) Die standardisierte Erfassung des Behandlungs- und Unterstützungsbedarfs bei schweren psychischen Erkrankungen (The standardized assessment of the need for treatment in severe mental illness). Psychiat Prax 28 (Sonderheft 2):S79–S83.

Kilian R, Roick C, Bernert S, Matschinger H, Mory C, Becker T, Angermeyer MC (2001b) Instrumente zur gesundheitsökonomischen Evaluation psychiatrischer Versorgungssysteme: Methodische Grundlagen der europäischen Standardisierung und der deutschsprachigen Adaptation. (Instruments for the economical evaluation of psychiatric service systems.) Psychiat Prax 28 (Sonderheft 2):S74–S78.

Knapp M (2000) Schizophrenia cost and treatment cost-effectiveness. Acta Psychiatr Scand 102 (suppl. 407):15–18.

Knapp M, Beecham J (1990) Costing mental health services. Psychol Med 20:893–908.

Knapp M, Chisholm D, Leese M, Amaddeo F, Tansella M, Schene A, Vázques-Barquero JL, Knudsen HC, Becker T, and the EPSILON Study Group (2002) Comparing pattern and costs of schizophrenia care in five European countries: The EPSILON study. Acta Psychiatr Scand 105:42–54.

Knapp M, Marks I, Wolstenholme J, Beecham J, Astin J, Audini B, Connolly J, Watts V (1998) Home based versus hospital-based care for serious mental illness. Controlled cost-effectiveness study over four years. Brit J Psychiatry 172:506–512.

Lave JR, Frank RG, Schulberg HC, Kamlet MS (1998) Cost-effectiveness of treatments for major depression in primary care practice. Arch Gen Psychiatr 55:645–651.

McCrone P, Leese M, Thornicroft G, Schene A, Knudsen HC, Vázques-Barquero JL, Tansella M, Becker T, Chisholm D, for the EPSILON Study Group (2001) A comparison of needs of patients with schizophrenia in five European countries: the EPSILON Study. Acta Psychiatr Scand 103:370–379.

Mory C, Matschinger H, Roick C, Kilian R, Bernert S, Angermeyer MC (2001) Die deutsche Version der Verona Service Satisfaction Scale (VSSS-EU). (The German adaptation of the Verona Service Satisfaction Scale.) Psychiat Prax 28 (Sonderheft 2):S91–S96.

Reinharz D, Lesage AD, Contandriopoulos AP (2000) Cost-effectiveness analysis of psychiatric deinstitutionalization. Can J Psychiatry 45:533–538.

Roick C, Kilian R, Matschinger H, Bernert S, Mory C, Angermeyer MC (2001) Die deutsche Version des Client Sociodemographic Service Receipt Inventory (CSSRI-EU). (German adaptation of the Client Sociodemographic and Service Receipt Inventory.) Psychiat Prax 28 (Sonderheft 2):S84–S90.

Rosenheck R, Cramer J, Xu W, Grabowski J, Douyton R, Thomas J, Henderson W, Charney D (1998) Multiple outcome assessment in a study of the cost-effectiveness of clozapine in the treatment of refractory schizophrenia. Health Serv Res 33:1237–1261.

Ruggeri M, Lasalvia A, Dail'Agnola R, van Wijingaarden B, Knudsen HC, Leese M, Gaite L, Tansella M (2000) Development, internal consistency and reliability of the European Version of the Verona Service Satisfaction Scale. Br J Psychiatry 177(suppl 39):S41–S48.

Salize HJ, Rössler W (1996) The cost of comprehensive care of people with schizophrenia living in the community. A cost evaluation from a German catchment area. Br J Psychiatry 169:42–48.

Seshamani M (2002) Is clozapine cost-effective. Unanswered issues. Eur J Health Econ 3:S104–S113.

UK700 Group (2000) Cost-effectiveness of intensive v. standard case management for severe psychotic illness. UK700 case management trial. Br J Psychiatry 176:537–543.

van Wijingaarden B, Schene AH, Koeter MWJ, Vázques-Barquero JL, Knudsen HC, Lasalvia A, McCrone P (2000) Caregiving in schizophrenia: Development, internal consistency and reliability of the Involvement Evaluation Questionnaire – European Version. Br J Psychiatry 177(suppl 39):S21–S27.

Ventura J, Green MF, Shaner A, Lieberman RP (1993) Training and quality assurance with the Brief Psychiatric Rating Scale: The drift busters. Int J Meth Psychiatr Res 3:221–244.

Wasem J, Hessel F, Kerim-Sade C (2001) Methoden zur vergleichenden ökonomischen Evaluation von Therapien und zur rationalen Ressourcenallokation über Bereiche des Gesundheitswesens hinweg. Einführung, Vorteile, Risiken. (Methods of comparative economic evaluations of therapies and for rational allocation of ressources across sectors of healthcare systems. Introduction, advantages, risks.) Psychiat Prax 28 (Sonderheft 1):S12–S20.

Hypertension and diabetes care among primary care doctors in Germany: results from an epidemiological cross-sectional study

DAVID PITTROW · WILHELM KIRCH · HANS-ULRICH WITTCHEN
for the Hydra Study Group*

Introduction

Significance of hypertension and diabetes

In the industrialized countries, both arterial hypertension and diabetes mellitus are highly prevalent disorders that lead to a high incidence of cardiovascular disease, cutting across all ethnic, racial and gender groups (Benjamin 2002). This in turn is the leading cause of death and disability, and outnumbers deaths from all sorts of cancers combined (AHA 2001). Consequently, hypertension and diabetes are among the most valuable targets of health care activities. This is particularly important for diabetic patients, whose main problems are macrovascular and not primarily microvascular complications. For example, in the United Kingdom Prospective Diabetes Study (UKPDS) fatal cardiovascular events were 70 times more frequent than fatal microvascular complications (Turner 1996). An analysis from the Tecumseh study estimated that the elimination of the cardiovascular risk from diabetes in just 60% of the affected population – an achievable goal – would reduce the 8-year predicted incidence of coronary heart disease as much as would the combined elimination of hypertension, hypercholesterolemia, and smoking in the diabetic populations (Smith 1996). In other words, the risk factor diabetes itself is of much greater importance than the other factors mentioned.

Epidemiology of hypertension and diabetes

Nonetheless, the situation for both diseases remains suboptimal: As for hypertension, over decades the high prevalence has been confirmed in numerous epidemological studies around the world with prevalence estimates of up to 27 per cent in adults (Hyman 2001). There is unequivocal evidence that a substantial proportion of patients with hypertension remain unrecognized, poorly treated, and uncontrolled in the industrialized nations (Burt 1995; Mancia 1997; Colhoun 1998; Thamm 1999; Joffres 2001). The picture is very similar for diabetes: type 2 diabetes has become epidemic in the past few decades owing to the advancing age of the population, a substantially increased prevalence of obesity, and de-

---

* The authors wrote on behalf of the HYDRA study group. HU Wittchen is the principal investigator of the HYDRA study, Peter Bramlage, Petra Krause, Michael Höfler, Hildegard Pfister, and Beate Küpper are members of the study group. The following experts serve as additional scientific consultants on various aspects of the project: Hendrik Lehnert, Magdeburg; Burkhard Göke, Munich; Eberhard Ritz, Heidelberg; Diethelm Tschöpe, Bad Oeynhausen; Arya M. Sharma, Hamilton/Canada. HYDRA is supported by an unrestricted educational grant from Sanofi-Synthelabo, Berlin.

reased physical activity, all of which have been attributed to a Western lifestyle (Nathan 2002). It is estimated that situation will even substantially deteriorate, with an estimated doubling in incidence of diabetes in the next 10 years (Amos 1997).

Not surprisingly therefore, improved recognition, diagnosis, and treatment of hypertension ranks among the most common clinical responsibilities of the primary health care system. Numerous national and international initiatives and programs have been launched to increase awareness and rates of detection, treatment and effective control of high blood pressure and diabetes in the population (Bodenheimer 1999, WHO 1999).

Outdated data

Unfortunately, most of the recent major reports on the prevalence and management of hypertension and diabetes are based on data collected over half a decade ago. Thus, the reports on the 3rd US National Health and Nutrition Examination Survey (NHANES III) (Burt 1995, Hyman 2001) or the Health Survey for England (Colhoun 1998), although published recently, are based on outdated data collected between 1991 and 1995. More recent surveys such as the assessment of self-reported hypertension treatment practices among primary care physicians in the US are often compromised by low response rates of the order of a third of all addressees (Hyman 2000). Data on the prevalence and treatment modalities of diabetes are also sparse, particularly in primary care (Thefeld 1999; Newnham 2002).

Improvement of therapy

Recent years have seen a number of important new data stemming from randomized, multicenter trials, which have resulted in substantial modification of international and national hypertension or diabetes guidelines regarding blood pressure targets and management issues in subgroups such as patients with diabetes, systolic hypertension, or the elderly (JNC-VI 1997, WHO-ISH 1999, DDG 2002). Furthermore, new classes of antihypertensive medications such as angiotensin receptor blockers have recently been introduced into therapy, while the role of older agents such as fast-acting calcium antagonists or a-adrenergic blockers has been reassessed (JNC-VI 1997, WHO-ISH 1999, German Hypertension League 2002). Numerous intervention studies have proved the protective effect of antihypertensive therapy (Neal 2000; ALLHAT Officers 2002) and antidiabetic therapy (UKPDS 1998; Turner 1996; DCCT 1993). New treatment concepts such as first-line combination therapy (JNC-VI 1997) or intensified multi-drug treatment in the Hypertension Optimal Treatment Study (Hansson 1998) have been explored in order to improve response rates. Several new drug classes (glitazones, glinidines) or new insulins have been added to the therapeutic arsenal for diabetes, and improved integrated treatment concepts have been reported to substantially improve outcomes (Gaede 2003).

Rationale for the study

Hypertension and diabetes as highly prevalent diseases are among the most common reasons for seeing primary care physicians. They serve as a barometer for the effectiveness of public health education, professional education, and health care effectiveness (Hyman 2001). Therefore, current reliable data derived from the primary care sector are a prerequisite for designing appropriate interventions.

In the light of the potentially significant beneficial effects of more aggressive and early treatment of hypertension or diabetes on the further development and course of complications as well as the overall costs of health care, efforts to improve recognition and management of the diseases must be based on a thorough understanding of the characteristics of the patient, the doctors and the system that contribute to poor control. Such studies should focus primarily on the primary care system as the central gatekeeper for hypertension management. This prompted us to initiate a nationally representative epidemiological study on "Hypertension and Diabetes Screening and Awareness" (HYDRA) to assess the prevalence as well as characteristics, comorbidities and management issues in patients with hypertension and diabetes in primary care.

In this chapter we present the background, design and methods of the HYDRA study; report results on the prevalence of hypertension, diabetes, their co-existence (comorbidity), as well as concomitant diseases, based on doctors' diagnoses; and report on the prevalence of microalbuminuria as a marker for early cardiovascular diseases in the sample population.

Study design

HYDRA is a cross-sectional point prevalence study of primary care attendees recruited from a representative nationwide sample of primary care practices in Germany. Primary aims of the study were: (1) to investigate the prevalence of hypertension, diabetes mellitus, and their comorbid presentation, (2) to identify the proportion and characteristics of high-risk patients, (3) to evaluate met and unmet needs for pharmacological and non-drug interventions, and (4) to identify characteristics and predictors of patients with poor hypertension and diabetes care.

HYDRA is based on a two-step epidemiological design (Fig. 1). In step one, we carried out a nation-wide recruitment of primary care practices, in which participating doctors completed a prestudy questionnaire regarding personal and structural characteristics of each practice and to assess self-perceived qualifications and attitudes related to recognition, diagnosis, and care of patients with hypertension and diabetes. The second step consisted of a target day assessment (half-day) of all patients attending the doctor's office on this day. All attending patients filled out a self-report patient questionnaire, and this was followed by a structured doctor's clinical appraisal, including documentation of lab test findings from the charts, blood pressure measurements, and assessment of microalbuminuria and urine glucose in spot samples.

Sampling of primary care doctors

HYDRA is based on a nation-wide sample of doctors with primary care functions (medical practitioners, generalists, general internists). Sampling was based on 1060 regional segments (according to the criteria of the Institute for Medical Statistics, Frankfurt am Main, Germany), clustered into geographical areas for which primary care doctor addresses were available. A total of 302 study monitors was responsible for recruiting the doctors into the study. Each monitor received a list of 24 randomly chosen doctors from the assigned region and was asked to recruit up to eight doctors (primary list), strictly following the order on the list. In the event of unwillingness of the doctor to participate, or because of impracticability, the monitor was instructed to proceed with subsequent addresses from the sampling list (supplementary list). All participating doctors signed the study enrolment

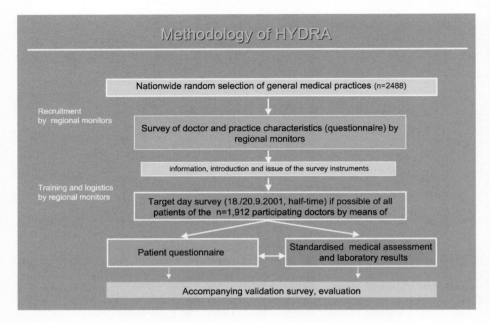

Fig. 1. Two step epidemiological design of HYDRA

form, and were offered remuneration of 15 DM (about 7.50 Euro) for each patient documented in the main study. Upon recruitment, all participating doctors also completed the pre-study doctor's questionnaire.

Participating doctors were trained by the study monitors regarding the study procedures and were instructed to screen all patients presenting in their practice on the forenoon of either the 18th or 20th September 2001, using the study instruments. The protocol specifically demanded inclusion of all attendees and prohibited any systematic choice of patients except for the following exclusion criteria: age below 16 years, acute medical condition making the screening procedure unacceptable on ethical grounds, dementia or other cognitive or sensory deficits that would make it unlikely that the self-reported measures could be completed or would provide meaningful information. Monitors also cautioned doctors to neither change their routine practice behaviour nor to selectively invite patients for participation on the target day, so as to provide a typical picture of their everyday practice and to avoid major selection effects.

Study participation of doctors

Out of a maximum total of 2416 primary care physicians, 1912 doctors were successfully recruited. This constitutes a conditional response rate of 79% (upper-bound estimate). Due to unwillingness of the primary doctor of choice to participate in the survey, 580 of the total of 1912 recruited doctors were sampled from the supplementary list, resulting in a lower-bound estimate for the response rate of 64%. Overall, this constitutes an acceptable response rate for a national sample. Reasons for non-participation included lack of time (23%), unavailability due to vacation (20%), lack of interest (11%), unspecified (35%) or other (11%). Based on the findings of the pre-study questionnaire, the study sample of doctors can be regarded as nationally representative in terms of regional distribution, age, years of experience, specialty orientation, and patient load per day.

Instruments

The prestudy questionnaire consisted of a self-report questionnaire asking for the qualification and specialization level of the doctor, number of patients seen per day, their most frequent disorders, doctor's most frequent diagnostic, drug and non-drug interventions (by type of disorder), and referral patterns. Further, attitudes towards the treatment and management of hypertension, diabetes, and associated illnesses, doctors' attitude towards guidelines and disease management programs, and perceived barriers to improved care were assessed. These variables were primarily intended for use as predictors in (future) secondary analyses.

The patient questionnaire consisted of three parts: In part I was assessed biosocial characteristics, service utilization, disability and quality of life measures. Part II assessed life-style and behavioural risk factors and current health status, self-reported illnesses, and past and current treatments. Part III, completed only if the patient had ever been diagnosed for hypertension or diabetes or was believed to have either condition, assessed age at first diagnoses and first treatment, as well as type of past and current treatments of hypertension and diabetes and their effects. In adition, most frequent problems with regard to health care providers and treatment and unmet needs were assessed, and knowledge about hypertension and diabetes and appropriate control measures and values ascertained.

The doctor's clinical appraisal asked for rating of the current presence of hypertension and diabetes as well as for 22 other specific somatic and mental disorders. All disorders were rated by severity using the Clinical Global Impression Scale (CGI; NIMH 1976). All past and current diagnostic measures for each patient were recorded in addition to the standardized measures required by the protocol (last recorded blood pressure values, total cholesterol, HDL and LDL cholesterol, serum creatinine, triglycerides, fasting blood glucose, HbA1c). Emphasis was further placed upon patient-specific evaluation of the degree to which the doctor believed that the current diabetes and/or hypertension was controlled, his drug and non-drug interventions (past and current) and his typical profile of problems in managing the patient.

Blood pressure and laboratory measures

Systolic and diastolic blood pressure was measured by indirect cuff sphygmomanometry after a 10-minute rest in sitting position in analogy to the American Society of Hypertension recommendations. A spot urine sample was tested for glucose and microalbuminuria. For the detection of microalbuminuria, the semi-quantitative dipstick Micral-Test II (Roche Diagnostics GmbH, Mannheim, Germany) was used. This test shows sensitivity down to 20 mg/L of albumin. Compared to Radio Immuno Assay (RIA) as the reference in random samples, the sensitivity of the Micral-Test II is 93% and the specifity 94%. It is important to note that this test was performed only once. For confirmation of the diagnosis microalbuminuria, it is required by standard guidelines that the test be positive on three different occasions (DDG 2002). However, a single test has, despite physiologic day-to-day variations in albuminuria, high diagnostic accuracy (Vestbo 1995, Zelmanovitz 1997). Urine glucose was measured semi-quantitatively with a reagent strip test (Combur-

E 9, Roche Diagnostics, Germany). HbA1c and selected other values (cholesterol, fasting blood glucose, etc.) were taken from the patients' charts.

Diagnostic conventions

In general, diagnostic findings reported here rely on the doctor's clinical diagnoses as reported and coded in the clinical appraisal form. More detailed analyses on selected topics also include the comparisons between clinical diagnoses and the results of blood pressure measurements (or laboratory evaluations), and information given by patients (Sharma 2003).

Statistical analyses

Prevalence estimates derived from the study are based on total assessment of all unselected consecutive primary care attendees of participating doctors during the relevant time period of the study assessment day and are thus point prevalence estimates. Descriptive statistics were used to compare the distributions of variables among all categories. Cross tables, frequency distributions and descriptive statistics were used to compare the distributions of variables among all categories. All analyses were conducted with the Stata 7 software package.

Results

Study Participation

On the two predetermined half-day recruitment periods, an estimated total of 66 920 patients attended the participating practices (mean number of patients per doctor: 35). Because of logistical problems resulting from high patient load, 53% of participating doctors were unable to successfully screen all eligible patients. Thus, only a total of 51,905 questionnaires were distributed to patients attending the clinic, of which 6,780 were excluded from further analyses, leaving a total numer of 45 125 patients (conditional response rate 87%) for the subsequent analyses. The following reasons led to exclusion of a submitted questionnaire: 2986 (5.8%) refusal or withdrawal of consent, 387 (0.8%) lack of basic demographic or psychosocial information (age and gender), 224 (0.5%) did not meet the minimum age criterion, 2179 (2.2%) stopped completing the questionnaire after the basic questions (sociodemographical characteristics, reasons for consulting etc.), and 1004 (2.2%) had no or largely incomplete doctor's clinical appraisal.

Diagnostic spectrum in primary care

On the study target day physicians were requested to rate all patients as to the presence of 24 common, predefined concomitant diseases. In contrast to many other studies, the focus was not just on pre-eminent diseases in connection with the main diagnosis, but on all syndromes and diagnoses applicable for the individual patient. In Figure 2a, the first 20 diagnoses are listed, and the remainder category *other* (frequency: 16.9%) has been left

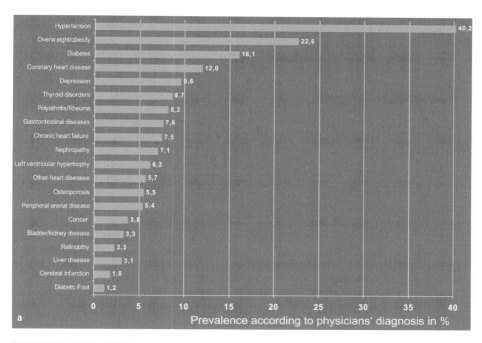

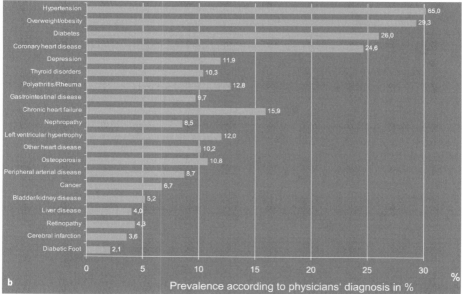

Fig. 2 a, b. Diagnostic spectrum of hypertension, diabetes, and further diseases that were explicitly listed on the physician's questionnaire. Top: All patients. Bottom: Patients over 60 years

out. The figure shows that the clinical diagnosis *hypertension* is by far the most common (40.2%), followed by *overweight/obesity* (22.6%), *diabetes mellitus* (16.1%), *coronary heart disease*, and *depresion* (9.6%). It is important to note that cardiac diseases (*chronic heart failure, left ventriular hypertrophy, other heart diseases*) account for over 30%. Figure 2b shows that the elderly patients (i.e., over 65 years) overproportionally contribute to the high prevalence rates. Almost all diseases were diagnosed twice as frequently in the elderly. The ranking of diseases remains unchanged at least for the 4 most common diseases. The frequency of hypertension is remarkably high in this age category (65.0%), as is the frequency of diabetes (26.0%). The steep increase in the prevalences occurs in almost all diseases. The prevalence for hypertension, for example, is relatively low (albeit remarkable) in patients below 30 years (3–9%), moderate in the 30- to 50-year-olds (10–32%), while very high in the elderly. The distribution pattern is similar among patients with diabetes: frequency rates are very low in patients below 45 years, while they drastically inrease to over 30% in patients over 65 years. The low rates in the young patient group give rise to the suspicion that a substantial number of those cases are not recognized.

Prevalence rates of hypertension and diabetes

According to the diagnosis of physicians (clinical global impression [CGI] at least 'mild'), rates of hypertension were 38.8%. Even in young patients (30–44 years), rates were considerable (13.3%), and steeply increased in elderly patients (60–74 years: 61.1%). This makes hypertension the most frequent condition seen in primary care. Point prevalence of diabetes was 18% in males and 14% in females (30 and 26% respectively among those aged over 60 years). Further details are displayed in a later section of this chapter (see East vs. West).

Multimorbidity is the rule

In the present sample, the very high rate of co-existing diseases (i.e., comorbidity) is striking. Among all patients, 2.8 additional diagnoses were given; in the over 60-year-old patients, as many as 4.2 diagnoses. Because of their high frequency as the primary diagnosis, both hypertension and diabetes, naturally contribute substantially to this comorbidity. For example, according to the physicians' ratings, almost two thirds of all diabetics suffer from hypertension. Figure 3 shows the frequency of associated and concomitant diseases in individuals without the diagnosis hypertension or diabetes, in comparison to those with hypertension or diabetes alone, or both diagnoses concomitantly. It is striking that in the first group the number of comorbidities is very low, but increases steeply in the latter groups.

For example, the proportion of patients with 2–3 additional diagnoses doubles when hypertension and/or diabetes are present. Even more important, in patients with both hypertension and diabetes the extent of multimorbidity is much more severe than in the other groups. Every fifth patient with hypertension and every fifth patient with diabetes have more than four additional diagnoses, whereas the respective rate in patients with both hypertension and diabetes is almost 40%.

This means that substantial multimorbidity is the rule, not the exception, in the primary care setting. In comparison to individuals without diabetes and hypertension (controls), there are multiple risk elevations (adjusted for age and gender) especially for atherosclerotic diseases such as left ventricular hypertrophy, particularly in the high risk con-

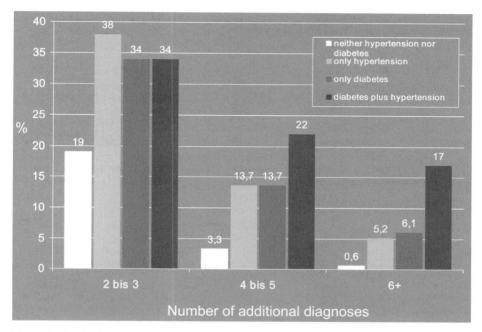

Fig. 3. Number of additional diagnoses assigned by physicians to patients with neither hypertension nor diabetes, hypertension or diabetes alone, or both diseases concomitantly. For details, refer to text

stellation of diabetes with hypertension (controls: 0.8%, hypertension: 14%, diabetes: 5.6%, diabetes and hypertension: 22.6%; odds ratios [OR] range: 3.5–15.6), coronary heart disease (controls: 4.2%, hypertension: 22.1%, diabetes: 17.9%, diabetes and hypertension: 36.9%; OR range: 2.0–4.9) and cardiac heart failure (controls: 2.4%, hypertension 13.9%, diabetes: 11.8%, diabetes and hypertension: 24.3%; OR range: 1.6–2.9); peripheral arterial disease (controls: 1.5%, hypertension 6.6%, diabetes: 8.6%, diabetes and hypertension: 16.7%; OR range: 2.1–5.2) und stroke (controls: 0.7%, hypertension 3.5%, diabetes: 3.0%, diabetes and hypertension: 5.1%; OR range: 2.2–5.1) As typical diabetes-associated and concomitant diseases there are the diabetic feet (9.6%), retinopathy (15.4%), neuropathy (22.0%), obesity (51.2%), amputations (1.3%) as well as nephropathy (12.5%).

The true prevalence of hypertension, diabetes and concomitant diseases has most likely been underestimated

It is likely that the physicians' ratings on many diseases are rather conservative estimates, as obviously a substantial number of diagnoses were either not given or were misclassified, as can be derived from the comparison of laboratory parameters or the results of other tests with the diagnoses assigned to patients.

The diagnosis 'nephropathy' serves as an example:

On the study target day all patients were to be tested for the presence of microalbuminuria with a urine test stick, and test results were obtained for 39 025 patients. 19.0% of these patients had a positive dipstick test for albuminuria in the microlbuminuric range, with a slight increase in the age groups above 40 years.

In patients without hypertension or diabetes, the rate was 14.6%, in patients with hypertension alone 21.2%, in patients with diabetes alone 30.2%. In patients with both hypertension and diabetes, however, the rate increased to 37.8%. These differences were noted for all age groups. The rate of positive test results was consistently higher in men than in women, most prominently in the group of patients with both hypertension and diabetes: 41.8% of men and 34.5% of women had a positive test result on the study day. These patients very often had assoiated cardiovascular diseases such as coronary heart disease (36.9%), heart failure (24.3%), left ventricular hypertrophy (22.6%), or peripheral arterial disease (16.7%). Obesity was diagnosed in 51.2% of these patients, and retinopathy in 15.4%.

The prevalence rates of a positive test on albuminuria in the microalbuminuric range also strongly depend on the severity on the underlying disease. For example, patients with mild or moderate severity of both hypertension and diabetes have a positive test result in 33%, while those with severe or extreme severity in 51.4%. Those patients with severe/extreme hypertension, but without diabetes, had a positive test result in 33.3%.

As physicians in their diagnostic questionnaire could tick – besides 24 other diagnoses – *nephropathy/dialysis,* it is possible to compare this clinical diagnosis with the test result for microalbuminuria as an established early manifestation of nephropathy (incipient nephropathy). A substantial discrepancy was found between both approaches: The number of patients with a positive test for albuminuria in the microalbuminuric range (37.5%) far exceeded the number with an assigned nephropathy diagnosis (12.5%). This discrepancy was consistently found across patients with neither hypertension nor diabetes, those with hypertension alone, those with diabetes alone, and those with hypertension plus diabetes. Many physicians are not in a position to weight lab findings against their clinical judgement: according to the findings of the prestudy practice characterisation questionnaire, more than a third reported that they *never or occasionally* conduct a test for microalbuminuria (3% never, 34.5% occasionally). On the other hand, 32.6% reported testing *frequently*, and 29.8% performing the test *always*.

Treatment patterns

Almost all patients with hypertension and/or diabetes receive therapy with at least one non-pharmacological measure and/or drug treatment. Non-pharmacological interventions are infrequently and indifferently used in hypertensive individuals. Only 63% received those at some time point during their disease history, and they are usually limited to counselling. According to the doctors' reports, 52.0% received *nutritional counselling,* but only 15.6% the more effective measures *nutritional training* and *counselling on physical activity.* Other established behaviour-modifying measures such as stress coping are rarely used. Conversely, pharmacological interventions were used in nearly all hypertensive patients: 96.6% received one ore more drugs. The spectrum of drugs used is within expectations. ACE inhibitors and beta-blockers are each taken by 44% of patients, diuretics by 34%, calcium antagonists by 25%, and AT_1 receptor blockers by 17%. Drugs capable of preventing the progression of nephroathy in patients at risk (AT_1 blockers, ACE inhibitors) seem – in view of the high frequency of albuminuria in the microalbuminuric range – to be underutilized. In concordance with clinical experience (Hanson 1998, ALLHAT Officers 2002), the majority of patients received two or more antihypertensive drugs at the same time. Almost all patients (nearly 90%) with hypertension plus diabetes received treatment with at least two drugs from different classes.

In patients with diabetes only or with diabetes and hypertension combined, non-pharmacological measures are used more frequently than in patients who are hypertensive only (about 90%); however, only for every second patient were specific types of training reported. Adjuvant strategies such as *antihypoglycaemic training* or *training on adequate drug* usage are rare. Further, less than 3% report *participation in patient groups*. Many patients reported that they had received one or more non-pharmacological interventions only once during the often protracted course of their disease: only 26% of patients said they had received such an intervention in the previous year. Almost all diabetic patients (86.7%) were on one or more antidiabetic drug. Sulfonylureas (30.9%), insulin (26.8%), and metformin (23.9%) were most frequently used, as opposed to the newer drug classes (glitazones, 4.6%, other: 11.8%).

East vs. West differences in diagnosis and treatment

In an ancillary analysis of the data, it was also investigated whether there are differences between the federal states formerly belonging to East Germany, and the West German states. We aimed to investigate the current situation on hypertension and diabetes mellitus in both regions. The population-based 1998 German Health Interview and Examination Survey had revealed marked differences with regard to the prevalence of both conditions between former East and West Germany (Thefeld 1999, Thamm 1999). In this population survey, for hypertension rates among males were 34.5% (East) and 28.5% (West) (females: 30.1% versus 26.1%).

For diabetes mellitus, total prevalence among 18 to 79-year-old males was 6.5% (East) and 4.3% (West) (females: 6.9% versus 5.2%).

In HYDRA, according to the diagnosis of physicians (clinical global impression [CGI] at least 'mild'), rates of hypertension were 40.4% (East) and 31.7% (West; OR: 1.4, CI: 1.3–1.6). However, there was no clinically relevant difference between measured mean blood pressures: 132.1/80.0 mmHg (East) versus 133.4/80.6 mmHg (West). Diabetes rates were: 15.9% (East) and 11.3% (West; OR: 1.4, CI: 1.2–1.6).

The rates of comorbidity of hypertension plus diabetes were: 15.9% (East) and 11.3% (West; OR: 1.9; CI: 1.7–2.1).

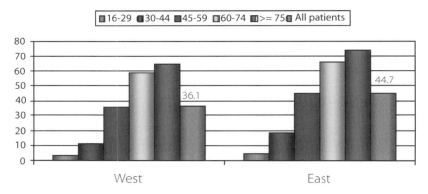

Fig. 4. Prevalence of hypertension in East versus West Germany according to age groups. According to general practitioners ratings, the prevalence of hypertension is substantially higher in the East (44.7 versus 32.1%). This finding is consistent across age groups

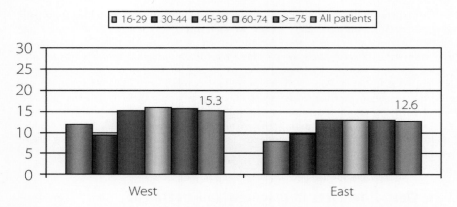

Fig. 5. Severity of hypertension according to physicians' ratings in East versus West Germany according to age groups. According to general practioners ratings, of all diagnosed cases – across age categories – the proportion of 'severe hypertension' is consistently slightly higher in the West

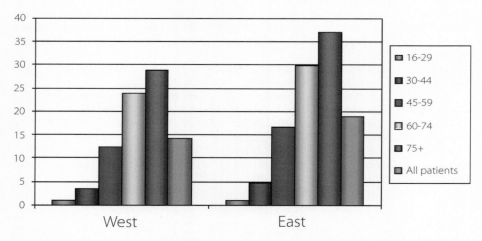

Fig. 6. Prevalence of diabetes in East versus West Germany according to age groups. According to doctors' ratings, the prevalence of DM was lower in the West than in the East. The prevalence was higher in men than in women (West: 16.9% M, 12.1% F; East: 22.1% M, 16,9% F)

Control of hypertension was rated as 'good' in 66.2% (East) and 60.0% (West), control of diabetes as 'good' in 61.6% (East) and 56.3% (West). Concomitant diseases significantly more frequently cited in the East were left ventricular hypertrophy (OR: 1.5, CI: 1.2–1.7) and coronary artery disease (OR: 1.5, CI: 1.3–1.6). Significantly less frequently cited in the East were: heart failure (OR: 0.8, CI: 0.6–0.8), depression (OR: 0.7, CI: 0.6–0.8) and sexual dysfunction (OR: 0.7, CI: 0.6–0.8).

Turning to intervention, 93% of all patients with the diagnosis of hypertension reeive pharmacological treatment. The following groups are most frequently used (odds ratios in brackets indicate likelihood of significantly increased prescription rates in East as compared to West; when ORs are missing, there was no significance): ACE inhibitors 45.3% (OR: 1.1), beta blockers 40.0% (OR: 1.3), diuretics 35.2% (OR: 0.8), calcium antagonists 24.8% (1.4), AT_1 blockers 15.7%, alpha blockers 3.1% (OR: 1.3), others 4.9%. Most frequently prescribed medications for diabetes were (OR: significantly inreased use in East vs. West): sulfonylureas 30.9%, insulin 26.8% (OR: 0.8), metformin 23.9% (OR: 0.7), glucosidase inhibitors 11.2%, glitazones 4.6%, others 11.6. Important non-pharmacological measures were used in 72.2%, nutritional counselling 63.0% (OR: 1.2), nutritional training 27.4%, and physiotherapy 7.1 (OR: 1.8).

Conclusion

The present study aims to describe representatively the prevalence, duration and severity of hypertension and diabetes in the primary care sector in Germany. At the same time it is possible to describe the actual health practice for these imporant indications and to compare the actual situation with the optimal one, as defined in clinical guidelines or similar guidance documents.

An important characteristic about the German health care system is its high frequency, short-duration visits to primary care physicians, which leads to a considerable shortage of time for a given individual patient. In our study, an average patient load of over 73 patients per physician and day gives an arithmetic mean contact time of 6.5 minutes. Against this background it is not surprising that we found a number of quantitative and qualitative shortcomings in the health practice. There are indicators of a substantial rate of under-diagnosed hypertensive or diabetic patients (e.g. when comparing blood pressure values with doctors' diagnoses). As for intervention, non-pharmacological interventions appear to be underused or often deficient, if used, and pharmacological treatment in many cases does not lead to the normalisation of target parameters. On the other hand, the individual targets agreed upon between physician and patient (or unilaterally defined by one of both) are likely to deviate in many cases from the stipulations laid down in clinical guidelines. For example, recent research in the US indicates that a significant proportion of primary care physicians have higher blood pressure thresholds for diagnosis and treatment than the criteria recommended by the actual JNC guidelines (Hyman 2001). The effect of practice guidelines in changing the attitude and performance of physicians is obviously limited due to a variety of reasons, such as the unstructured pattern of clinical practice that is unlike the strictly structured situation when a patient is enrolled in a clinical trial, the perception that primary care patients substantially differ from highly selected study patients, or simple disagreement or distrust of guidelines written by experts (Lomas 1989, Greco 1993, Dowie 1996, Allery 1997, Marshall 1998).

The HYDRA study for the first time displays the magnitude and complexity of the co- and multimorbidities in primary care, which is diametrical to the high grade of time efficiency, which is considered a prerequisite in primary care. Obviously this crucial factor has been underestimated so far. Subsequent analyses from the study dataset will probably help to formulate proposals for integrated coordinated improvement measures. The reality in primary care should be the yardstick at which these measures should be targeted.

References

Allery LA, Owen PA, Robling MR. Why general practitioners and consultants change their clinical practice: critical incident study. BMJ 1997; 314:870–874.

American Heart Association. 2002 Heart and Stroke Statistical Update. Dallas, TX: American Heart Association, 2001.

Amos AF, McCarthy DJ, Zimmer P. The rising global burden of diabetes and its complication: estimates and projections to the year 2010. Diabetes Med 1997; 14 (Suppl 5):S1–85.

Benjamin EJ, Smith SC Jr, Cooper RS, Hill MN, Luepker RV. Task force #1 – magnitude of the prevention problem: opportunities and challenges. 33rd Bethesda Conference. J Am Coll Cardiol 2002; 40:588–603.

Bodenheimer T. The American health care system – the movement for improved quality in health care. N Engl J Med 1999; 340:488–492.

Burt VL, Cutler JA, Higgins M, Horan MJ, Labarthe D, Whelton P, Brown C, Roccella EJ. Trends in the prevalence, awareness, treatment, and control of hypertension in the adult US population. Data from the Health Examination Surveys, 1960 to 1991. Hypertension 1995; 26:60–69.

Colhoun HM, Dong W, Poulter NR. Blood pressure screening, management and control in England: results from the health survey for England 1994. J Hypertens 1998; 16:747–752.

Diabetes Control and Complications Trial Research Group: The effect of intensive treatment of Diabetes on the development and progression of long-term complications in insulin-dependent diabetes mellitus. N Engl J Med 1993; 329:977–986.

Dowie J. The research-practice gap and the role of decision analysis in closing it. Health Care Anal 1996; 4:5–18.

Empfehlungen zur Diagnostik bei arterieller Hypertonie. Deutsche Hochdruckliga, November 2002.

Gaede P, Vedel P, Larsen N, Jensen GV, Parving HH, Pedersen O. Multifactorial intervention and cardiovascular disease in patients with type 2 diabetes. N Engl J Med 2003; 348:383–393.

Greco PJ, Eisenberg JM. Changing physicians' practices. N Engl J Med 1993; 329:1271–1273.

Hyman DJ, Pavlik VN. Self-reported hypertension treatment practices among primary care physicians: blood pressure thresholds, drug choices, and the role of guidelines and evidence-based medicine. Arch Intern Med 2000; 160:2281–2286.

Joint National Committee on Prevention, Detection, Evaluation, and Treatment of High Blood Pressure. The Sixth Report of the Joint National Committee on Prevention, Detection, Evaluation, and Treatment of High Blood Pressure. Arch Intern Med 1997; 157:2413–2445.

Lomas J, Anderson GM, Domnick-Pierre K, Vayda E, Enkin MW, Hannah WJ. Do practice guidelines guide practice? The effect of a consensus statement on the practice of physicians. N Engl J Med 1989; 321:1306–1311.

Mancia G, Sega R, Milesi C, Cesana G, Zanchetti A. Blood-pressure control in the hypertensive population. Lancet 1997; 349:454–457.

Marshall MN. Qualitative study of educational interaction between general practitioners and specialists. BMJ 1998; 316:442–445.

Nathan DM, Meigs J, Singer DE. The epidemiology of cardiovascular decease in type II diabetes mellitus: How sweet it is or is it? Lancet 1997; 350 (Suppl. I):4–9.

National Institute of Mental Health. Clinical Global Impressions. In: Guy, W. (Ed.): ECDEU Assessment for Psychopharmacology, Rev. Ed. Rockville, MD (1976), 221–227.

Neal B, MacMahon S, Chapman N. Effects of ACE inhibitors, calcium antagonists, and other blood-pressure-lowering drugs: results of prospectively designed overviews of randomised trials. Blood Pressure Lowering Treatment Trialists' Collaboration. Lancet 2000; 9, 356:1955–1964.

Newnham A, Ryan R, Khunti K, Majeed A. Prevalence of diagnosed diabetes mellitus in general practice in England and Wales 1994 to 1998. Health Statistics Quarterly 2002; 14:5–13.

Praxis-Leitlinien der Diabetes-Gesellschaft (DDG). Diabetes und Stoffwechsel 2002; 11 (Suppl 2):1–40.

Sharma AM, Wittchen HU, Krause P, Kirch W, Pittrow D et al. High Prevalence and Poor Control of Hypertension in Primary Care in Germany. In press.

Smith DA. Comparative approaches to risk reduction of coronary heart disease in Tecumseh non-insulin-dependent diabetic population. Diabetes Care 1996; 9:601–608.

Thamm M. Blutdruck in Deutschland – Zustandsbeschreibung und Trends. Gesundheitswesen 1999; 61 Suppl:S90–S93.

The ALLHAT Officers and Coordinators for the ALLHAT Collaborative Research Group. Major outcomes in high-risk hypertensive patients randomized to angiotensin-converting enzyme inhibitor or calcium channel blocker vs Diuretic: the antihypertensive and lipid lowering treatment to prevent heart attack trial (ALLHAT). JAMA 2002; 288:2981–2997.

Thefeld W. Prävalenz des Diabetes mellitus in der erwachsenen Bevölkerung Deutschlands. Gesundheitswesen 1999; 61:S85–S89.

Turner R, Cull C, Holman R. United Kingdom Prospective Diabetes Study 17: a 9-year update of a randomized controlled trial on the effect of improved metabolic control and complications in non-insulin-dependent diabetes mellitus. Ann Intern Med 1996; 124:136–145.

UK Prospective Diabetes Study Group. Intensive blood-glucose control with sulphonylureas or insulin compared with conventional treatment and risk of complications in patients with type 2 diabetes (UKPDS 33). Lancet 1998; 352:837–853.

Vestbo E, Damsgaard E, Froland A, Mogensen C. Urinary albumin excretion in a population based cohort. Diabet Med 1995; 12(6):488–493.

WHO/ISH Hypertension Guidelines Subcommittee. 1999 WHO-ISH guidelines for the management of hypertension. J Hypertens 1999; 17:151–183.

Zelmanovitz T, Gross J, Oliveira J, Paggi A, Tatsch M, Azevedo M. The receiver operating characteristics curve in the evaluation of a random urine specimen as a screening test for diabetic nephropathy. Diabetes Care 1997; 20(4):516–519.

Cardiac rehabilitation

Piotr Dylewicz · Slawomira Borowicz-Bieńkowska · Ewa Deskur-Śmielecka
Izabela Przywarska

> *"In the 21st century, all patients who can benefit from*
> *cardiac rehabilitation services should receive them."*

Wenger NK et al. Cardiac Rehabilitation. New York. Basel 1999 [28]

Definition of cardiac rehabilitation

It will soon be 40 years since the World Health Organization Expert Committee was appointed in 1963 to lay the foundations of modern cardiac rehabilitation [29].

The Committee worked out the first definition of cardiac rehabilitation:
Definition of cardiac rehabilitation (WHO Expert Committee 1964) [30]
The *rehabilitation of cardiac patients can be defined as the sum of activities required to ensure them the best possible physical, mental and social conditions so that they may, by their own efforts, resume as normal a place as possible in the life of the community.*

As it follows from the given text, the statement enumerates all postulates of modern cardiac rehabilitation. The importance of multifactorial nature of cardiac rehabilitation, encompassing influence on physical, psychological and social status of the patient, has been highlighted. Moreover, it has been emphasized that patient's involvement is pivotal in the rehabilitation process. The definition concludes that the ultimate purpose of cardiac rehabilitation is to help the patients in achieving the best possible place in the community.

In the 1960s the target population for cardiac rehabilitation was predominantly limited to survivors of uncomplicated myocardial infarction. The unquestionable achievement of cardiac rehabilitation in this period was its fundamental contribution to important shortening of immobilization after myocardial infarction and advancing of noninvasive and subsequently invasive diagnostic procedures, which resulted in considerable reduction in the duration of the hospital stay. These changes in the management of myocardial infarction had measurable physical, psychological and social effects as well as favourable economic outcomes.

In this period several original conceptions of phase II cardiac rehabilitation were elaborated. In many countries, e.g. Germany, Austria, Swiss, France, Spain, the Czech Republic, Slovakia, Hungary, Romania, Bulgaria, Slovenia, Croatia, Poland and Lithuania, stationary models were preferred. The development of stationary cardiac rehabilitation systems in these countries was probably facilitated by traditions of spa treatment and the availability of infrastructure and personnel suitable for this new domain of rehabilitation. In other countries, such as USA, GB, Holland, Sweden and Finland, ambulatory form was predominant. Special rehabilitation centres came into being, offering supervised programs and coordinating unsupervised, home-based rehabilitation [11].

In the 1980s the purposes of cardiac rehabilitation evolved gradually. These changes were due to evidence provided by meta-analyses of Oldridge et al. [21] and O'Connor et al. [20] published in 1988 and 1989. These investigations have proved that cardiac rehabilitation not only improves the quality of life, but also reduces mortality. These effects were shown despite several drawbacks of the studies included into the meta-analyses: the duration of the diagnostic procedures was limited, and the programs did not address the issues concerning secondary prevention.

Based on these premises, the U.S. Department of Health and Human Services formulated in 1988 a new definition of cardiac rehabilitation. In the author's opinion, this statement should be a message for all public health professionals in the coming years.

Definition of the Cardiac Rehabilitation (US. Department of Health and Human Services, Public Health Service. 1988) [9].

Comprehensive, long-term programs involving medical evaluation, prescribed exercise, cardiac risk factor modification, education, and counselling. These programs are designed to limit the physiological and psychological effects of cardiac illness, reduce the risk of sudden death or reinfarction, control cardiac symptoms, stabilize or reverse the atherosclerotic process, and enhance the psychosocial and vocational status of selected patients.

Analysing this statement one should notice the postulated long duration of rehabilitation service, going far beyond the acute phase of cardiac illnesses. The obligations of health care providers participating in the rehabilitation process have been enumerated: careful medical assessment of the patients, detection and effective modification of risk factors, education and counselling regarding healthy lifestyle. The importance of interventions designed not only to minimize rapidly consequences of cardiac illnesses, but most of all to slow the disease progression, reduce the risk of sudden death and maintain patient's optimal status in all fields of life as long as possible has also been addressed.

The benefits of cardiac rehabilitation

The results of several important studies published during the past 15 years confirmed wide-ranging efficacy of rehabilitation practice in a broad spectrum of cardiovascular diseases.

The benefits of cardiac rehabilitation

1. reduction in overall mortality and in mortality from cardiovascular causes [20, 21]
2. slowing of the atherosclerotic process [24, 27]
3. decreasing of rates of subsequent coronary events and hospitalisation [15, 25].

The cardiovascular illnesses considered eligible for and likely to benefit from cardiac rehabilitation

1. in the early 60s
   ▶ mainly younger patients recovering from uncomplicated myocardial infarction
2. at present also:
   ▶ the elderly
   ▶ patients with complications of myocardial infarction
   ▶ patients with compensated heart failure
   ▶ patients with arterial hypertension under pharmacological control
   ▶ patients after myocardial revascularization procedures
   ▶ patients with valvular heart disease
   ▶ patients after surgical correction of congenital heart disease

> ▶ patients with implanted cardiac pacemakers or cardioverter-defibrillators
> ▶ patients following cardiac transplantation
> ▶ patients with comorbidities [11, 18, 28].

It should be emphasized that rehabilitation programs have been proven to be highly effective in the management of cardiovascular risk factors.

Beneficial effects of cardiac rehabilitation programs

1. increase in exercise capacity [10, 19]
2. improvement in physical activity [14]
3. smoking cessation [4, 7]
4. decrease in blood pressure [13]
5. reduction of body weight [15]
6. correction of lipid profile [15, 27]
7. improvement in blood glucose control [6]
8. decrease in insulin resistance [5]
9. improvement in psychosocial well-being [2, 12, 22]
10. higher return to work rate [3, 16].

Cost-effectiveness of cardiac rehabilitation

There is some evidence to indicate favourable relation between costs and effectiveness of cardiac rehabilitation. Nevertheless, the number of studies, particularly those conducted in Europe, is insufficient.

Costs

1. Rehabilitation procedures are cost-effective as other treatment forms of cardiovascular diseases
2. The cost savings by reduced rehospitalisation and a higher return to work rate may even prevail over the initial costs of rehabilitation [11, 23].

On the strength of the evidence derived from numerous studies, carefully carried out according to evidence-based medicine principle, the WHO group formulated the following thesis in 1993:
"Rehabilitation is considered to be an essential part of the care that should be available to all cardiac patients" [31].

Cardiac rehabilitation – the cornerstone of secondary prevention

The development of invasive cardiology and its spectacular short-term successes diverted the attention of many health-care managers from issues regarding secondary prevention. The EUROASPIRE I and II studies, conducted in Europe in 1995–1996 and 1999–2000, have shown that preventive cardiology has not improved over this time [8].

Table 1. The results of EUROASPIRE I and II Trials [8]

	EUROASPIRE I (1995–1996)	EUROASPIRE II (1999–2000)
Smoking	19%	21%
BMI > 30 kg/m²	25%	33%
BP ≥ 140/90 mmHg	55%	54%
Total cholesterol ≥ 5.0 mmol/L	86%	59%

BMI body-mass index; BP blood pressure

Comparison of the results of EUROASPIRE I and II trials reveals that the prevalence of cardiovascular risk factors was similar in both studies, with the only exception of high total cholesterol concentrations (≥5.0 mmol/L), which decreased significantly from 86 to 59% (Table 1). Nevertheless, the proportion of patients with hypercholesterolemia is still disturbingly high (59%), as is the prevalence of obesity, hypertension and smoking.

Cardiac rehabilitation could be one of the possible ways to improve this situation, and the shortage of rehabilitation services can be a reason why the effects of secondary prevention are unsatisfactory. Therefore, the necessity of compiling preventive and rehabilitation interventions is addressed more and more frequently [1, 28]. J. Perk, the president of the Working Group on Rehabilitation and Exercise Physiology during meeting of the Group in 1999 considered cardiac rehabilitation to be a cornerstone of secondary prevention [26].

The current availability of cardiac rehabilitation is highly insufficient. Only small proportion of appropriate patients – about 15% – takes part in formal rehabilitation programs. A number of reasons contributes to this unfavourable situation.

The reasons for low participation rates in rehabilitation programs

1. geographic barrier
2. weak motivation to change lifestyle habits
3. failure of physicians to refer patients, particularly elderly persons, women, those with less education and the unemployed [1, 28].

Cardiovascular diseases become more and more serious problem in developing countries. In addition, in such countries as well as in less developed regions the access to rehabilitation services is the most difficult.

Poor motivation to change one's lifestyle, frequently observed in most social groups, is another important challenge. It may result from common belief that achievements of contemporary cardiology are so mighty that modification of lifestyle habits is no longer necessary. It is much easier to take a pill than start exercising regularly or limit the consumption of favourite delicacies. Nowadays, in the era of stents and statins, people are willing to forget obvious fact that these modern therapies do not solve the problem of disease progression and do not prevent completely its recurrence.

Many physicians underestimate the importance of counselling regarding lifestyle. Moreover, healthcare professionals seem to be particularly reluctant to discuss such issues with the elderly, women and individuals with lower socio-economic status – that is in groups of patients requiring special attention because of the poorest knowledge of the disease [17].

Challenge for the nearest future

A new statement of the Working Group of Rehabilitation and Exercise Physiology of the European Society of Cardiology concerning cardiac rehabilitation is expected in the nearest months to be published. Groups working on this statement have to face new challenges given to the contemporary cardiac rehabilitation. Of course, even now several purposes can be formulated on the basis of the analyses of recently reported studies as well as the experience of groups involved in rehabilitation [1, 28].

The goals of cardiac rehabilitation and secondary prevention for the 21st century

1. the number of patients participating in cardiac rehabilitation programs should be increased
2. an individualized program should be developed (in cardiac-rehabilitation centres, particularly for those with complications and who are elderly, or home-based, as well as for some uncomplicated younger patients)
3. life-long prolongation of the rehabilitation/secondary prevention strategies is necessary
4. system of care that can effectively reduce risk in patients with coronary heart disease should be established, comprising the following important components of rehabilitation procedures:
   - determination of metabolic risk factors,
   - optimising of physical activity prescription,
   - effective weight-loss programs and nutritional counselling,
   - optimising preventive procedures (also pharmacological),
   - optimising hypertensive and diabetic, and other metabolic disorders care,
   - recognizing and treating depression.

The research work performed during the past four decades has provided evidence that cardiac rehabilitation is purposeful and effective. Decision-makers in the area of public health should be aware that number of patients participating in cardiac rehabilitation programs must increase. Rehabilitation should be compiled with secondary prevention, and the duration of many interventions should be life-long. Fulfilling of these postulates would be associated with higher costs. Therefore, rehabilitation should be individualized and rationalized. Stationary rehabilitation should be reserved for patients with complicated disease, the elderly, those with severe deconditioning, subjects with lower socio-economic status and living in places distant from medical centres. Other patients, particularly younger and those willing to return to work rapidly, should be offered various models of ambulatory and home-based rehabilitation, with special emphasis put on the detection and management of risk factors. Modern rehabilitation system should provide not only exercise-based programs, but also education and counselling concerning weight reduction, dietary habits, optimal management of hypertension and diabetes as well as assessment and intervention for psychosocial risk factors, including depression. Cardiac rehabilitation programs could also provide education regarding preventive pharmacotherapy.

Summary

During the past four decades, cardiac rehabilitation has proven its usefulness in modern healthcare system – in the public health system. In the 21st century, new principles will be introduced into the health policy. Unfavourable economic situation, observed in the whole world, may prevent realization of many justified postulates. We should hope that the postulate formulated by N. Wenger [28], expressing the need for advancing of cardiac rehabilitation programs to eligible patients, will not be realized on paper only.

References

Ades PA. (2001) Cardiac rehabilitation and secondary prevention of coronary heart disease. N Engl J Med 345:892–902

Bar F et al. (1992) Cardiac rehabilitation contributes to the restoration of leisure and social activities after myocardial infarction. J Cardiopulmonary Rehabil 12:117–125

Boudrez H et al. (1994) return to work after myocardial infarction: results of a longitudinal population based study. Eur Heart J 15:32–36

DeBusk RF et al. (1994) A case-management system for coronary risk factor modification after acute myocardial infarction. Ann Intern Med 120:721–729

Dylewicz P et al. (1999) The influence of short-term endurance training on the insulin blood level, binding, and degradation of ^{125}I-insulin by erythrocyte receptors in patients after myocardial infarction. J Cardiopulmonary Rehabil 19:98–105

Dylewicz P et al. (2000) Beneficial effect of short-term endurance training on glucose metabolism during rehabilitation after coronary bypass surgery. Chest 117:47–51

Engblom E et al. (1992) Exercise habits and physical performance during comprehensive rehabilitation after coronary artery bypass surgery. Eur Heart J 13:1053–1059

EUROASPIRE I and II Group. European Action on Secondary Prevention by Intervention to Reduce Events (2001) Clinical reality of coronary prevention guidelines: a comparison of EUROASPIRE I and II in nine countries. Lancet 357:995–1001

Feigenbaum E, Carter E (1988) Cardiac rehabilitation services. Health technology assessment report No 6 U.S. Department of Health and Human Services, Public Health Service, National Center for Health Services Research and Health Care Technology Assessment. DHHS publication No. PHS 88-3427, Rockville

Froelicher V et al. (1984) A randomized trial of exercise training in patients with coronary heart disease. JAMA 252:1291–1297

Gohlke H, Gohlke-Bärwolf C (1998) Cardiac rehabilitation. Eur Heart J 19:1004–1010

Gulanick M. (1991) Is phase 2 cardiac rehabilitation necessary for early recovery of patients with cardiac disease? A randomized, controlled study. Heart Lung 20:9–15

Hamalainen H et al. (1989) Long-term reduction in sudden deaths after a multifactorial intervention programme in patients with myocardial infarction: 10-year results of a controlled investigation. Eur Heart J 10:55–62

Hambrecht R et al. (1993) various intensities of leisure time physical activity in patients with coronary artery disease: effects on cardiorespiratory fitness and progression of coronary atherosclerotic lesions. J Am Coll Cardiol 22:468–477

Haskell WL et al. (1994) Effects of intensive multiple risk factor reduction on coronary atherosclerosis and clinical cardiac events in men and women with coronary artery disease. The Stanford Coronary Risk Intervention Project (SCRIP). Circulation 89:975–990

Hedback B et al. (1993) Long-term reduction of cardiac mortality after myocardial infarction: 10-year results of a comprehensive rehabilitation programme. Eur Heart J 14:831–835

Kędzierski A, Dylewicz P (2000) Knowledge about ischaemic heart disease in healthy subjects and in patients after myocardial infarction Kardiol Pol 52:118–122

Lear SA, Ignaszewski A (2001) Cardiac rehabilitation: a comprehensive review. Curr Control Trials Cardiovasc Med 2:221–232

Miller NH et al. (1984) Home versus group exercise training for increasing functional capacity after myocardial infarction. Circulation 70:645–649

O'Connor GT et al. (1989) An overview of randomized trials of rehabilitation with exercise after myocardial infarction. Circulation 80:234–244

Oldridge NB et al. (1988) Cardiac rehabilitation after myocardial infarction. Combined experience of randomized clinical trials. JAMA 260:945–950

Oldridge N et al. (1991) Effects on quality of life with comprehensive rehabilitation after acute myocardial infarction. Am J Cardiol 67:1084–1089

Oldridge NB (1998) Comprehensive cardiac rehabilitation: is it cost-effective? Eur Heart J 19(Suppl O):042–049

Ornish D et al. (1990) Can lifestyle changes reverse coronary heart disease? The Lifestyle Heart Trial. Lancet 336:129–133

Ornish D et al. (1998) Intensive lifestyle changes for reversal of coronary heart disease. JAMA 280:2001–2007

Perk J (1999). Cardiac rehabilitation – the cornerstone of secondary prevention.1999. Working Group on Cardiac Rehabilitation and Exercise Physiology Balatonfüred, Hungary 1999. Avaible at: http:// www.escardio.org/society WG/Balatonfured/cardiac_rehabilitation

Schuler G et al. (1992) Regular physical exercise and low-fat diet. Effects on progression of coronary artery disease. Circulation 86:1–11

Wenger NK et al. (1999) Cardiac Rehabilitation. Marcel Dekker INC, New York Basel

World Health Organization (1964) Rehabilitation of patients with cardiovascular diseases. Report of a WHO Expert Committee. WHO Technical Report Series, No 270

World Health Organization Regional Office for Europe (1969) The rehabilitation of patients with cardiovascular disease. Report on a Seminar Noordwijk aan Zee. Copenhagen

World Health Organization Expert Committee on Rehabilitation after Cardiovascular Diseases, with Special Emphasis on Developing Countries (1993) Rehabilitation after cardiovascular diseases, with special emphasis on developing countries: report of a WHO expert committee. WHO, Geneva

Spatial patterns of cancer mortality in Europe

Carolyn A. Davies · Alastair H. Leyland

Introduction

The high number of cancer deaths in the Western World is of growing concern. There were an estimated 2.6 million new cases of cancer in Europe in 1995, representing over one quarter of the world burden of cancer despite Europe's inhabitants comprising only approximately one-eighth of the world's population. The corresponding number of deaths from cancer was around 1.6 million [1]. It has been predicted that in 2020, 3.4 million new cases of cancer will occur in Europe [2]. These figures demonstrate the very substantial burden of cancer in Europe, and the scope for prevention. Previous studies of geographic variation in cancer rates have provided important clues to the role of lifestyle factors and cancer risk.

The relationship between dietary components and cancer is not fully established; however, the overall impact of diet on cancer mortality appears to be significant. Evidence that diet is a determinant of cancer risk comes from several sources, including: correlation between national and regional food consumption data and the incidence of cancer in the population; studies on the changing rates of cancer as they migrate from a region or country of one dietary culture to another; case-control studies of dietary habits of individuals with and without cancer; prospective studies; intervention studies. While it is not yet possible to provide quantitative estimates of the overall risks, it has been estimated that 35 percent of cancer deaths may be related to dietary factors [3]. The association between dietary components and cancers differs among different cancers or groups of cancers.

A recent study into the estimates of cancer incidence and mortality in Europe [1] showed that the most common cause of death in Europe in 1995 among cancers was lung cancer with 330 000 deaths, representing about one fifth of the total number of cancer deaths. Deaths from cancer of the colon and rectum (189 000) ranked second. Breast cancer was the most common cause of cancer in females, representing 17% of all female cancer deaths and lung cancer the most common in males (29%). Most countries in Europe have shown a rising trend in oesophageal cancer over the last thirty years, especially in males [4]. In 1990, oesophageal cancer accounted for 3% of male cancer deaths [5]. The rising trend and poor prognosis (five-year survival in Europe is less than 10 percent [6]), makes this disease of growing concern in cancer research. Further details of the specific relationships in these cancer groups (breast, colon, oesophageal, and lung) are summarised in Table 1. Note that the blank areas in the table indicate that there is insufficient evidence of a relationship.

Breast cancer is a common cause of death in woman throughout Europe. The EURO-CARE II study recently estimated survival rates of incident cases between 1985 and 1989 in 17 countries in Europe [6] in which breast cancer was shown to have a five-year survival rate of 75%. One of the most often studied cancer associations is breast cancer risk and dietary fat. Earlier studies have supported the causal association between dietary fat and

Table 1. Association between dietary components and selected cancers

Dietary component	Site of cancer			
	Breast	Colorectal	Oesophageal	Lung
Animal Fats	+	+		+
Vegetables	–	–	–	–
Fruit	–	–	–	–
Fish/Fish Oil	–	–		
Alcohol	+	+	+	
Coffee	–			
Cheese	+			

+ = positive association; increased intake with increased cancer mortality
– = negative association; increased intake with decreased cancer mortality

breast cancer; however, many recent studies have been uncertain. Research suggests that these conflicting results are due to concentration on dietary fat as opposed to a more specific focus on content of saturated fat in the diet along with fruit and vegetable consumption [7]. Saturated fat, found mainly in animal fats, has been found to be positively related to risk of breast cancer. A recent ecologic study conducted using breast cancer mortality rates and dietary supplement data confirmed results from other studies showing that animal products are associated with risk for breast cancer and that fish intake and vegetable consumption are associated with risk reduction [8]. There is strong and consistent evidence that increased consumption of fruit and vegetables is associated with reduced risks of many common forms of cancer including breast cancer [9]. A meta-analysis of studies on breast cancer risk and diet confirmed the association between intake of vegetables and, to a lesser extent, fruits and breast cancer risk [10]. There has been much research focusing on dairy foods specifically. However, the only conclusive results regarding breast cancer risk appears to be a positive association with cheese intake [11]. Many case-control and cohort studies have found an association between alcohol use and breast cancer. A study found risk of breast cancer was increased by 40–45% for woman ever drinking versus never drinking [12]. The ecologic study examining breast cancer mortality rates [8] found alcohol to be an associated risk factor.

Colon cancer is the third most common form of cancer with particularly high incidence rates in Western Europe. Colorectal cancer is a leading cause of cancer mortality in the industrialised world. More literature is available examining relationships between diet and colon cancer incidence rather than mortality, however incidence should reflect colon mortality mortality as survival of cancer of the colon is fairly poor because most cases are diagnosed at an advanced stage [13]. The EUROCARE II project [6] showed colorectal cancer to have a five-year survival rate of 50%. Almost all the specific risk factors of colon cancer are of dietary origin. International comparisons indicate diets low in dietary fibre (low in vegetable and fruit consumption) and high in animal fat increase the risk of colon cancer [14]. The large majority of studies in humans has found a protective effect of fibre from vegetables and possibly fruits [15]. Willett et al. showed that animal fat from red meat intake was positively associated with colon cancer but dairy foods, which contributed to total animal fat intake, were not significantly related to the risk of colon cancer [16]. Fernandez et al. suggested that fish consumption has a protective effect against colon cancer [17]. Tavani confirmed coffee to be a risk factor showing an inverse association between coffee intake and risk of cancer of the colon [18]. A prospective study of cancers of the colon and rectum confirmed a positive association between alcohol use and cancer of the colon [19].

Cancer of the oesophagus is generally characterised by relatively low mortality rates in Europe with incidence in most Western European countries also being low [20]. Several studies have demonstrated a positive association between oesophageal cancer and several dietary factors including low intakes of vitamin A, C, riboflavin, nicotinic acid, calcium and zinc [21]. In dietary terms the associations are with low intakes of lentils, green vegetables, fresh fruits and animal protein. Fernandez et al. found a significant negative relationship with fish consumption and oesophageal cancer [17]. Alcohol appears to play a major risk in many of the epidemiological studies examining risk factors for oesophageal cancer with intake of alcohol appearing to be an independent risk factor [21]. A fairly recent study looking at oesophageal cancer mortality in Spain found similar results to other studies, supporting a role of alcohol in causation of oesophageal cancer [22].

Lung cancer is the most common cause of cancer mortality among men in Europe, and is becoming an increasingly important cause of cancer mortality among women [1]. During the last 25 years it has become apparent that diet is the other major cause of cancer, but theories have moved steadily from a search for causal agents (e.g., too much fat) to protective agents (e.g., too little fruit and vegetables) [23]. Mortality studies have shown excess risk to be associated with consumption of saturated fats (red meat) [24, 25] and protective effects associated with the intake of vegetables [26] and fruit [27]. Evidence of dairy fats having a particular effect on lung cancer is inconclusive [11].

Other lifestyle factors such as smoking and socio-economic status are commonly associated with the risk of cancers. It has been shown that people with high socio-economic status are at a greater risk from some cancers; however, evidence of an association with cancer mortality is sometimes inconclusive. Smoking is well known to be a major risk factor for many common cancers. The relationship between such lifestyle factors and the four cancers previously discussed are shown in Table 2.

Earlier evidence that breast cancer risk is unlikely to be affected by cigarette smoking continues to be challenged by recent findings. Although no definite conclusions can be made, several recent studies have reported findings that strongly hinted at such a relationship. A recent survival study found smoking to be a significant risk factor for breast cancer mortality [28]. However, a recent collaborative reanalysis of individual data from 53 epidemiological studies [29] showed smoking has little or no independent effect on the risk of developing breast cancer. Some recent studies have established passive exposure to environmental tobacco smoke (ETS) as a risk factor for breast cancer [30], yet, another study looking at breast cancer mortality found no relationship with ETS [31]. It appears that results from studies into the effect cigarette smoking has on breast cancer mortality are equivocal and need further examination.

Socio-economic status is thought to influence the risk of breast cancer. A study of breast cancer in young women showed that, compared with controls, cases were significantly more educated [32], with breast cancer incidence being most frequently reported in

Table 2. Association between other lifestyle factors and cancer mortality

Lifestyle factor	Site of cancer			
	Breast	Colon	Oesophageal	Lung
Smoking			+	+
High socio-economic status	–	–		–

those with greater than thirteen years education. Few studies have shown such a relationship with breast cancer mortality, and many conflicting results have appeared. However, a recent study showed a clear gradient in survival, with better survival for women with higher socio-economic status [33].

Colon cancer also appears to be clearly affected by socio-economic status. Tavani showed that the number of years of education was strongly associated with colon cancer with a significant trend in risk when comparing those with the highest level of education to those with less than seven years education [32]. There is little evidence to suggest that this association is also apparent with colon cancer mortality but incidence, again, may be viewed as an indicator of mortality due to the poor survival rates. There also appears to be no evidence of an association between cigarette smoking and colon cancer mortality.

Many studies have consistently identified smoking as a risk factor for oesophageal cancer. A recent mortality study confirmed this by showing the role of cigarette consumption on causation of oesophageal cancer [22]. There is little evidence of an association between socio-economic status and deaths from oesophageal cancer.

It is well known and accepted that tobacco smoking is the main risk factor for lung cancer. Evidence of a causal relationship between cigarette smoking and lung cancer mortality has been accumulating since the 1950's. In recent years more attention has been focused on the potential health effects of ETS. Numerous studies have now led to the expectation that exposure to ETS also entails some increase in lung cancer risk [34]. There is little evidence of a relationship between socio-economic status and lung cancer mortality. The prognosis of lung cancer is generally poor due to the carcinomas being diagnosed at an advanced stage. In Europe, the 5-year survival from 1985–1989 is reported to be 10% for woman and 9% for men [35], therefore there is less scope, in terms of time, for inequalities in survival by socio-economic group to occur. However, due to the poor prognosis, relationships with lung cancer incidence and socio-economic status are likely to reflect mortality rates as well. In most countries, lung cancer incidence in men and woman shows a social class gradient, with those from higher social classes having lower incidence than lower social classes [36].

Studies of the continuity of mortality rates across national borders and an evaluation of the distribution between national and regional variations in health status have revealed large spatial mortality variation both within and between countries in Europe [37]. This paper shows such patterns in relation to cancer mortality in the EU. Variation in cancer mortality often reflects differences in demographic structure, socio-economic conditions or lifestyle factors such as those previously discussed. We are interested in the quantification of the effect of such factors on cancer mortality patterns and also in examining any relationships that exist after taking these factors into account. Trends or patterns still existing suggest other factors, including genetic predisposition, have a discernible effect on the pattern of cancer mortality.

Data and methods

Population data

The World Health Organisation recently published an atlas of mortality in Europe [37]. Population and mortality information was collected for the periods 1980/1981 and 1990/1991, co-ordinating with two recent censuses, in an attempt to identify differences in trends in mortality at the subnational level in Europe. The data collected by WHO have been made available and provide the main source of information for this study. A subset of these data has been used and the population data include the number of residents, according to midyear estimates, per region of residence in 11 European Union countries for the year 1991. Four of the 15 current EU countries have data missing due to either the mortality or population data not being available for the time point being examined here. The countries with missing data are Ireland, Belgium, Italy and Spain. The data have been broken down into 5-year age bands (up to the 80–84 age band and then all aged 85 and over) for both sexes. Region of residence was defined according to the EUROSTAT nomenclature of administrative units. Where available, the units of analysis were level II NUTS (standard nomenclature of territorial units for statistics). This sub-national level is that just below the country level such as county in the UK or *département* in France. The total population for the 11 EU countries (Austria, Denmark, Finland, France, Germany, Greece, Luxembourg, Netherlands, Portugal, Sweden and UK) was 257 075 105 with a mean of 23 370 464, ranging from 38,7100 (Luxembourg) to 80 013 896 (Germany). Population data are available at a sub-national level for 10 of the EU countries (not Luxembourg) in 1991. The mean population for a region was 2 734 842 with a range from 24 734 (Ahvenanmaa in Finland) to 17 429 759 (North Rhine-Westphalia in Germany).

Mortality data

Cause-specific death data by gender and region of residence were available for population groups aged 0, 1–14, 15–34, 35–64, 75–79, 80–84 and 85 and over. The causes of deaths were based on the Ninth Revision of the International Classification of Diseases (ICD-9) [38]. The causes of death considered in this paper are malignant neoplasms (ICD-9 140–208). In 1991 the total number of recorded deaths from cancer in these 11 countries was 654 126. The directly standardised mortality rates were calculated based on the standard European age and sex specific population. A summary of these is given in Table 3. The average standardised death rate for all countries is 297 per 100 000, ranging from 163 (Finland and Sweden) to 267 (Denmark). At the regional level standardised death rates range from 125 (Epirus in Greece) to 320 (Copenhagen and Frederiksberg city in Denmark).

Risk/protective factor data

Since there is strong evidence of relationships between diet and other lifestyle factors and mortality from some cancers it is important that we should adjust for these factors as necessary before examining spatial patterns of cancer mortality. We are also interested in quantifying what effect these factors have on mortality rates, and so need measures relating to diet and lifestyle.

Data were obtained from various sources to allow the potential causal factors to be included. A summary of the data is given in Table 4. To take into account the dietary factors, information was obtained from the Food and Agriculture Organisation (http://apps.fao.org). The aggregated nutritional data provided the amounts of the commodity in question available for human consumption in a given country during a specific year. Average consumption data for animal fats, alcoholic beverages, fruit and vegetables were obtained for the period 1991. These cover the dietary components that appear to be related to the most common cancer mortalities. The data are measured in kilograms per year per head of population for each of the EU countries being examined.

WHO collected smoking data for the Tobacco or Health programme, 1997, and provided figures for the annual average consumption of manufactured cigarettes per adult (+15)

Table 3. Summarised Cancer Mortality data

Country	Total deaths	Standardised death rate (per 100 000)	If regional data available: min (region)	max (region)	No. of regions
Austria	19 317	196	181 (Tirol)	224 (Burgenland)	9
Denmark	17 764	267	228 (Sonderjylland)	320 (Copenhagen and Frederiksberg city)	15
Finland	9626	163	151 (Kuopio)	172 (Ahvenanmaa)	12
France	139 310	212	182 (Midi-Pyrénées)	251 (Nord-Pas-de-Calais)	22
Germany	210 537	206	187 (Brandenburg)	221 (Bremen)	16
Greece	19 945	164	125 (Epirus)	192 (Macedonia East and Thrace)	13
Luxembourg	957	208	–	–	–
Netherlands	35 645	209	197 (Friesland)	223 (Groningen)	12
Portugal	18 230	165	150 (Centro)	189 (Azores)	7
Sweden	20 406	163	148 (Kristianstad)	196 (Gävleborg)	24
UK	162 389	218	186 (Gloucestershire)	264 (Tyne and Wear)	56

Table 4. Summarised Risk Factor Data

Risk/protective factors	Median	Minimum	Maximum
Animal Fat kg/year/capita	16.4 (France)	2.3 (Greece)	26.8 (Luxembourg)
Fruit kg/year/capita	100.8 (Sweden)	74.5 (UK)	142.6 (Greece)
Vegetables kg/year/capita	80.6 (Austria)	58.8 (Finland)	300.4 (Greece)
Alcohol kg/year/capita	123.20 (UK)	60.0 (Greece)	173.9 (Germany)
Smoke cigarettes/year/adult	2210 (UK & Austria)	1550.0 (Sweden)	3590.0 (Greece)
GDP (region level) ECU/inhabitant	17 136 (Lorraine – France)	5611 (Ipeiros – Greece)	44 711 (Copenhagen and Frederiksberg city – Denmark)

(http://www.cdc.gov/tobacco/who/whofirst.htm). The figures for the time period 1990–1992 have been used to reflect the average level of smoking in each of the EU countries.

To take into consideration the differences in socio-economic status between the countries of the EU, data were obtained from Eurostat (http://europa.eu.int/comm/eurostat). The data used to represent this risk factor were gross domestic product (GDP). The data are available for each region (NUTS II) within each country. GDP is measured in ECU (European currency unit) per inhabitant in 1995.

It should be noted that the time periods used for each of the risk/protective factors might not be ideal. It is difficult to determine at which time period each exposure should be measured, for example at which period of a person's life their diet most affects their risk of cancer. For a population it is clearly impossible to consider accumulated lifetime exposure to such factors. Also, there is sometimes a lack of availability of risk/protective factor data at specific time periods. For these reasons, data that exists from approximately the same period as our mortality data have been used for the modelling in an attempt to reflect the cultures of the different countries or regions. However, it is important to remain aware that if the change over time in patterns of exposure to risk or protective factors has differed substantially between these regions or countries then this will impact upon both the estimated relationship with such risk factors and the estimated adjusted risk of mortality in these countries.

Disease mapping

Disease mapping is a growing area in the field of public health with a variety of methods in use. A recent book edited by Lawson et al. [39] illustrates many such methods, giving a useful review of them and their importance. Producing accurate maps of disease incidence and mortality allows the assessment of the true underlying distribution of a disease. In doing so the aim is to produce a map 'clean' of random noise and any natural variation in the human population, identifying areas with high or low rates. These types of maps can be used, for example, to assess the need for geographical variation in health resource allocation. Including additional information into the analysis such as covariates can be useful in research examining the relation of incidence or mortality to factors that could possibly be affecting the prevalence of the disease.

To assess the health status of an area with respect to disease incidence or mortality it is appropriate to examine what disease rates should be expected in a given area and then compare the observed rate with the 'expected' rate. This standardised mortality and morbidity approach is commonly used for the analysis of counts and traditionally maps of such ratios have been examined. However, when examining SMRs, the ratios for small or sparsely populated areas will often dominate the map as there are few or no observations. Modern approaches use methods that make use of interpolation methods to provide estimates of the rates in such areas. One common approach is to map standardised rates based on Poisson inference [40]. Mapping the modelled standardised rates has the advantage of providing estimates of the disease rates but does have some disadvantages.

Firstly, when observing numbers of events, whether these are disease mortality or incidence, the variation often exceeds that expected from Poisson inference especially when considering rare diseases or areas with small populations. In such cases, variation in the observed number of events is due partly to Poisson sampling, but is also due to extra-Poisson variation. Another problem in using conventional Poisson based methods is that it they do not take account of any spatial pattern of disease, i.e. they ignore the fact that areas geographically close to one another share similar disease rates and common factors which influence the incidence and outcome of disease.

There is a large amount of literature examining Bayesian and empirical Bayes approaches to disease mapping which overcome such problems. Tsutakawa considered an approach using normally distributed logits of disease risk [41]. Mollié gives a fairly in depth overview of empirical Bayes and fully Bayesian approaches to disease mapping [42]. Clayton and Kaldor used hierarchical models and empirical Bayesian inference for region-specific SMRs, which allows spatial correlation between neighbouring regions [43]. Besag et al. furthered this approach to a fully Bayesian method using Markov chain Monte Carlo algorithms [44]. Another extension is to model geographically distributed data using multilevel modelling techniques based on iterative generalised least squares procedures [45]. The geographically distributed data described earlier where we have counts of cancer deaths within regions within countries exemplify the type of data appropriate for a multilevel analysis.

Multilevel modelling

Firstly, if we consider a population of regions, i, $i = 1, \ldots, I$, with observed (O_i) and expected (E_i) counts of deaths. E_i are often calculated through standardisation based on the number of deaths in the population N_i. This standardisation is conducted for age and sex bands k and calculated as

$$E_{ik} = N_{ik} \frac{\sum O_{ik}}{\sum N_{ik}}$$

$$E_i = \sum E_{ik}$$

The relative risk of the mortality from the disease of interest is then

$$\theta_i = \frac{O_i}{E_i} \, .$$

A basic single level Poisson model can be written as [46]:

$$O_i \sim Poisson\,(\mu_i)\,,$$

$$log\,(\mu_i) = log\,(E_i) + a + x_i\beta + u_i\,,$$

$$[u_i] \sim N\,(0, \Omega_u), \; \Omega_u = [\sigma_u^2]\,.$$

Where $log\,(E_i)$ is treated as an offset and is included to account for the different populations at risk of death from cancer in each area. a is a constant and x is an explanatory variable with coefficient β (this may be generalised to a number of explanatory variables). We assume that the number of counts within each area follow a Poisson distribution. The u_i represent heterogeneity effects between areas [47] which can be viewed as having extra Poisson variation caused by the variation among underlying populations at risk in the areas considered. This can be extended to a simple spatial model by adding further random effects [45].

$$log\,(\mu_i) = log\,(E_i) + a + x_i\beta + u_i + v_i\,,$$

$$v_i = \sum_{j \neq i} z_{ij} v_j^*\,,$$

$$\begin{bmatrix} u_i \\ v_j^* \end{bmatrix} \sim N\,(0, \Omega_{uv})\,, \; \Omega_{uv} = \begin{bmatrix} \sigma_u^2 & \\ \sigma_{uv} & \sigma_v^2 \end{bmatrix}.$$

The v_i are spatially dependent random effects, and may have any one of a number of structures describing adjacency or nearness in space [48]. The spatial effects v_i are considered to be the weighted sum of a set of independent random effects v_i^*. The v_i^* can be considered to be the effect of area upon other areas, moderated by a measure of proximity of each pair of areas z_{ij}. There are many ways in which z_{ij} can be formulated, in general it is written [49]

$$z_{ij} = w_{ij}/w_{i+} ,$$

In this case the w_{ij} are either 1's or 0s representing an adjacency matrix and

$$w_{i+} = \sum_j w_{ij} .$$

The v_i^* can then be estimated directly from the model. Therefore we have a multilevel model where within-area effects are modelled with a Poisson distribution and relative risks between areas are considered as having a lognormal distribution. The full details of the iterative procedure to fitting such models can be found in Goldstein, 1995 [50].

Results

The expected number of events in the ith region, E_i, has been calculated based on the 1990 European age and sex specific mortality rates. The variance component model with all explanatory variables fitted took the form

$$O_i \sim Poisson\,(\mu_i)$$

$$\log\,(\mu_i) = \log\,(E_i) + \beta_{0i} + \beta_{1i} FRU_i + \beta_{2i} VEG_i + \beta_{3i} ANF_i +$$
$$+ \beta_{4i} ALC_i + \beta_{3i} SMO_i + \beta_{6i} GDP_i$$

$$\beta_{0i} = \beta_0 + u_i$$

$$[u_i] \sim N(0, \Omega_u)\,,\ \Omega_u = [\sigma_u^2]\ .$$

A variance components model describes the random variation in the data by a set of variances. Looking at this model it can be seen that all the variance is at a single level, i, which is region. There is only one random parameter, σ_u^2. Potentially, and more appropriately, this model can be expanded by partitioning the variance into that which is attributable to random variation between countries and that which arises due to differences between regions within countries, i.e. adding a further level. However, looking at the preliminary model, the response, O_i is the number of observed cancer deaths, and this can be assumed to be Poisson distributed. This model allows us to take account of Poisson variation at a regional level plus extra Poisson variation, taking into account the fact that the expected number of deaths, E_i, are heterogeneous [47]. β_0 is the intercept term and $\beta_{1...6}$ are the mean (fixed) effects of the factors fruit consumption, vegetable consumption, animal fat consumption, alcohol consumption, cigarette consumption and gross domestic product respectively. The results of the variance components models are shown in Table 5. Model A shows the null model with no explanatory variables included and model B is the results from the full model shown above.

Firstly, looking at model B, the overall intercept β_0 represents an average number of cancer deaths in all regions included in the study in addition to the (centred) logarithm of the expected cases, when all other fixed coefficients are zero. The estimates of the intercept

Table 5. Results from Variance Components and Spatial Models

	Model A estimate (95% C.I.)	Model B estimate (95% C.I.)	Model C estimate (95% C.I.)
Fixed Part			
β_0	7.53 (7.50, 7.56)	6.83 (6.68, 6.99)	6.83 (6.53, 7.13)
β_1 (FRU)		−7.58 (−8.65, −6.50)	−7.51 (−9.67, −5.36)
β_2 (VEG)		−1.12 (−1.69, −0.55)	−1.11 (−2.25, 0.04)
β_3 (ANF)		26.36 (19.28, 33.42)	25.98 (11.72, 40.23)
β_4 (ALC)		0.64 (−0.17, 1.45)	0.71 (−0.91, 2.33)
β_5 (SMO)		0.49 (0.39, 0.59)	0.49 (0.29, 0.69)
β_6 (GDP)		0.20 (−4.61, 5.01)	0.33 (−9.40, 10.06)
Random Part			
σ_u^2	0.040 (0.032, 0.048)	0.014 (0.011, 0.017)	0.002 (−0.014, 0.017)
σ_{uv}			0.011 (−0.001, 0.023)
σ_v^2			0.044 (0.011, 0.077)

are not particularly informative in these models as they reflect an unlikely situation whereby an area has zero exposure to any of the risk or protective factors. Before examining the other fixed parameter estimates it should be noted that for the purpose of interoperability the explanatory variables were re-based. The consumption variables were modelled in terms of 1000 kgs consumed per person per year, smoking was scaled to how many 1000 cigarettes were smoked per person per year, and GDP was examined as millions of ECUs per inhabitant per year. The estimate of β_1 is the mean, or fixed slope for the explanatory variable fruit and it can be seen the estimate is negative and, judging significance by approximate 95 per cent confidence intervals, significant. This implies that when taking the other variables into account, an increase in fruit consumption decreases cancer mortality on average in the EU. The parameter estimate of −7.58 is a log relative risk of cancer mortality for each 1000 kg increase in fruit consumption per person per head. This suggests that every 10 kg increase in fruit consumption per person per year is associated with a decrease in the risk of cancer mortality of about 7% ($RR = \exp\{-0.0758\} = 0.927$). It can be seen that the other variables which significantly affect cancer mortality are vegetable consumption, showing an inverse association, animal fat consumption showing to be a significant risk factor and smoking again showing to significantly heighten the risk of cancer mortality. The actual effect size of these variables will be discussed further on. There has been no partitioning of variance yet so all the variation here is due to differences between regions ($\sigma_u^2 = 0.014$). If we compare this value to the variance under model A ($\sigma_u^2 = 0.040$) it can be seen there has been a 66% reduction in variation after adding the explanatory variables. Due to the significant explanatory variables being at country level, this shows that these factors are helping to explain the differences in cancer mortality between regions

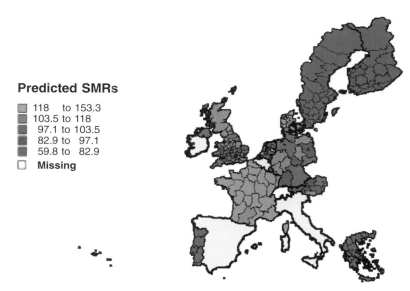

Predicted SMRs

- 118 to 153.3
- 103.5 to 118
- 97.1 to 103.5
- 82.9 to 97.1
- 59.8 to 82.9
- ☐ Missing

Fig. 1. Mapped SMRs from Model A

and countries. To show these differences visually, the predicted SMRs from model A have been mapped and are shown in Figure 1.

The main features of the map indicate that France and Denmark have particularly high cancer mortality rates. Cancer mortality rates in these regions are between 18 and 53% higher than expected if the European age and sex specific mortality rates had been applied to that area. Greece, Portugal, Finland and Sweden appear to have the lowest rates. The pattern suggests that there is lower cancer mortality in the east and higher in the west with the exception of Portugal. However, data are missing for 4 EU countries, illustrated in yellow here, so it is difficult on the basis of these data to tell if this pattern is consistent across the whole EU. These results do not take into consideration the effects of the risk and protective factors shown to have a significant effect on cancer mortality rates. The map seems fairly smooth, indicating that it is clean of any random noise or any artefacts of population variation and suggesting that even the initial models have been effective at smoothing geographic variation.

However, the modelling so far doesn't take into account the geographical structure (the fact that areas close to each other in geographical space may share common factors that influence cancer mortality). Fitting the spatial model to the data allows us to take this into account. This extension to the variance components models is as follows

$$\beta_{0i} = \beta_0 + u_i + v_i$$

$$v_i = \sum_{j \neq i} z_{ij} v_j^*$$

$$\begin{bmatrix} u_i \\ v_j^* \end{bmatrix} \sim N\left(0, \Omega_{uv}\right), \quad \Omega_{uv} = \begin{bmatrix} \sigma_u^2 & \\ \sigma_{uv} & \sigma_v^2 \end{bmatrix}.$$

Now we have a slightly more complex covariance structure. The variance has been partitioned with σ_u^2 referring to the variance that arises due to heterogeneity between regions and σ_v^2 referring to that which arises due to the spatial structure. The random effect has now been written as the sum of the heterogeneity effect, u_i, and a correlated spatially structured component, v_i. The model takes on similar structure to a simple autocorrelation model. The weights, z_{ij} can be thought of as spatial explanatory variable, and represent a measure of the relevance of area j to area i. The results for the more complex model C are shown in Table 5.

Firstly, comparing the fixed parts results from the variance components model and this model, the estimates change very little after including the spatial component. However, looking at the standard errors, they almost double for each term in the spatial model. The probable reason behind this is that areas geographically close tend to display positive dependence or positive autocorrelation, but when this is ignored as in the variance components model, incorrect inference will result, in particular standard errors of explanatory variables will be too small. Fitting the spatial model here has improved the accuracy of the model. Using the variance terms, the total variance can be calculated. The spatial part is dependent on the number of neighbours an area has, and taking this into account implies a total variance of 0.0124. 85% of this variance now arises from spatial effects, confirming the importance of the spatial part in the model.

We are also interested in quantifying the effect size of the risk or protective factors when examining cancer mortality. The relative risks have been calculated for each of the significant variables and are given in Table 6. Firstly, for the consumption of fruit, the table shows that Greece has the highest level of consumption in these 11 countries and the UK has the lowest. The relative risk of 0.58 shows that a population consuming, on average, the same amount of fruit as Greece has a risk of cancer mortality that is 42 per cent lower than if consumption was on the same level as the UK. Also, consuming the same level of vegetables as Greece leads to a risk of cancer mortality that is 28% less than if consumption was at the same level as Finland or Sweden. Luxembourg consumes the most animal fat in the EU countries being examined and this level of consumption leads to a RR over 2 times as high as if consumption was on the same level as Greece. Finally, the inhabitants of Greece, on average, smoke the most cigarettes. This level of smoking leads to a RR of cancer mortality 3 times as high as if cigarette consumption was at the same level as Sweden (where cigarette consumption is the lowest).

To examine visually the apparent effect of risk factors and also to compare the different models fitted, plots of the predicted relative risks from the three models are given in Figure 2. A measure of latitude (south to north positioning) has been plotted against the predicted relative risks for each region in the EU for the three models. This is an alternative to mapping the results and prevents the loss of information that occurs when grouping mortality rates in ranges. A relative risk of 1 on the plot indicates a region where the number of cancer deaths is as expected. The region in France with the highest relative risk, of about 1.5, is an area where cancer mortality is 50% higher than expected. Looking at the

Table 6. Variable effect sizes

Variables	Area with		
	highest consumption	lowest consumption	relative risk
Fruit	Greece	UK	0.58
Vegetables	Greece	Finland & Sweden	0.72
Animal Fat	Luxembourg	Greece	2.03
Cigarettes	Greece	Sweden	2.99

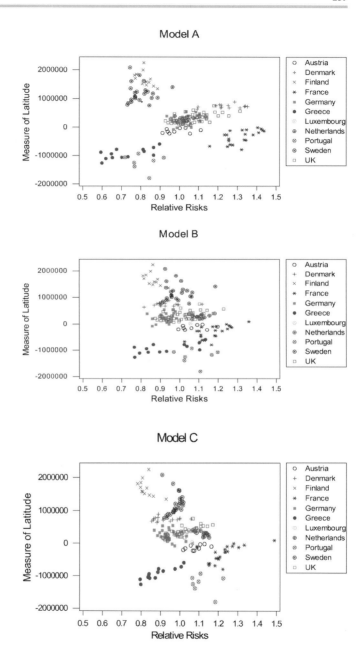

Fig. 2. Relative Risks from
three models

plot for model A, the variance components model with no explanatory variables included, it is obvious that there is definite clustering, with mortality rates for regions within each country being very similar. There also appears to be evidence of a negative slope, with the exception of Greece and Portugal, suggesting that rates tend to be highest in Southern Europe and lowest in Northern Europe. Examining the plot of model B, the variance component model including the explanatory variables, it can be seen that the spread decreases. The relative risks for countries with low relative risks are higher than in model A and those that previously had high relative risks are lower. This is because the risk or protective factors included are measured at the level of country and are therefore explaining differences between countries. The key features from fitting this model are that regions in Portugal, which were previously shown to have low cancer mortality rates, now appear to have a risk of cancer mortality that is higher that expected given the lifestyle factors. Portugal has fairly high consumption of fruit and vegetables and very low animal fat consumption, so after taking these into consideration they have above average mortality. Also, looking at Denmark, the cancer mortality risks are high under model A but under model B for most regions they are below average. So, taking into account the fact that Denmark has high animal fat consumption and low fruit and vegetable consumption, the rates are actually lower than expected. Finally, moving onto the estimates obtained from model C, there is more distinction between countries. In the previous plot they were clustered but showed more variation within each country and more overlap between countries. With the spatial model the relative risks are more tightly clustered within countries. This is due to the mean for each area being centred on the mean of its neighbours. This plot also shows the model is also predicting some more extreme relative risks, e.g. a region in France having a fairly high value. With the variance components model, the area effects are shrunk towards a mean effect of zero; however, the spatial model shrinks the results towards a local mean which is obviously going to be high for France. In effect this pattern is what provides greater smoothing to a map.

Discussion

It has been shown that spatial variation in cancer mortality exists both within and between countries throughout the EU. Whilst a large part of the variation between countries can be accounted for by adjusting for known risk and protective factors for cancer mortality, variation still clearly exists throughout these European countries. Through examination of the relationship cancer mortality has with latitude, there appears to be some evidence of a negative gradient, with adjusted mortality being lower in Northern Europe.

Fruit and vegetable consumption appear to have a strong protective association with cancer mortality and animal fat consumption and smoking are seen to be strong risk factors at the population level, complementing previous research in cancer mortality. It was seen that around two thirds of the variation that exists between regions in the EU can actually be explained by taking into account fairly crude measures of exposure to the above significant risk and protective factors.

Further modelling provided evidence that the remaining variation between regions is not random. It can be seen that about 85% of the variation is spatially patterned, suggesting that there are other factors not included in this study which are spatially patterned that also influence cancer mortality. Such factors which may be affecting these spatial patterns of mortality include genetic predisposition to cancer, other measures of socio-economic status such as education or employment, and health care provision. It is also important to note that at this stage most of the variables used in our modelling (and all the significant variables) are measured at country level, resulting in model estimates which may not have taken into account differences in exposure between regions within countries. Therefore, it is possible that part of the spatial patterning that exists is reflecting different patterns of these factors at a sub-national level.

Grouping all cancers may be seen as a fairly crude form of analysis, however, we believe that we have shown the potential for further investigations of the association of cancer with various dietary, lifestyle and socio-economic factors. Given that the literature suggests that these relationships vary for different cancers the next logical step would be to consider the different cancers individually. We can also look to generalise the results further by including more European countries and data from other years. In addition to allowing us to explore the patterns in Eastern Europe, data from other countries may provide further evidence of any relationship between cancer mortality and latitude, and may also provide clues as to the extent to which mortality rates in Greece differ from the patterns existing in the rest of the EU.

Summary

Background – Previous research in cancer mortality has revealed large spatial variations within and between countries and that factors associated with the aetiology of most cancers include diet, socio-economic status, smoking and genetic predisposition. Without detailed data on individual mortality and exposure to risk factors it is still possible to explore the geographical variations in cancer mortality and their relationships with population characteristics. **Data and Methods** – Cancer mortality data and population data are available for 187 regions in 11 EU countries by age and sex. All deaths from neoplasms are examined for 1991 and standardised mortality rates have been calculated. Other data available are consumption (per head) of fresh fruit, vegetables, animal fats, alcohol and cigarettes for each country and GDP per head at a regional level. Spatial multilevel models were used to examine the distribution of cancer mortality. Mapping the mortality rates from these models allows visual exploration of patterns across Europe. The addition of covariates in the models allows the associations with causal factors to be examined. **Results** – After taking into account the spatial structure of the data and adjusting for significant causal factors, France has the highest mortality rates and Greece and Finland have the lowest, with mortality appearing highest in the West. Univariate analyses of the effect of the covariates on cancer mortality suggest fruit and vegetable consumption are negatively associated with the risk of all cancer mortality and animal fat consumption is positively associated. Smoking appears to show no association with cancer mortality. When examining the factors together, the positive association between smoking and cancer mortality becomes apparent. **Conclusions** – High variability in cancer mortality between and within countries in EU is evident. Lifestyle factors have strong influences on the risks of cancer mortality. Estimates are improved by taking into account spatial relationships and relationships with covariates.

References

1. Bray, F., et al., Estimates of cancer incidence and mortality in Europe in 1995. European Journal of Cancer, 2002. 38:99–166.
2. Parkin, D.M., Global cancer statistics in the year 2000. The Lancet Oncology, 2001. 2:533–443.
3. Doll, R. and R. Peto, The Causes of Cancer – Quantitative Estimates of Avoidable Risks of Cancer in the United-States Today. Journal of the National Cancer Institute, 1981. 66:1191.
4. Survival of Cancer Patients in Northern Ireland 1993–1996. 2001, N. Ireland Cancer Registry: Belfast.
5. Facts and Figures of Cancer in the European Community. 1993, International Agency for Research on Cancer, Commission of the European Communities, WHO "Europe Against Cancer".
6. Berrino, F., et al., Survival of Cancer Patients in Europe: The EUROCARE-2 Study. 1999, IARC Scientific Publications.
7. Lee, M.M. and S.S. Lin, Dietary fat and breast cancer. Annual Review of Nutrition, 2000. 20:221–248.

8. Grant, W.B., An ecologic study of dietary and solar ultraviolet-B links to breast carcinoma mortality rates. Cancer, 2002. 94:272–281.

9. Boyle, P., P. Maisonneuve, and P. Autier, Update on cancer control in women. International Journal of Gynecology & Obstetrics, 2000. 70:263–303.

10. Gandini, Meta-analysis of studies on breast cancer risk and diet: the role of fruit and vegetable consumption and the intake of associated micronutrients (vol 36, pg 636, 2000). European Journal of Cancer, 2000. 36:1588–1588.

11. Jain, M., Dairy foods, dairy fats, and cancer: A review of epidemiological evidence. Nutrition Research, 1998. 18:905–937.

12. Bowlin, S.J., et al., Breast cancer risk and alcohol consumption: Results from a large case-control study. International Journal of Epidemiology, 1997. 26:915–923.

13. Dove-Edwin, I. and H.J.W. Thomas, Review article: The prevention of colorectal cancer. Alimentary Pharmacology & Therapeutics, 2001. 15:323–336.

14. Detels, R., et al., eds. Oxford Textbook of Public Health. 1997, Oxford Medical Publications.

15. Willett, W., The Search for the Causes of Breast and Colon Cancer. Nature, 1989. 338(6214):389–394.

16. Willett, W.C., et al., Relation of Meat, Fat, and Fiber Intake to the Risk of Colon Cancer in a Prospective-Study among Women. New England Journal of Medicine, 1990. 323:1664–1672.

17. Fernandez, E., et al., Fish consumption and cancer risk. American Journal of Clinical Nutrition, 1999. 70:85–90.

18. Tavani, A., et al., Coffee and tea intake and risk of cancers of the colon and rectum: A study of 3530 cases and 7057 controls. International Journal of Cancer, 1997. 73:193–197.

19. Klatsky, A.L., et al., The Relations of Alcoholic Beverage Use to Colon and Rectal-Cancer. American Journal of Epidemiology, 1988. 128:1007–1015.

20. Schouten, L.J., Oesophageal and stomach cancer, in Gastrointestinal Cancer in the Netherlands 1989–1992, R.A.M. Damhuis, L.J. Schouten, and O. Visser, Editors. 2001, Netherlands Cancer Registry: Netherlands. p. 1–8.

21. Shetty, P.S. and J. W.P.T, Nutrition, in Oxford Textbook of Public Health, R. Detels, et al., Editors. 1997, Oxford University Press. p. 157–174.

22. Cayuela, A., J. Vioque, and F. Bolumar, Esophageal Cancer Mortality – Relationship with Alcohol Intake and Cigarette-Smoking in Spain. Journal of Epidemiology and Community Health, 1991. 45:273–276.

23. Hill, M.J., Changes and developments in cancer prevention. Journal of the Royal Society for the Promotion of Health, 2001. 121:94–97.

24. Mulder, I., et al., Role of smoking and diet in the cross-cultural variation in lung-cancer mortality: the Seven Countries Study (vol 88, pg 665, 2000). International Journal of Cancer, 2001. 91:901–901.

25. Breslow, R.A., et al., Diet and lung cancer mortality: a 1987 National Health Interview Survey cohort study. Cancer Causes & Control, 2000. 11:419–431.

26. Kubik, A.K., et al., Lung cancer risk among Czech women: A case-control study. Preventive Medicine, 2002. 34:436–444.

27. Chow, W.H., et al., A Cohort Study of Tobacco Use, Diet, Occupation, and Lung- Cancer Mortality. Cancer Causes & Control, 1992. 3:247–254.

28. Manjer, J., et al., Survival of women with breast cancer in relation to smoking. European Journal of Surgery, 2000. 166:852–858.

29. Collaborative Group on Hormonal Factors in Breast Cancer, Alcohol, tobacco and breast cancer – collaborative reanalysis of individual data from 53 epidemiological studies, including 58515 women with breast cancer and 95067 women without the disease. British Journal of Cancer, 2002. 87:1234–1245.

30. Rookus, M.A., et al., Passive and active smoking and the risk of breast cancer. American Journal of Epidemiology, 2000. 151:109.

31. Wartenberg, D., et al., Does passive smoking exposure increase female breast cancer mortality? American Journal of Epidemiology, 2000. 151:110.

32. Tavani, A., et al., Risk factors for breast cancer in women under 40 years. European Journal of Cancer, 1999. 35:1361–1367.

33. Schrijvers, C.T.M., et al., Deprivation and Survival from Breast-Cancer. British Journal of Cancer, 1995. 72:738–743.

34. Baynard, S.P., et al., Respiratory Health Effects of Passive Smoking: Cancer and Other Disorders. 1992, Office of Health and Environmental Assessment: Washington DC.

35. Janssen-Heijnen, M.L.G., et al., Variation in survival of patients with lung cancer in Europe, 1985–1989. European Journal of Cancer, 1998. 34:2191–2196.

36. Schrijvers, C.T.M., et al., Socioeconomic Variation in Cancer Survival in the Southeastern Netherlands, 1980–1989. Cancer, 1995. 75:2946–2953.
37. Atlas of Mortality in Europe: subnational patterns, 1980/81 and 1990/1991. European Series, No. 75. 1997: WHO regional publications.
38. Manual of the International Statistical Classification of Diseases, Injuries and Causes of Death. Ninth revision. 1997: WHO: Geneva.
39. Lawson, A., et al., eds. Disease mapping and risk assesment for public health. 1999, John Wiley & Sons Ltd.
40. Lawson, A., et al., Disease Mapping and Its Uses, in Disease Mapping and Risk Assessment for Public Health. 1999, John Wiley & Sons Ltd. p. 3–13.
41. Tsutakawa, R.K., Estimation of Cancer Mortality-Rates – a Bayesian-Analysis of Small Frequencies. Biometrics, 1985. 41:p. 69–79.
42. Mollie, A., Bayesian and Empirical Bayes Approaches to Disease Mapping, in Disease Mapping and Risk Assessment for Public Health. 1999, John Wiley & Sons Ltd. p. 15–29.
43. Clayton, D. and J. Kaldor, Empirical Bayes Estimates of Age-Standardized Relative Risks for Use in Disease Mapping. Biometrics, 1987. 43:671–681.
44. Besag, J., J. York, and A. Mollie, Bayesian Image-Restoration, with 2 Applications in Spatial Statistics. Annals of the Institute of Statistical Mathematics, 1991. 43:p. 1–20.
45. Langford, I.H., et al., Multilevel modelling of the geographical distributions of diseases. Journal of the Royal Statistical Society Series C-Applied Statistics, 1999. 48:253–268.
46. Langford, I.H. and R.D. Day, Poisson Regression, in Multilevel Modelling of Health Statistics, A.H. Leyland and H. Goldstein, Editors. 2001, John Wiley & Sons, Ltd. p. 45–57.
47. Langford, I.H., Using Empirical Bayes Estimates in the Geographical Analysis of Disease Risk. Area, 1994. 26:p. 142–149.
48. Besag, J. and J. Newell, The Detection of Clusters in Rare Diseases. Journal of the Royal Statistical Society Series a-Statistics in Society, 1991. 154:p. 143–155.
49. Langford, I.H., et al., Multilevel Modelling of Area-Based Health Data, in Disease Mapping and Risk Assesment for Public Health, A. Lawson, et al., Editors. 1999, John Wiley & Sons Ltd. p. 218–228.
50. Goldstein, H., Multilevel Statistical Models. 1995, London: Edward Arnold.

Evidence-based dentistry and dental Public Health: a German perspective

Klaus W. Böning · Burkhard H. Wolf · Michael H. Walter

Introduction

In recent years Dental Public Health gained increased attention in Germany. Evidence-based Dentistry is a subject closely related to Dental Public Health and must be considered an essential but still underestimated tool for professionals working in the field of Public Health.

In the context of Dental Public Health, Evidence-based Dentistry (EBD) has practical as well as political impact such as the delivery of structured information in a user-friendly format for patients, professionals and other people involved in dental health care, quality management, validation of the benefit of diagnostic tests or therapies and on optimising the allocation of the declining resources in the health care systems [56–58, 60, 62]. Last not least neglecting the instruments of EBD in Dental Public Health results in an enormous waste of resources, because frequently we see the following scenario: An expensive study is conducted, financed through grants by the tax payer. After publication in a sophisticated international journal the study results remain hidden to the ordinary practitioner due to the enormous bulk of dental and medical literature. The intention, to make the relevant information accessible to the public is one major task of EBD.

Even before the publication of the classic book on Evidence-based Dentistry by David Sackett et al. [50], the necessity of a dentistry based on evidence was pointed out in English dental journals already in 1996 [11, 28]. Subsequently many authors contributed to this topic in editorials and overviews. For example the December issue of the Quintessence International 1998 dedicated most of its space to contributions on Evidence-based Dentistry and the Journal of Prosthetic Dentistry published between January and July 2000 a sequence of eight articles which made the principles of EBD accessible to the readers.

With some delay Germany has recognised the importance of EBD [37, 44, 47, 48]. This article shall represent the present state of EBD, its possible impact on clinical decision making in prosthetic dentistry and its importance to future dental education.

The scientific environment in German dentistry

About 500 dental journals and periodicals world-wide publish approximately 42 000 articles annually [9]. Despite this high number of publications the number of clinical studies of high level of evidence is very limited. Dumbrigue et al. [18] found that of 3631 articles, published between 1988 and 1997 in three leading international prosthetic journals (Journal of Prosthetic Dentistry, International Journal of Prosthodontics, Journal of Prosthodontics) only 62 (1,7%) were randomised controlled trials. In addition, MEDLINE based bibliometric studies [3, 42] pointed out, that between 1995 and 1997 clearly less randomised controlled trials and meta-analyses were conducted in dentistry compared to medical fields. The average number the meta-analyses per year in dentistry amounted to 8, compared to 38 in the medical fields (average value of seven fields considered) [42].

One or more of the following reasons may be responsible for this discrepancy between medicine and dentistry [7]:

In clinical dental education the students work independently with their patients; at German universities this is the case in the last four out of ten semesters. The necessary high intensity of surveillance in these clinical courses is binding faculty resources.

The pressure on young researchers to "publish or perish" is contra productive with regard to long-term trials and follow-ups. To compete successfully, young researchers aiming at a university career, are forced to publish a high number of articles in a relatively short time frame. So, ironically the quality and longevity of dental restorations become a problem: True end points like tooth loss, breakdown of a restoration or prosthetic concept may not occur until many years of service. For this reason prospective long-term studies are avoided, not only due to their costs, but also for their extraordinary time frame [59]. Researchers in dentistry favourably conduct retrospective studies or use early measurable, but less powerful surrogate criteria instead of true end points.

In Germany, dental materials are not controlled by the legal regimes for pharmaceuticals. Hence there is no necessity enforced by law to conduct phase II, III and IV studies, which are mandatory when introducing new pharmaceutics.

Due to marketing-strategies of the dental industry the time periods between the introduction of new or changed products become shorter and shorter. This makes clinical studies absurd, if products under investigation are replaced shortly after publication or even within the time frame of the study. Therefore, dental researchers are cautious to conduct studies beyond laboratory tests, short-term observations or case reports, if the long-term availability of the product is doubtful.

Difficulties and problems of finding evidence and critical appraisal

There are various difficulties in finding strong evidence in the field of dentistry. According to estimates by Richards [49] presently only 8% of dental therapies are based on results from randomised controlled studies. With regard to the lack of strong evidence from clinical studies clinicians, faculty and students are dependent on consensus-statements or expert opinions as the best evidence available in most areas of dentistry.

Among others the following data sources are available for a fast access to summarised information at different levels of evidence:

The systematic reviews of the Oral Health Group of the Cochrane Collaboration, which can be considered the most reliable evidence in dentistry (Table 1).

Since November 1998 the journal *Evidence-Based Dentistry* searches the international dental literature for relevant randomised controlled trials (RCTs) and systematic reviews and publishes them in summarised form. To these summaries a comment from an expert in the field of EBD is added.

Since June 2001 the Journal of Evidence-Based Dental Practice is available, which also reviews and comments primary literature.

There are different Web sites with EBD topics to relevant questions (Table 2).

A comprehensive data base of medical guidelines is published by the Association of the Scientific Medical Societies in Germany (140 societies). In the data base guidelines relevant for dentistry are included. They were developed by the German Society for Maxillo-Facial Surgery. The guidelines are based mainly on the instruments of formal consensus or Delphi conferences. Evidence in form of systematic reviews normally is not included.

Table 1. Systematic reviews published by the Cochrane Collaboration (January 2003)

Fluoride gels for preventing dental caries in children and adolescents
Fluoride varnishes for preventing dental caries in children and adolescents
Guided tissue regeneration for periodontal infra-bony defects
Interventions for preventing oral candidiasis for patients with cancer receiving treatment
Interventions for preventing oral mucositis or oral candidiasis for patients with cancer receiving chemotherapy (excluding head and neck cancer)
Interventions for replacing missing teeth: hyperbaric oxygen therapy for irradiated patients who require dental implants
Interventions for replacing missing teeth: preprosthetic surgery versus dental implants
Interventions for replacing missing teeth: maintaining and re-establishing healthy tissues around dental implants
Interventions for replacing missing teeth: different types of dental implants
Interventions for the treatment of burning mouth syndrome
Interventions for treating oral mucositis for patients with cancer receiving treatment
Interventions for treating oral leukoplakia
Interventions for treating oral candidiasis for patients with cancer receiving treatment
Interventions for treating oral lichen planus
Orthodontic treatment for posterior crossbites
Potassium nitrate toothpaste for dentine hypersensitivity

Table 2. Internet-Links to web sites with topics concerning Evidence-based Dentistry, guidelines and scientific statements

Institution	Web-Address
Centre for Evidence-Based Dentistry	http://www.ihs.ox.ac.uk/cebd/
Cochrane Oral Health Group	http://www.cochrane-oral.man.ac.uk/
Dental Health Services Research Unit	http://www.dundee.ac.uk/dhsru/
Health Evidence Bulletins Wales	http://hebw.uwcm.ac.uk/oralhealth/index.html
German Society of Dentistry and Oral Medicine	http://www.dgzmk.de
Association of the Scientific Medical Societies in Germany	http://www.awmf-online.de/

Scientific statements with evidence levels ranging from formal consensus to expert opinion are published by the German Society of Dentistry and Oral Medicine. These statements are published in the journals *Zahnärztliche Mitteilungen* and *Deutsche Zahnärztliche Zeitschrift* and are also available online (http://www.dgzmk.de).

A peculiar problem in Evidence-based Dentistry is the step of critical appraisal within the literature review process. Standards and procedures generally accepted in Evidence based Medicine [29, 38] are of limited validity in dentistry. For instance in dentistry blinding or even double blinding is not possible in most clinical trials (e.g., comparison of different dentures, different therapeutic strategies or different surgical treatments). In other cases randomisation is not feasible ethically, because patient desire must be part of the decision-making process (example: after loss of a central incisor the dentist must inform the patient about therapeutic alternatives like implants, adhesive bridges or conventional bridges). Hence, according to the evaluation standards set for Evidence based Medicine, clinical trials in dentistry are more prone to poor quality ratings.

Other problems of a critical appraisal in dental literature lie in the large variation of end points and surrogates, different social and ethnic backgrounds, in which the studies were conducted, the high drop out rates in dental long-term studies as well as in differences with regard to the nomenclature of the therapeutic appliances. For instance in many anglo-american publications the term removable partial denture describes simple resin based prostheses with wrought wire clasps, while European publications (especially papers from Germany) describe removable partial dentures with cast clasps, telescopic crowns or precision attachments [34].

These problems are partially due to the fact that so far there are no generally accepted standards for the publication of clinical studies. On the other hand attempts have been made recently to standardise the quality of publications of clinical studies (CONSORT-STATEMENT [63]).

Guideline equivalents in Germany

The general discussion on quality management, the international acceptance of guidelines as instruments of the quality assurance and the advanced guideline development in medicine led to the understanding, that guidelines in dentistry might be useful [8]. So the German federal dentists' chamber advocated for a development of guidelines in their September 2000 statement concerning quality assurance. Nevertheless, a development of guidelines in dentistry is still in "statu nascendi".

Scientific statements are developed, published and maintained by the German Society of Dentistry and Oral Medicine (DGZMK) (Table 2). Arguments for and against a systematic development of guidelines in dentistry are discussed controversially within the scientific societies. First of all there is the argument of the absence of high-level evidence from clinical studies in most fields in dentistry. Furthermore there is a fear among dentists, that guidelines might be misinterpreted as directives by lawyers and judges and misused by health insurance companies as an instrument to reduce costs. Whether the implementation of guidelines in dentistry would lead to a significant reduction in costs or to an increase of normative treatment need remains unclear. If guidelines are able to maintain or even accelerate the increasing success in primary and secondary prevention, edentulousness in the elder population will decline and prevalence of partial or even full dentition increase. Hence, a rise of normative dental treatment need such as periodontal treatment, root caries treatment, fixed or removable partial dentures would be conceivable and expected especially in geriatric dentistry.

Application of evidence-based dentistry in the decision making process in prosthetic dentistry

Prosthetic dentistry probably is the field of dentistry requiring the most sophisticated treatment decisions. However, trying to implement evidence based approaches in every day decision-making the committed dentist fairly often encounters problems that might finally lead to disillusionment and disappointment. Due to a lack of high-level evidence concerning most concrete questions he still has to rely on traditional paradigms and his own expertise. Even a thorough and time-consuming literature search will not provide a solution to his problem in many cases. Furthermore, clinical decision-making is based on a number of criteria that are handled and weighed in astonishingly diverse ways leading to the well-known phenomenon of abundance of treatment variations. There have been only few attempts to score prosthetic treatment need, sometimes using complicated algorithms [20]. Realising these shortcomings, the authors proposed an index system that is intended to serve as a clinical tool in need assessment and decision-making [61]. It bases on a multidimensional understanding of prosthetic treatment need. Simplicity and universal applicability were given highest priority. The system was designed to systematise the

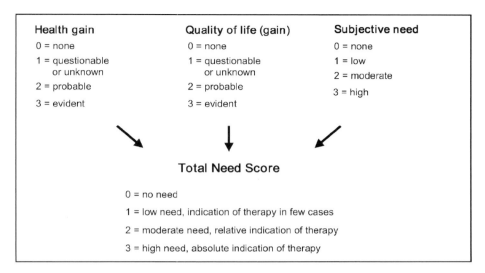

Fig. 1. Prosthetic Treatment Need Index. Rating of components and total need

clinical decision-making process by considering always the same and most important components of prosthetic treatment need: health gain, gain in oral health-related quality of life (QOL), and patient's perception, i.e. subjective need. Thus, our system comprises these three basic components (Fig. 1). All components are scored 0 to 3. The parameters health gain and QOL are evaluated by professional assessment on the basis of best available evidence. With the parameter health gain aspects of (physical) health are taken into account such as tissue preservation, risk-benefit ratio, and longevity. Aspects to be considered with the parameter QOL are psychosocial well-being, masticatory ability, phonetics, esthetics etc. Subjective need is scored by the patient. This component reflects the necessity of considering patient perception, which is approved by most modern prosthodontists who advocate a patient-centered approach. The components may be regarded separately. Alternatively, a total (e.g. mean) score can be calculated from the three basic components. The index may be used for general need assessment. However, because of a strong dependence of need on the available treatment the instrument is especially suitable for need assessment regarding a certain treatment in a certain clinical situation.

The index is by no means an expert system for decision-making. It is basically a structured framework. The user has to collect and appraise knowledge to assign a treatment to one of the ratings in each component. It shall help to systematise clinical decision-making and will whenever used require a structured decision-making process. By asking for scores the question of the available evidence rises almost automatically, brings the lack of it home to the user frequently and by this strengthens critical thinking. It has to be emphasised that rating certain clinical treatments have to be subject of steady adjustment because of the change of our knowledge base with time.

As a matter of course, the index systems needs more development and evolution for being applicable in dental routine work. As a first step in that direction we conducted a pilot study to pretest the system with special focus on practicability and inter-individual variability of the professionally assessed parameters health gain and QOL.

For pretesting, 20 dentists from a dental school setting were asked to participate. None of them had his main interest or focus in prosthodontics. There were no further inclusion

Table 3. Ratings for index components health gain and QOL (in parantheses) for 18 treatments made by 20 dentists. Median, range, and interquartile range for the different therapy options. For description of cases and therapy options see Table 2

Therapy option	1.1	1.2	1.3	2.1	2.2	2.3	3.1	3.2	3.3	4.1	4.2	4.3	5.1	5.2	5.3	6.1	6.2	6.3
Median	2	1	3	1	1	3	2	2	1	2	2	2	2	2	2	2	2	2
	(2)	(2)	(3)	(2)	(2)	(3)	(2)	(2)	(1)	(2)	(3)	(3)	(2)	(2)	(3)	(3)	(2)	(3)
Range	2	3	1	2	2	1	3	3	2	3	2	2	1	2	3	3	2	3
	(2)	(2)	(1)	(2)	(3)	(1)	(2)	(2)	(3)	(2)	(1)	(2)	(2)	(2)	(2)	(1)	(2)	(3)
Inter-quartile range	1	1	1	0.75	1	1	1	1.5	1	1	1	1	0.75	1	1	0	1	1
	(1)	(1)	(1)	(1)	(0)	(1)	(1)	(1.75)	(1)	(1)	(1)	(1)	(1)	(1)	(1)	(1)	(1)	(1)

and exclusion criteria because of the explorative feature of the study. The subjects received information on the index system. They further got standardized information on six common clinical cases including history, intraoral photographs, clinical assessment, and additional case dependent findings. For each of these cases three different treatment options were offered. The participants were asked to score all treatment options for health gain and QOL resulting in a total of 18 assessments per person.

Table 3 gives the results for all 18 treatment options. The results indicated substantial inter-individual variations in health gain and QOL ratings among dental professionals displayed by high ranges. For both components the ranges were up to the highest possible value 3 and never 0, i.e. within the 18 therapy options there was not one, which was scored unanimously. For health gain, an interquartile range 1 was found 14 times out of 18. For QOL, an interquartile range 1 was found 16 times out of 18.

To score the treatment options on a more systematic and evidence-based basis, scientific literature was searched using EBM-principles in Medline and by full-text examination with the following question: Which knowledge base exists for the clinical cases and treatment options respectively regarding health gain and QOL? Exclusively meta-analyses and randomised controlled trials (RCTs) were included and served as indicators for the available knowledge based on high level evidence. The search was terminated in January, 2002. 98 meta-analyses were found. After full-text examination the number of the suitable meta-analyses decreased to 8. 486 randomised clinical trials were identified. After full-text examination only 29 papers remained.

The number of the relevant publications for the cases # 1, 2, and 3 is shown in Table 4. High level evidence was lacking concerning the health gain aspects tissue preservation and risk-benefit-ratio. Furthermore, evidence was lacking concerning QOL aspects. Only one RCT could be found.

The results of the systematic search of the prosthetic literature for the cases # 4, 5, and 6 are given in Table 5. The best knowledge base was found for the edentulous mandible.

Within the limits of this explorative study, it was concluded that high-level evidence is rare or lacking regarding questions related to health gain and QOL in most common prosthetic cases. This finding may partially explain the substantial inter-individual variations in rating health gain and QOL among dental professionals and, more in general, the well-known and ubiquitous therapy variations in dentistry. Great efforts are needed to transfer the available knowledge to the dental practitioner. Within the scientific community the focus should be laid on high quality studies on health gain and QOL aspects.

Provided further development, the index system could be transferred from the individual patient level to a populational level for example to identify under-treatment, false, or over-treatment. By this, a strong Public-Health dimension is obvious.

Table 4. Results of a systematic search of the literature for relevant meta-analyses and randomized controlled trials (RCTs). Cases # 1–3

Case	Therapy options		Number of relevant publications				
			Health gain				QoL
			Tissue preservation	Secondary damage/prevention	Risk-benefit-ratio	Longevity	Masticatory ability, phonetics, physiognomy, esthetics
#1 Missing central incisor (maxilla)	#1.1 Resin bonded bridge	Meta-analyses	–	–	–	[16]	–
		RCTs	–	–	–	–	–
	#1.2 Fixed partial denture	Meta-analyses	–	[51]	–	[15, 51]	–
		RCTs	–	–	–	–	–
	#1.3 Implant	Meta-analyses	–	[19, 54]	–	[14, 33]	–
		RCTs	–	–	–	[52]	–
#2 Missing first pre-molar (maxilla)	#2.1 Fixed partial denture	Meta-analyses	–	[15, 51]	–	–	–
		RCTs	–	–	–	–	–
	#2.2 Cantilever fixed partial denture	Meta-analyses	–	[10, 51]	–	[15, 51]	–
		RCTs	–	–	–	–	–
	#2.3 Implant	Meta-analyses	–	[19]	–	[14, 33]	–
		RCTs	–	–	–	[52]	–
#3 Uni-laterally missing molars (mandible)	#3.1 Cantilever fixed partial denture	Metaanalyses	–	[51]	–	[15, 51]	–
		RCTs	–	–	–	–	[39]
	#3.2 Two implants	Meta-analyses	–	[19]	–	[14, 33]	–
		RCTs	–	–	–	[27]	–
	#3.3 Removable partial denture	Meta-analyses	–	–	–	–	–
		RCTs	–	–	–	–	–

Dissemination and implementation of EBD in dental education

The curriculum in German dental education is still based on legislation from the year 1955 with a strong focus on technical and manual training. In recent years paradigms in dentistry have shifted from the traditional curative approach towards prevention orientated dentistry. Furthermore half-life periods of medical knowledge are getting shorter and shorter and it is easy to predict that the field of geriatric dentistry will be a main future challenge. Hence future dental education must also strengthen the students' ability for continuing self-education, handling of electronic data bases and critical appraisal of information [45].

To meet these demands, numerous international dental schools implemented the concept of Problem Based Learning (PBL). By an active integration of the students into the learning process PBL focuses on the transfer of knowledge as well as on teaching how to gather and critically appraise information from textbooks, journals and electronic databases.

Table 5. Results of a systematic search of the literature for relevant meta-analyses and randomized controlled trials (RCTs). Cases #4–6

Case	Therapy options		Number of relevant publications				
			Health gain				QoL
			Tissue preservation	Secondary damage/ prevention	Risk-benefit-ratio	Longevity	Mastica-tory ability, phonetics, physio-gnomy, esthetics
#4 Edentulous mandible	#4.1 Complete denture	Meta-analyses	–	–	–	–	–
		RCTs	–	–	[12]	[2, 12, 17 26, 46]	[1, 2, 5, 6, 22–26, 46]
	#4.2 Implant overdenture	Meta-analyses	–	[19, 54]	[54]	[14, 19, 54]	–
		RCTs	–	[12, 41, 55]	–	[4, 35, 36, 43, 52, 55]	[2, 5, 6, 13, 17, 21–26, 46, 53]
	#4.3 Implant bridge	Meta-analyses	–	[19, 54]	–	[14, 54]	[13, 17, 21]
		RCTs	–	[41, 43, 55]	[55]	[30–32, 40, 52, 64]	
#5 Multiple tooth loss (mandible)	#5.1 Removable partial denture (telescopic)	Meta-analyses	–	–	–	–	–
		RCTs	–	–	–	–	–
	#5.2 Removable partial denture (Dolder bar)	Meta-analyses	–	–	–	–	–
		RCTs	–	–	–	–	–
	#5.3 Implant bridge (after tooth extraction)	Meta-analyses	–	–	–	[14]	–
		RCTs	–	–	–	–	–
#6 Multiple tooth loss (maxilla)	#6.1 Fixed partial denture	Meta-analyses	–	[51]	–	[15, 51]	–
		RCTs	–	–	–	–	–
	#6.2 Removable partial denture	Meta-analyses	–	–	–	–	–
		RCTs	–	–	–	–	–
	#6.3 Implants	Meta-analyses	–	[19]	–	[14, 33]	–
		RCTs	–	–	–	[52]	–

In PBL tutorials with small students groups (8 to 10) medical or dental problems are presented on the basis of adapted patient cases. The students compile data and facts from the cases, analyse the complaints and draw hypotheses. In a discussion guided by a tutor they decide which further information is needed to support or reject their hypotheses.

Between single tutorials the students search and compile information needed independently. The independent search for information and knowledge confronts the students with the problems of search strategies in dental journals and electronic databases and also with the problem to handle the growing information overload.

The discussion of divergent information from textbooks, journals or electronic databases rises questions about validity and reliability and ultimately leads to the hierarchy of levels of evidence. So the concept and philosophy of Evidence-based Dentistry can be considered an integral component of the method of Problem Based Learning.

Future perspectives of evidence-based dentistry

The future success of Evidence-based Dentistry depends on the question whether its concepts can be integrated in every day practice. Currently the discussions and activities are theoretical and limited mainly to academic platforms. The following suggestions might be crucial for a successful implementation.

► Systematic training of dental students and dentists with the purpose of learning the principles of EBD and how to convert them into practice. Dentists should be offered more EBD courses as it is already the case in Great Britain (e.g. from the Cochrane Oral Health Group [www.cochrane-oral.man.ac.uk] and from the University of Oxford [www.conted.ox.ac.uk/health/htmlfiles/dentistry/dentfr.htm]).

► Implementation of EBD should be made easy for the dentist. Practitioners who spent a ten-hour working day in their private practice cannot be expected to read sophisticated English literature in the evening, neither will they browse through English EBD databases. Translation of summaries, systematic reviews, guidelines or other sources of high level evidence already existing into native language and a broad publication of these articles are crucial.

► Systematic compilation of the relevant clinical studies from the different disciplines of dentistry that have been published in German speaking journals. These efforts are time consuming. However, unfortunately many German speaking dental journals, even premium journals like the Deutsche Zahnärztliche Zeitschrift are not listed in the Medline data base, maintained by the U.S. National Library of Medicine. By a separate compilation of German studies, these would be much easier accessible.

A positive aspect is the integration of dentistry into the co-ordination circle of the German network for Evidence based Medicine (www.ebm-netzwerk.de). This acknowledges the importance of Evidence-based Dentistry within the entire field of dentistry and within the overall development of Evidence-based Medicine.

References

1. Awad MA, Feine JS (1998) Measuring patient satisfaction with mandibular prostheses. Community Dent Oral Epidemiol 26:400–405.
2. Awad MA, Locker D, Korner-Bitensky N, Feine JS (2000) Measuring the effect of intra-oral implant rehabilitation on health-related quality of life in a randomized controlled clinical trial. J Dent Res 79:1659–1663.
3. Badovinac R., Conway S., R. N (1999) Bibliometric analysis of evidence-based dental therapeutics literature. J Dent Res (spec issue) 78:124 (abstr. 148).
4. Bergendal T, Engquist B (1998) Implant-supported overdentures: a longitudinal prospective study. Int J Oral Maxillofac Implants 13:253–262.
5. Boerrigter EM, Geertman ME, Van Oort RP, Bouma J, Raghoebar GM, van Waas MA, et al. (1995) Patient satisfaction with implant-retained mandibular overdentures. A comparison with new complete dentures not retained by implants – a multicentre randomized clinical trial. Br J Oral Maxillofac Surg 33:282–288.
6. Boerrigter EM, Stegenga B, Raghoebar GM, Boering G (1995) Patient satisfaction and chewing ability with implant-retained mandibular overdentures: a comparison with new complete dentures with or without preprosthetic surgery. J Oral Maxillofac Surg 53:1167–1173.

7. Böning K (2000) Leitlinien in der Zahnmedizin? In: Walter M, Böning K (eds). Public Health und Zahngesundheit. Mundgesundheitsziele. Workshop Freiburg 1999. Roderer, Regensburg. pp. 55–77.
8. Böning K (2000) Leitlinien in der Zahnmedizin? [Editorial]. Dtsch Zahnärztl Z 55:293–294
9. Böning K, Walter M (2000) Evidenz-basierte Zahnmedizin. ZMK 16:290–293.
10. Budtz-Jorgensen E, Isidor F (1990) A 5-year longitudinal study of cantilevered fixed partial dentures compared with removable partial dentures in a geriatric population. J Prosthet Dent 64:42–47.
11. Burke FJT (1996) Finding the evidence. Dental update 23:269.
12. Burns DR, Unger JW, Elswick RK, Beck DA (1995) Prospective clinical evaluation of mandibular implant overdentures: Part I – Retention, stability, and tissue response. J Prosthet Dent 73:354–363.
13. Burns DR, Unger JW, Elswick RK, Giglio JA (1995) Prospective clinical evaluation of mandibular implant overdentures: Part II–Patient satisfaction and preference. J Prosthet Dent 73:364–369.
14. Cochran DL (1999) A comparison of endosseous dental implant surfaces. J Periodontol 70:1523–1539.
15. Creugers NH, Kayser AF, van't Hof MA (1994) A meta-analysis of durability data on conventional fixed bridges. Community Dent Oral Epidemiol 22:448–452.
16. Creugers NH, Van't Hof MA (1991) An analysis of clinical studies on resin-bonded bridges. J Dent Res 70:146–149.
17. de Grandmont P, Feine JS, Tache R, Boudrias P, Donohue WB, Tanguay R, et al. (1994) Within-subject comparisons of implant-supported mandibular prostheses: psychometric evaluation. J Dent Res 73:1096–1104.
18. Dumbrigue HB, Jones JS, Esquivel JF (1999) Developing a register for randomized controlled trials in prosthodontics: results of a search from prosthodontic journals published in the United States. J Prosthet Dent 82:699–703.
19. Esposito M, Hirsch JM, Lekholm U, Thomsen P (1998) Biological factors contributing to failures of osseointegrated oral implants. (II). Etiopathogenesis. Eur J Oral Sci 106:721–764.
20. Falcon HC, Richardson P, Shaw MJ, Bulman JS, Smith BG (2001) Developing an index of restorative dental treatment need. Br Dent J 190:479–486.
21. Feine JS, de Grandmont P, Boudrias P, Brien N, LaMarche C, Tache R, et al. (1994) Within-subject comparisons of implant-supported mandibular prostheses: choice of prosthesis. J Dent Res 73:1105–1111.
22. Fontijn-Tekamp FA, Slagter AP, van't Hof MA, Kalk W, Jansen JA (2001) Pain and instability during biting with mandibular implant-retained overdentures. Clin Oral Implants Res 12:46–51.
23. Fontijn-Tekamp FA, Slagter AP, van't Hof MA, Geertman ME, Kalk W (1998) Bite forces with mandibular implant-retained overdentures. J Dent Res 77:1832–1839.
24. Geertman ME, Boerrigter EM, Van Waas MA, van Oort RP (1996) Clinical aspects of a multicenter clinical trial of implant-retained mandibular overdentures in patients with severely resorbed mandibles. J Prosthet Dent 75:194–204.
25. Geertman ME, Slagter AP, van't Hof MA, van Waas MA, Kalk W (1999) Masticatory performance and chewing experience with implant-retained mandibular overdentures. J Oral Rehabil 26:7–13.
26. Geertman ME, Slagter AP, van Waas MA, Kalk W (1994) Comminution of food with mandibular implant-retained overdentures. J Dent Res 73:1858–1864.
27. Gunne J, Astrand P, Lindh T, Borg K, Olsson M (1999) Tooth-implant and implant supported fixed partial dentures: a 10-year report. Int J Prosthodont 12:216–221.
28. Hargreaves JA (1996) Evidence-based dentistry. J Can Dent Assoc 62:947–956.
29. Jadad AR, Cook DJ, Jones A, Klassen TP, Tugwell P, Moher M, et al. (1998) Methodology and reports of systematic reviews and meta-analyses: a comparison of Cochrane reviews with articles published in paper-based journals. Jama 280:278–280.
30. Kapur KK (1989) Veterans Administration Cooperative Dental Implant Study – comparisons between fixed partial dentures supported by blade-vent implants and removable partial dentures. Part II: Comparisons of success rates and periodontal health between two treatment modalities. J Prosthet Dent 62:685–703.
31. Kwakman JM, Voorsmit RA, Freihofer HP, Van Waas MA, Geertman ME (1998) Randomized prospective clinical trial of two implant systems for overdenture treatment: a comparison of the 2-year and 5-year results using the clinical implant performance scale. Int J Oral Maxillofac Surg 27:94–98.
32. Kwakman JM, Voorsmit RA, van Waas MA, Freihofer HP, Geertman ME (1996) Transmandibular implant versus intramobile cylinder implants: a randomized, prospective clinical trial. Int J Oral Maxillofac Surg 25:433–438.

33. Lindh T, Gunne J, Tillberg A, Molin M (1998) A meta-analysis of implants in partial edentulism. Clin Oral Implants Res 9:80–90.
34. Luthardt R, Spieckermann J, Böning K, Walter M (2000) Therapie der verkürzten Zahnreihe. Dtsch Zahnärztl Z 55:592–609.
35. Meijer HJ, Geertman ME, Raghoebar GM, Kwakman JM (2001) Implant-retained mandibular overdentures: 6-year results of a multicenter clinical trial on 3 different implant systems. J Oral Maxillofac Surg 59:1260–1268.
36. Meijer HJ, Raghoebar GM, Van't Hof MA, Visser A, Geertman ME, Van Oort RP (2000) A controlled clinical trial of implant-retained mandibular overdentures; five-years' results of clinical aspects and aftercare of IMZ implants and Branemark implants. Clin Oral Implants Res 11:441–447.
37. Meyle J (2000) Evidence based medicine (EBM) in der Parodontologie. In: Heidemann D (ed). Deutscher Zahnärzte Kalender 2000. Deutscher Zahnärzte Verlag, Köln. pp. 33–44.
38. Moher D, Jadad AR, Nichol G, Penman M, Tugwell P, Walsh S (1995) Assessing the quality of randomized controlled trials: an annotated bibliography of scales and checklists. Control Clin Trials 16:62–73.
39. Moynihan PJ, Butler TJ, Thomason JM, Jepson NJ (2000) Nutrient intake in partially dentate patients: the effect of prosthetic rehabilitation. J Dent 28:557–563.
40. Naert IE, Duyck JA, Hosny MM, Quirynen M, van Steenberghe D (2001) Freestanding and tooth-implant connected prostheses in the treatment of partially edentulous patients Part II: An up to 15-years radiographic evaluation. Clin Oral Implants Res 12:245–251.
41. Narhi TO, Geertman ME, Hevinga M, Abdo H, Kalk W (2000) Changes in the edentulous maxilla in persons wearing implant-retained mandibular overdentures. J Prosthet Dent 84:43–49.
42. Niederman R, Badovinac R (1999) Tradition-based dental care and evidence-based dental care. J Dent Res 78:1288–1291.
43. Payne AG, Solomons YF (2000) The prosthodontic maintenance requirements of mandibular mucosa- and implant-supported overdentures: a review of the literature. Int J Prosthodont 13:238–243.
44. Prchala G (2000) Evidence-Based Dentistry. Nachweis und Orientierung für die Praxis. Zahnärztl Mitt 90:106–111.
45. Priehn-Küpper S (2000) Modellkurs in Dresden. Problemorientiert erarbeiten Zahnmedizin-Studenten ihren Lernstoff. Zahnärztl Mitt 90:2162; 2164–2165.
46. Raghoebar GM, Meijer HJ, Stegenga B, van't Hof MA, van Oort RP, Vissink A (2000) Effectiveness of three treatment modalities for the edentulous mandible. A five-year randomized clinical trial. Clin Oral Implants Res 11:195–201.
47. Reich E (2000) Evidenzbasierte Kariologie. In: Heidemann D (ed). Deutscher Zahnärzte Kalender 2000. Deutscher Zahnärzte Verlag, Köln. pp. 1–32.
48. Reinert S (2000) Evidence based medicine in der Mund-Kiefer-Gesichtschirurgie. In: Heidemann D (ed). Deutscher Zahnärzte Kalender 2000. Deutscher Zahnärzte Verlag, Köln. pp. 45–52.
49. Richards D (1999) Evidence-based Dentistry International Collaborative Group. Evidence-Based Dentistry 2:3–4.
50. Sackett DL, Richardson WS, Rosenberg W, et al. (1997) Evidence-Based Medicine. How to Practice and Teach EBM. Churchill Livingstone, New York.
51. Scurria MS, Bader JD, Shugars DA (1998) Meta-analysis of fixed partial denture survival: prostheses and abutments. J Prosthet Dent 79:459–464.
52. Sethi A, Kaus T, Sochor P (2000) The use of angulated abutments in implant dentistry: five-year clinical results of an ongoing prospective study. Int J Oral Maxillofac Implants 15:801–810.
53. Tang L, Lund JP, Tache R, Clokie CM, Feine JS (1999) A within-subject comparison of mandibular long-bar and hybrid implant-supported prostheses: evaluation of masticatory function. J Dent Res 78:1544–1553.
54. Taylor TD (1998) Prosthodontic problems and limitations associated with osseointegration. J Prosthet Dent 79:74–78.
55. Tinsley D, Watson CJ, Russell JL (2001) A comparison of hydroxylapatite coated implant retained fixed and removable mandibular prostheses over 4 to 6 years. Clin Oral Implants Res 12:159–166.
56. Türp JC (2000) Symposium „Evidenzbasierte Zahnmedizin". Cochrane Netzwerk Deutschland: Rundbrief Nr. 6 für den deutschsprachigen Raum. www.cochrane.de/deutsch/pnews6/htm.
57. Türp JC (2000) Warum brauchen wir eine auf Evidenz basierende Zahnmedizin? [Editorial]. Quintessenz Zahntechn 26:547–549.
58. Türp JC (2001) Klinische Erfahrung und evidenzbasierte (Zahn-)Medizin – ein Widerspruch? [Editorial]. Quintessenz 52:5–6

59. Türp JC, Antes G (2000) EbM in der Zahnmedizin – Beispiel „Myoarthropathien des Kausystems". In: Kunz R, Ollenschläger G, Raspe HH, et al. (eds) Lehrbuch Evidenzbasierte Medizin in Klinik und Praxis. Deutscher Ärzte-Verlag, Köln. pp. 330–338.
60. Türp JC, Antes G (2000) Evidenzbasierte Zahnmedizin. Dtsch Zahnärztl Z 55:394–400.
61. Walter M, Wolf B, Rieger C, Boening K (2001) The Prosthetic Treatment Need Index PTNI: a new multidimensional approach. Community Dental Health 18:195.
62. Walther W, Micheelis W (2000) Evidence-Based Dentistry. Evidenz-basierte Medizin in der Zahn-, Mund- und Kieferheilkunde. Deutscher Zahnärzte Verlag DÄV-Hanser, Köln.
63. Windeler J, Koch A (2000) CONSORT – was eine ordentliche wissenschaftliche Publikation leisten muss. Med Klin, pp 91–97.
64. Wismeijer D, Van Waas MA, Vermeeren JI, Mulder J, Kalk W (1997) Patient satisfaction with implant-supported mandibular overdentures. A comparison of three treatment strategies with ITI-dental implants. Int J Oral Maxillofac Surg 26:263–267.

Part IV Information
         and Promotion

Public Use Files – The dissemination of empirical research data of the German Research Associations Public Health via the Internet

Dirk Meusel · Peggy Göpfert · Wilhelm Kirch

Introduction

Dibona, Stone & Ockman (1999) compare the general scientific practice with the Open Source movement in computer science. Counterpart to the commercial software model that created software giants like Microsoft, the Open Source movement has been matured to considerable importance since the advent of the Internet. In the here used sense, an open source describes a software development process, where all resources including the so called source code is shared and distributed for free within the framework of a GPL (General Public Licence). Nothing that contributed to a final software will be handled as a secret. The authors state:

Science, after all, is ultimately an Open Source enterprise. The scientific method rests on a process of discovery, and a process of justification. For scientific results to be justified, they must be replicable. Replication is not possible unless the source is shared: the hypothesis, the test conditions, and the results. The process of discovery can follow many paths, and at times scientific discoveries do occur in isolation. But ultimately the process of discovery must be served by sharing information: enabling other scientists to go forward where one cannot: pollinating the ideas of others so that something new may grow that otherwise would not have been born (Dibona, Stone, & Ockman 1999: 2).

Transforming this ideal type of scientific methodology into Public Health research practise provokes serious questions. On one hand, data sets in Public Health research often contain sensible patient data, which have to fulfil data privacy restriction guidelines. The Internet, on the other hand, has the distinction of being most non-restrictive in providing access to information. This sharp contrast, among others, leads to further questions: Does it match the research subject's interest that data (even if completely anonymous) is given to third parties (even if scientific). For which information of research practice does it seem meaningful to provide them on the Internet? In what respect could an advantage be seen for Open Source handling of research data in Public Health science?

The here given research practise report outlines issues connected to the creating of Public Use Files on the background of Public Health research in Germany. Benefits and obstacles in archiving and disseminating research data within Public Use files will be discussed.

Background

Since 1991, German research in Public Health was funded with approximately 50 million Euros of public tax incomes by the Federal Ministry of Education and Research (Bundesministerium für Bildung und Forschung, BMBF). Almost 200 research projects have been carried out with the objective to analyse health risks in the population and to develop strategies for prevention and health promotion. As one result, an enormous pool of research data has been created that addresses Public Health relevant topics. These topics comprise health risks and health promotion, children's and elderly health, dental health, health care quality, quality assurance and economy of health services, nutrition as well as information and communication in health care.

The importance of giving a public account of research activities faces new attention in Germany as well. Researchers in many European or North American countries meet this demand of accountability by publishing so called Public Use Files. On one hand, as outlined further down, these files provide transparency of research practice as well as research results. On the other, they provide the opportunity of secondary analysis of scientific data. The compilation of Public Use Files furthermore implies the advantage of promoting research results without additional expenses as well as the opportunity of stimulating research in one's emphasised field of interest.

In accordance with the German Association of Public Health (Deutsche Gesellschaft für Public Health, DGPH) and the BMBF, a workgroup *Public Use Files* has been set up with the purpose of archiving and publishing data of German Public Health research. It is enclosed with the Research Association Public Health Saxony and located in its central office in Dresden, Germany. Members of this workgroup are, among others, the commission of Public Affairs of the DGPH and the German Coordinating Agency for Public Health in Freiburg. This workgroup chooses suitable research projects, designs the formal framework for the Public Use File creation, and preserves the interest of the particular research project groups. One of the main objectives within this PUF workgroup is the dissemination of Public Use Files via Internet.

Defining Public Use Files

Most generally, a Public Use File can be defined as a scientific data set, which is distributed to various users via a variety of media (e.g. CD-ROM, Internet, paper copy). Nevertheless, a Public Use File may serve many intentions and even might have various names, of which we try to outline a selection in the following typology. One reason to publish scientific data sets in form of a Public Use File may lie in the distinction between scientific *data production* and *data analysis*. We call this first case *governmental driven data production*.

Governmental population surveys, as for instance the *microcencus* in Germany, produce huge amounts of scientific vulnerable data sets. Since one of the strictest data privacy protection laws exist in Germany, we like to outline the example in more detail to show different strategies involved in providing scientific data sets to public or scientific users.

The microcensus is the official representative statistics of the population and the labour market, involving every year 1% of all households in Germany (continuous household sample survey). The total number of households participating in the microcensus is about 370 000 (820 000 persons), including about 70 000 households (about 160 000 persons) in the new Laender and Berlin-East. The organisational and technical preparation of the microcensus is done at the Federal Statistical Office, while actually conducting the survey and processing the data are tasks of the statistical offices of the Laender... The purpose of the microcensus is to provide statistical information on the economic and social situation of the population as well as on employment, the labour market, and education (multi-purpose sample). It also provides estimates updating the results of the population census. In addition, it is used to evaluate other official statistics such as the sample survey of household income and expenditure (Federal Statistical Office Germany 2003).

On one hand, the approach of the microcensus is broad, covering a multitude of issues interesting to scientists of many disciplines. Moreover it provides a substantial data basis to evaluate these topics in a regular form. On the other hand, financial and human resources of the Federal Statistical Office as well as the Statistical Offices of the Laender do not allow data analysis as extensive as the potential of the data sets might suggest. In addition, data privacy protection laws prohibit the passing on of these data sets in their original form. A fact that might be of benefit for the surveyed subjects consequently provides scientist a dilemma: To have far-reaching data sets, which can not be employed in scientific research. At this point, the term *Public Use File* comes into play.

In fact, data sets are passed on for data analysis reasons from the Federal and Laender Statistical Offices to the scientific community with plausible benefits for both, whereas the name of the passed file does describe the degree of anonymity creating procedures that has been performed on the original data. The Federal Statistical Office distinguishes *Scientific Use Files, on-Site Scientific Use Files, Public Use Files* and *Remote computing*. The *Public Use File* in this definition describes a data set of total anonymity that can be given to any interested party in society. No information that might be used to trace back a research subject's identity can be found in these files. This strict procedure of creating anonymity describes a significant drawback from the scientist's point of view since s/he is no longer able to correlate the effects examined with socio-demographic variables of interest.

For that reason the Federal Statistical Office issues *Scientific Use Files* that are made available to scientists for further analysis. The degree of anonymity employed here is called *de facto anonymity* being not as restrictive as total anonymity and consequently providing more socio-demographic variables. The underlying ratio of *de facto anonymity* is that the expenses of tracing back the research subject's identity must be higher than the prospective benefit a possible intruder might have from this misuse of the data. These files represent the best balance between comfortable use and scientific requirements.

One step further, *on-Site Scientific Use Files* provide the possibility of employing microcensus data sets in the least restrictive manner. A lot of socio-demographic variables that can not be found in the off-site version of the Scientific Use File are to be found in the on-site version. This advantage has to be paid for with several restrictions that apply to the scientific user on-site. As the name suggests, the on-Site file can only be used at special network isolated workstations in the Federal and Laender Statistical Offices. Additionally, data analysis is possible at the specific file only, no comparison with other data sets will be allowed. Likewise results derived from the work with the file will be controlled by the office stuff.

Remote Computing, as the fourth strategy of making governmental data sets available should be regarded as a very innovative approach, although some serious drawbacks remain with it as well. The core idea is as genius as it is straight forward: the public or scientific user writes the source code needed for her/his statistical analysis in the statistical software of his/her preference (e.g. SPSS, STATA, SAS). A dummy file can be accessed for this reason that contains merely the data set's structure with no specific data contents. The source code of the desired statistical analysis is sent to the Federal or Laender Statistical Office, where the source code is evaluated for compliance with data protection and performed on the real data set. The result is sent back to the user after a second check. This approach provides the user probably with the most non-restrictive data sets. On the other hand, a lot of workload is put on the Statistical Office's staff for evaluating and performing the source codes delivered to them, resulting in longer waiting times.

The second case of Public Use File typology we call *data production as scientific service*. A German example of this kind can be seen in the *General Social Survey (ALLBUS)* carried out by the Centre for Survey Research and Methodology in Mannheim (for more information see: [http://www.gesis.org/en/social_monitoring/allbus/index.htm]) as a nongovernmental initiative.

The German General Social Survey (ALLBUS) is a biennial survey that has been conducted since 1980 on the attitudes, behaviour, and social structure of persons resident in Germany. A representative cross-section of the population is questioned using face-to-face interviews. As a service to social scientific research and teaching, ALLBUS data are disseminated to all interested persons and institutions as soon as the data and documentation have been prepared. ALLBUS is a substantively rich and methodologically sophisticated database which can be used for a variety of analytical purposes: (1) to describe and analyse attitudes, behaviour and social structure of Germans with up-to-date cross-sectional data; (2) for longitudinal analysis of German society (ALLBUS time series, replicated questions from other survey studies); and (3) for international comparative analysis. ALLBUS includes questions also asked in the American General Social Survey and the Polish General Social Survey (Centre for Survey Research and Methodology 2003).

Surveys, as resembled by ALLBUS, are carried out with the original intention to provide the scientific community with regular data sets for statistical analysis. Its aim is to make general variables available with a persistent quality to describe trends in the general population. Therefore the quality of data sets is tailored for being published as a Public or Scientific Use File from the beginning of fieldwork onwards. In this category, the use of the term *Public* or *Scientific* does not describe any difference in the data quality or the degree of anonymity of data sets, except that it highlights the targeted end user of the file. This practice is well known in Public Health science as well. The Robert-Koch-Institute in Berlin issues next to others the Federal Health Survey and the Health Survey East as Public Use Files (for more information see: [http://www.rki.de/gesund/daten/public/public.htm]).

In summarising, the criteria for the above mentioned Public or Scientific Use Files categories has been the separation of data accumulation and data analysis as well as the general population scope as a property of data quality. Drawing from the work done in the workgroup Public Use File with the Research Association Public Health Saxony in Dresden, we suggest a third type, named *data archiving as scientific service*. Here, Public or Scientific Use Files are produced out of scientific research projects posterior. Research projects are carried out using the conventional way of planning, data accumulation, data analysis and publication of results. However, afterwards the data sets of these projects get integrated in a Public Use File library, together with all resources and materials that accompanied the research team's work. This form of a Public Use File can be thought of as a collection of data sets, documentations, research reports, field instruments, coding and analysis instructions as well as publications. Clearly, as it provides advantages this type of issuing bears its own pitfalls as well and, thus, are outlined next.

Pro and contra of Public Use Files

Although research projects in German Public Health research have not been intended to publish data sets as Public Use Files, a fact that in turn produces sincere problems outlined further down, many positive factors support the collection, archiving and dissemination of research project's resources as Public Use Files.

First, the conception of Public Use Files provides the opportunity of *secondary analysis* as well as comparative analysis. The 'normal' course of research work could most conventionally be described by the conception of the research task, followed by data collection, data analysis and the publishing of results. Subsequently, data sets may be deleted to comply with data privacy guidelines, they may get simply lost or they may not be documented in detail to enable further use. The creation of a Public Use File out of the research project's resources can change such a lost of data, since data sets are being documented well, materials used in the original research are being stored together with the data sets and a recent overview of literature that has been published based on the data sets informs about the latest analysis carried out with the data set. If at all possible, the data set published in a Public Use File should be usable for secondary analysis even if the original research team finished its work or may no longer exist.

Second, additionally to the conventional publishing of research results in scientific literature, the publishing of data sets and research resources could contribute to more *transparency* and lucidity of research methods and designs, and therefore enabling other scientists to put scientific results better into order with the present body of knowledge in the field. Moreover, the publishing of Public Use Files supports the comprehensibility as well as the potential of the scientific results to add further research in the same direction. Therefore, as Public Use Files archived data sets may be used to perform follow-up studies to compare the original data with recently collected data.

Finally, Public Use Files may be used as study material to make Public Health training more attractive. Data sets may prove to be the optimal basis for the *instruction to scientific statistical analysis* by means of realistic data. Therefore, not only general survey data files could be used as study material, but also more specific data sets, which deal with individual populations. As a result, the training of statistical analysis could better approach the prospective fields of work for students involved in Public Health training.

There are, of course, contra arguments to the creating of Public Use Files. Firstly, as outlined in the second section of this article, the opportunity of violating data protection privacy requires data sets to be of a certain degree of anonymity. A supposed file user may use data sets under deceptive scientific reasons to trace back identity of research subjects. In turn, science would, at the very least, jeopardise the confidence between research and research subjects. At worst, a serious cut into the private sphere of research subjects would have been caused by publishing of data sets. However, not only the intended violating of data privacy might present a problem, but also the unauthorized passing of Public Use Files to third parties.

A second argument contra creating Public Use Files is the expenditure of designing and maintaining a data base. Because of its potential of being able to reproduce fast changing information instantly, access to information on the internet correlates to a considerable degree with the actuality of data. Nevertheless, the medium's potential fast changed into its prerequisite. Therefore, a constant updating is required for rapidly changing information, as there are contact details to research teams, literature information and subsequent research results. Public Use Files of smaller scale, as described here, are only useful in research practice, if that information is being provided in an up-to-date way.

Finally, an argument contra creating Public Use Files derives from the data quality in Public Health science. One central point of interest is the evaluation of medical or psychological diagnoses in relation to a specific or more general population. The interpretation of many of them requires a sound elementary knowledge in the constructs portrayed by the variables. A simple publishing of data sets might lead to misinterpretations or misjudgements of scientifically correct accumulated data by non-experienced third party analysts.

From ideal type to praxis

In the preceding sections, we gave a rough idea about categories of issuing scientific data sets as well as their pro and contras. We now like to move on discussing the potential of issuing Public Use Files in Public Health science and outlining the right approach for its realisation by referring to experiences made at our project's work. Since the workgroup's aim of creating a library with numerous Public Use Files of the type *data archiving as scientific service* can be seen as a relative novelty, little practical expertise could be shared with.

As Jacobi (2003) summarises, one of the classic problems in clinical psychology (and we propose in Public Health science more generally as well) is the extraction of a suitable sample. Common problems arise from the work with small sample sizes, as there are comparisons of one's own sample with population wide survey samples and the huge expenses of acquiring new samples for cross validation of results. These problems could be toned down if researchers were able to access data sets deriving from other studies in the field. Therefore, a prerequisite is a rather *standardised research approach*, especially in terms of socio-demographic variables. Herein we find the first quality a Public Use File of the *data archiving as scientific service* section should have as well as a worthwhile potential that the issuing bears if the prerequisite is realised.

The workgroup Public Use Files started with the selection of suitable projects out of a pool of about 200 Public Health research projects that had been funded by the Federal Ministry of Education and Research. The selection was done in the particular Research Associations because of their greater confidence with the projects methodology. Various criteria have been guiding the selection, as for instance whether there have been data accumulated in the research team's field work, the quality of the data sets and variables as well as the general suitability of the acquired data for publishing. Accordingly, the proposed working process at this stage has been contacting research teams, familiarising with data sets, documentation material and further resources as well as choosing suitable variables from data sets along with the appropriate strategy for realising the best level of anonymity. Subsequently, the creation, archiving and dissemination have been planned.

However, contacting research groups and communicating to them the idea of Public Use Files described further above proved to be one of the most difficult component of our mission. First, objectively based in the funded character of Public Health research, research teams get together in the research project's planning stage just as they break off when the research project is brought to an end. The chosen research projects had been in different levels of realization. Therefore, while some research teams could be contacted very easily, others just did not exit any more. As a result, no detailed resources, materials or documentations could be obtained from these research teams.

Since the creation of Public Use Files has not been in the original intention of the research groups, we faced many objections to the publishing or passing on of data sets within the research groups. The most common reasons for scepticism indicated to us have been doubts of maintaining data privacy, additional workload for the research team that could not be financially compensated by us, and, last but most important, a general distrust of publishing data. Here, we like to bring to a close the introductory metaphor from the beginning of this article.

The principle of free and open sharing of information, resources and data is still an ideal in science and even is well documented. Campell et al. (2002) reported 47 percent of geneticists being denied at least once with a request to another faculty for additional information, data or material in the preceding 3 years. The authors conducted a mailed survey in May to July 2000 of geneticists and other life scientists in the 100 US universities that received the most funding from the National Institutes of Health in 1998. Furthermore, 10 percent of all post-publication requests for additional information were reported of being denied in this study.

As reasons for withholding publication information, data or materials the authors mention in sequence of perceived importance: (1) effort required to actually produce materials or information; (2) need to protect a graduate student's, postdoctoral fellow's, or junior faculty member's ability to publish; (3) need to protect own ability to publish; (4) financial cost of actually providing the materials or information transfer; (5) likelihood that the other person will never reciprocate; (6) need to honor the requirements of an industrial sponsor; (7) need to preserve patient confidentiality; and (8) need to protect the commercial value of the results (Campbell et al. 2002).

The consequences of withholding research data and resources are best described with the words of Polanyi (1962), which the authors employ as introductory quote and which we liked to refer to again: "Without the free exchange of published scientific information and resources, researchers may unknowingly build on something less than the total accumulation of scientific knowledge or work on problems already solved" (Polanyi, cited in Campbell et. al. 2002: 473).

Out of the reasons for withholding data from the Campbell study, we experienced reasons (1) through (7) in sole occurrence as well as in mixed interplay. Furthermore, in Public Health research very often qualitative data is collected that are being obtained with personal interviews, subjective accounts or written statements from the research subjects. These data have to comply with data privacy restrictions in a particular way. Because of that reason and the reasons outlined above, we decided not only to provide the opportunity of publishing Public Use Files, but also to provide the opportunity of publishing, what we called, *Public Documentation Files*. These files follow the idea of Public Use Files, except that no specific data set is given away. Therefore, the Public Documentation File can be described as a collection of all resources that are produced during the research team's work, excluding the data sets. The latter have to be requested to the original research team directly, of which the recent contact details are stored with the Public Documentation File.

Quality criteria of Public Use Files

Quality criteria play a central role in the creation of Public Use Files, since it defines whether the file user is able to familiarize oneself with the presented data sets and documentation materials or whether additional help is required. Jacobi (2003) outlines six central criteria for proper documentation and provision of aiding materials that have to be included in a Public Use File: (1) background information about original aims and methods of the research project that collected the given data sets; (2) general information about handling the Public Use File, especially the file format and its evaluation; (3) Exact variable description and codebook with, as far as possible, the primary field instruments in form of questionnaires, interviewer guidelines etc.; (4) algorithms that have been employed to compute super ordinate variables, as for instance diagnoses computed out of symptom combinations, time criteria and exclusion criteria; (5) sample reference analysis for comparison that can be employed for a first controlled computation; and (6) a summary of recent analysis carried out using the data set (Jacobi 2003).

Within the *Public Use/Documentation File* library of Public Health research we tried to realise these criteria as best we could. Of course, creating multiple files simultaneously is making this task a difficult one. Therefore, especially concerning criteria (5) we work at a generalised routine that computes a standardised reference analysis to be performed on all files in the same way.

The realisation process

While we ran through the more theoretical parts of the Public Use File creation in the foregoing, we continue with the more technical side in the succeeding section. We start discussing the present situation and further describe the database design and data collec-

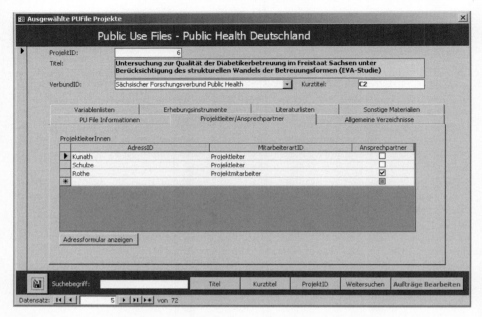

Fig. 1. Data base interface for managing the Public Use File documents, materials, and data sets

tion process. Section 8 will review the web interface as an innovative opportunity for research teams to work on their own Public Use/Documentation File online.

The present situation of the data base reflects an extensive information pool. The database comprises 76 Files in total, of which 31 files have been accepted as being published in form of a Public Use File. The remaining 45 files are being published as Public Documentation Files. Furthermore, 6 files are being published elsewhere (see for more details: Bavarian Research Association Public Health) and externally offered by the workgroup. The final research reports of 46 research projects have been scanned and are being provided in electronic form.

First step in realising the Public Use File database is collecting required data and documentations. These materials embrace five main areas: (1) *general information* about the research projects that are being evaluated using standardised describing categories; (2) *field instruments* as for example questionnaires, interview guidelines, research designs and research programmes; (3) *documentations* as for example variable descriptions and instructions for analysis; (4) *research reports* as for example final reports, literature listings, unpublished materials and further references; and (5) data files. Resources of all these categories are being collected in hard copy or electronically, depending on availability.

In a second step, all materials have been transferred into a local data base where information about research projects is associated with the research teams and stored in a relational data base structure. Figure 1 illustrates the user interface that has been programmed in the workgroup for managing all the data, documentations and data sets in both, the data base as well as the structured file system.

The data base not only serves the archiving of data and documentations, but also the complete work to create Public Use Files. Following the collection of materials and archiving them, various steps have to be performed: (1) analysis and description of data sets;

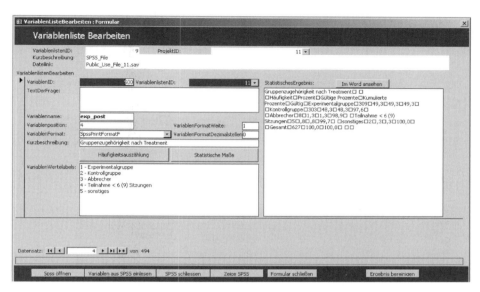

Fig. 2. Interface for working with data sets and performing simple statistical analysis

(2) the unified creation of files; and (3) providing information on the internet about the file and its contents. Since the workload increases with the number of Public Use Files to be created, an automatism had to be developed to handle all required working stages faster. Once the procedures that are necessary to create a Public Use File are programmed, several advantageous side effects can be benefited from. First, the Public Use Files are being created in a unified form, making navigation through multiple files easier to the final user. Second, Public Use Files can be created more easily in the future just using the already developed procedures. In the following, we outline some working stages of Public Use File creation in more detail.

Data sets are not being stored in the data base itself. Rather information about the data set's contents is stored in the data base for various purposes. On one hand, code books and variable descriptions can be created on the fly using that information. On the other hand, the information can be provided on internet in combination with a search engine, making the handling of code books or variable descriptions much easier and comfortable. Figure 2 illustrates the data working interface that transfers variable information from data sets into the data base. A SPSS® background procedure is used to obtain, among others, variable name, variable short description, value labels as well as a simple frequency statistics for each variable in the data set. The results are stored as a time stamp in the data base.

The same mechanism is used for creating the final hard copies of particular Public Use Files. In order to print the most updated information available, the procedure first involves updating the local data base with the latest information available from the web server. Afterwards the desired hard copies are created automatically using a MS Word® background procedure. Figure 3 demonstrates the interface used for this task, which in turn provides a pseudo programming strategy. An extensive expandable listing gathers prepared instructions, required parameters and file numbers. Afterwards, the listing is worked through by the underlying application resulting in the Public Use Files being written to a

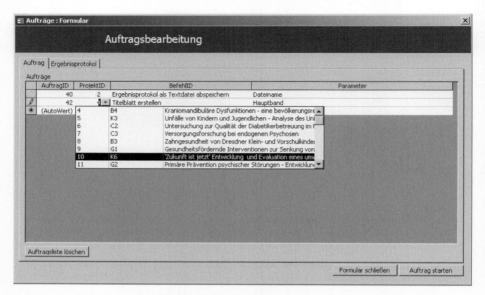

Fig. 3. Interface for creating hardcopy Public Use Files based on the latest available information

given directory or being sent to the printer. Performed actions and possible errors are written to a log file. Figure 4 illustrates the final design of an exemplary Public Use File main part.

The final file

Public Use or Documentation Files include several components and are being delivered either on CD-ROM only or as hard copy print out in combination with the CD-ROM. Additional costs for printing apply to the latter. Nevertheless, the given information in both is identical. The *main volume* contains all general information available about the research project: descriptive information, contact details, specific characteristics as well as latest literature and publication listings.

A second volume *field instruments* contains questionnaires, subscales as well as possible descriptions and instructions into these instruments. In case of a Public Use File, a third volume *variable description* encloses the code book with all the information about variables in the Public Use File's data sets. As the name suggests the fourth volume *final research reports* contains the electronically scanned final research reports.

Finally, on the delivered CD-ROM you find all volumes described above in form of an electronic *pdf* document (portable document format by Adobe) together with a free reader software. In case of a Public Use File, the CD-ROM furthermore contains the data set(s) in various file formats, above all a variety of SPSS® native formats, dBase formats and plain text formats. Moreover, the CD-ROM holds all associated data from the central data base in form of *html* tables that can be opened, read and searched through on every computing architecture without having installed additional software.

All volumes are identifiable by a unified design that helps to recognize different files as to belonging to the same library. Figure 4 illustrates the design on the basis of the main

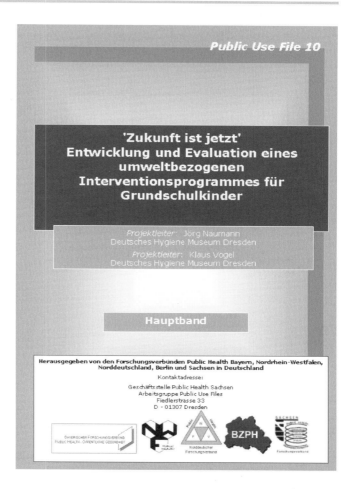

Fig. 4. The final design of a particular Public Use File

volume. Furthermore, the design is thought to communicate the idea of a similar navigation through the different volumes of a particular file as well as through the various files of the complete library. Identifying file number, file title and volume title is being made easier across all files.

The web interface

A central concern of the workgroup *PUF (Public Use File)* proved to be the handling of fast changing information as there are for instance contact details to research teams, publication information, research results etc. That information has to be handled dynamically instead of storing the information in static quality. Therefore, using the internet's potential to provide dynamically presented information presented itself as a first idea. Nevertheless, putting all data of potential Public Use Files to a web server conflicted with data security restrictions. A reasonable solution to this dilemma could be found in the conception of a *shared database*, which we intend to outline next.

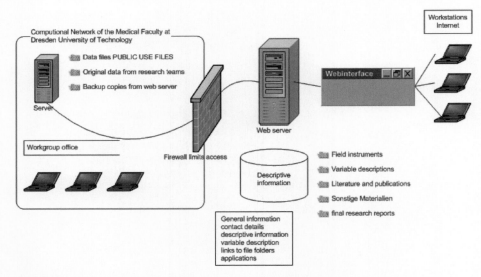

Fig. 5. Conception of a shared database using a internet web interface

The core idea behind the *shared database* conception is the demand for both, enabling writing data via internet as well as storing sensitive data in a restricted and secured computing area. While considering every data stored on a web server as being stored unprotected, the possible solution lies in two identical database systems that synchronise their database steadily. Two database systems have been set up as illustrated by Figure 5.

The first database serves for data writing capabilities on the web server in conjunction with a dynamic web application. Herewith, research teams are being provided with the opportunity of working on their own Public Use/Documentation File. Every descriptive data can be altered by means of a password secured area on the web directly, as there are contact details, research team members, recent literature and publications, general descriptions and new results.

The second database is the firewall secured computing network of the Medical Faculty at Dresden University of Technology. From workstations of the *PUF* workgroup the first web server database system can be synchronised with the local database system that serves the storing and creating of Public Use/Documentation Files with its complete data files and resources as it has been outlined above. Therefore, the creation of a new Public Use File bases on the most updated information available from the original research team. Latest discussion contributions are being enclosed with the file as well.

For dissemination of Public Use/Documentation Files via Internet, the *PUF* workgroup has set up a web application with a double purpose. On one hand, the prospective *PUF* user shall be able to access information regarding the files. On the other hand, the research teams shall be able to keep the information presented in the *PUF* up-to-date. The web application for disseminating Public Use/Documentation Files via the internet is accessible by URL [*http://www.public-health.tu-dresden.de*]. As the domain name suggests, the web application is embedded in the general Public Health Research Association Saxony's web site, which offers the possibility of sharing information. The web application is designed with portal characteristics, meaning that after a successful login by valid username and password, the client user is granted access to various functionalities within the web application depending of the user rights that have been set for the username. These func-

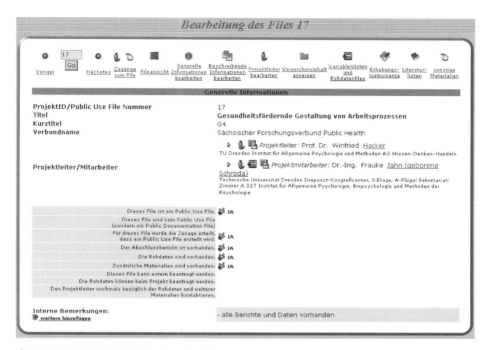

Fig. 6. The work on Public Use File web page dialog

tionalities are accessible by a personalised option page (to be found at the *people's* icon in the top right-hand corner).

The user of the described web application is being classified into the *public user* or the *authorised user*. The former either did not log in by a valid username and password or its user rights are being g set to *guest* (Gast_Allgemein). Clicking the index card *Public Use File* the public user is already able to access copious information. First, the public user can browse or search by single words the file archive for Public Use/Documentation Files of particular interest. Second, the public user is able to search all variables in all Public Use Files for specific terms or expressions (e. g. *child* or *alcohol*). Via the results listing the particular research project's description can be accessed. Thirdly, a forum on different issues regarding the work with Public Use/Documentation Files can be accessed for reading. Finally, the download area provides various resources for downloading. Once the public user is logged in as *guest* (a new username can be registered by clicking the *Registrieren* button) additional functions are accessible, as for instance, providing one's own contact details, news, event announcements and web links with Public Health relevance on the web site. Furthermore, both the extended online view as well as the use of particular files can be applied for. After approval of application the extended view is accessible on the personalised option page too.

The term *authorised users* applies to members of the research teams, whose research project has been compiled to a *Public Use/Documentation File*. After registering the username, the workgroup evaluates the purpose remarks in the registration form. Following a telephone contact the user rights are set to work on the corresponding file or files. Figure 6 shows the web page dialog that is accessible via the personalised option page. Every single information can be altered, deleted or added. General information concerning the research project, descriptive information, and information about research team members are to be changed directly via HTML forms. Additional files can be used to provide information about field instruments, questionnaires, published and unpublished literature etc. These files may have any file format that is supported by most of the prospective client users. Therefore, Acrobat's *portable document format (pdf)* is the most appropriate. Once the files are generated, research team members are able to upload theses file to the web server and to associate those with the corresponding *Public Use/Documentation File*. For the latter, a mere database entry by the authorised user (research team member) is sufficient to describe the file more detailed and to make it visible to client users.

We described elsewhere (Meusel, Göpfert, Wagner, Merker, Kirch 2002: pp. 377) the pilot web application that was used to test the general concept illustrated above. Presently, efforts are brought forward to enhance the web application and its handiness. For this reason, the data base structure is being worked over and integrated into new structured server side scripts. Furthermore, cooperation with the German Public Health internet portal (http://www.ph-portal.info/) is intended. An additional improvement of the web application shall be the translation into English. Finally, we work to provide the opportunity of remote computing, as outlined in section 3.

Getting the files

In summarising, free information on the file contents is available via the Internet. Nevertheless, using the Public Use/Documentation Files in hardcopy as well as using the extended view into a particular Public Use/Documentation File on the web site requires putting forward an application. The applications can be submitted using the Public Use File web application as well as by contacting the workgroup and requesting an application form. This formal application contains statements about the secondary research intentions, intentions of publications as well as a statement of commitment to general terms of use. Following the authorization of the application by a scientific board, the CD-ROM or/and hardcopies will be shipped to the prospective user. The targeted users of the Public Use/ Documentation Files are scientific institutions. Students are being requested to provide a confirmation of their scientific guidance by the institute's staff.

Prospects

Concluding this paper, some remarks on further prospects shall outline an approach to implement an *Open Source* strategy in Public Health science more broadly. To begin with, the shared database conception and design could be extended for European wide Public Health science and research. Therewith, a persistent research resource base might be set up and maintained to collect materials, results and data sets of all aspects of Public Health research in Europe. Little by little, the entirety approach and concept of issuing Public Use Files might even be left in favour of a more fluent approach that we may call *Open Source strategy*. Figure 7 demonstrates a possible way of realising that methodology.

The core idea would be a central data and/or resource base, where research teams are being provided with a unified way of documenting and publishing resources of their research project's work. Here, we like to stress that we do not mean to omit the conventional and well established publishing system of scientific journal contributions in the future, rather than having it interpreted as an add-on to it. These documentations may comprise research reports only in case the research design prevents publishing of research data sets

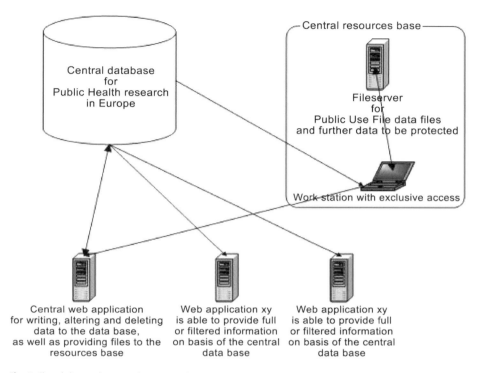

Fig. 7. Shared data and resource base conception

in general, but also may comprise all or parts of data sets and resources accumulated in the particular research project's work. The information given in the data and/or resource base could then be provided on different web applications or web sites in complete or in filtered form.

References

Bavarian Research Association Public Health (2003), "Public-Use Files des Bayerischen Forschungsver-bundes Public Health" [online accessed 12-01-2003] URL: http://mfv.web.med.uni-muenchen.de/pubusef.html.

Campbell, E. G., Clarridge, B. R., Gokhale, M., Birenbaum, L., Hilgartner, S., Holtzman, N. A., & Blumenthal, D. (2002), "Data Withholding in Academic Genetics", *JAMA*. 287, 473–479.

Centre for Survey Research and Methodology (2003), "German General Social Survey (ALLBUS)" [online accessed 12-01-2003] URL: http://www.gesis.org/en/social_monitoring/allbus/index.htm.

Dibona, Ch., Stone, M., & Ockman, S. (1999), Open Sources: Voices from the Open Source Revolution (O'Reilly Open Source) O'Reilly & Associates.

Federal Statistical Office Germany (2003), "Microcensus introduction" [online accessed 12-01-2003] URL: http://www.destatis.de/micro/e/micro_c1.htm.

Jacobi, F. (2003), "Public Use Files als Perspektive für die klinisch-psychologische Forschung," in Klinische Psychologie im Internet, C. Eichenberg & R, Ott, eds., Hogrefe, Göttingen.

Meusel, D., Göpfert, P., Wagner, N., Merker N., & Kirch, W. (2002), "Data Based Web Application for Public Health Relevant Research Data", Zschr. Gesundheitswiss. (J. Public Health), 10, 377–381.

The span in information from researching new tools to accessible presentation – experience from child and adolescent health

Michael Rigby · Sean Denyer · Aidan Macfarlane · Ann McPherson
Ailis Quinlan · Ulrike Ravens-Sieberer

Introduction

Children (inclusive of all young people up to the age of 18 years) form a significant part of the total population, not only in terms of numbers, but also in terms of significance. The health of children should therefore be seen as doubly important – because children are important individual citizens in their own right, and because of the importance of ensuring the continued health and well-being of society. This is further deepened by the fact that children are in general dependent upon the pattern of care and services provided for them, and are little able to influence their macro determinants of health.

However, the position of children and child health is something of a paradox. At the policy level, most countries and societies, particularly within Europe, claim to value children highly. At the international level the United Nations Convention on the Rights of Child, including the right to health, has been endorsed by virtually all nations (United Nations, 1989). Specialist services for children, particularly sick children, are beneficiaries of goodwill and support. At the individual level, children are generally valued within families and society. But this positive picture conceals serious hidden challenges to health and well-being – firstly, a small but significant group of children are not well respected at the individual level, due either to family dysfunction or because they come from particular marginalised groups, and these disadvantaged children tend to be lost and unnoticed. Secondly, and even more importantly, despite the general societal claims of support for children, in practice society and its policies and activities are highly focussed on adult interests and structures. They are adapted towards the economically and physically active adult, and access to services and presentation of need are potentially difficult for those who are dependent such as children (but also for other groups such as the frail elderly or those with intellectual disabilities). This invisibility is also true within information systems, which is the linking theme of this paper.

The challenge of child-focussed information

In any other form of public health activity, including health policy formulation, it is self-evident that appropriate information is needed. Yet finding this with regard to the child population can be surprisingly difficult. For instance, it is difficult to find the exact number of children. Most demographic systems analyse data in 5-year age bands, but the most widely recognised definition of children is those aged 0–17 years inclusive, and this is the definition adopted by the United Nations Convention, yet the number of persons aged 0–17 is not readily available from routine sources. Another example relates to census data, where most of the analyses are by household. Thus it is possible to identify a range of health determinant factors ranging from tobacco smoking or overcrowding through to income group or educational levels per household, but there are no routine analyses of the number of children, by age group, affected by each of the census-recorded determinants such as exposure to household tobacco smoke. Thus those working to develop child health services or otherwise promote the health of children are disadvantaged by lack of appropriate data.

Furthermore, it is important for some data systems to be designed specifically to capture information directly from children. Information supplied by adults about children will be biased according to the adult's view of what is appropriate, and is furthermore highly unlikely to include the child's own perspective or perception.

Yet, adequate balanced information is vital for forward planning, and policy determination. Rigby (1999) has previously highlighted this importance, and has emphasised that information requirements exist at five different levels (Rigby, 1998).

- ▶ Political
- ▶ Strategic Management
- ▶ Operational Management
- ▶ Case Load Management
- ▶ Individual or Case

The three central levels within this range are generally recognised even if poorly served within child health, but the importance of the first and last needs to be fully recognised. At the individual case level individuals look to information sources to influence their own patterns of behaviour and also health treatment, and professionals look for reference data. At the political level, many decisions are taken which determine policy or health in a direct or indirect way, and it is important that information is distilled and presented which is understood by the non-specialists at this level.

Thus there is a particular importance in developing information systems in child health, with a close link between information, evidence, and research. On the one hand, activity should be evidence-based, and in turn evidence should optimally be researched based (Sackett *et al.*, 1996; Roberts, 1999). In turn, the current limited availability of child-relevant information means that research into improved information systems, and particularly information gathering, is very important.

This chapter illustrates this continuum from research into information gathering methods through to making available robust information at the political level, taking child health as the important working domain. Four initiatives are highlighted – each has come about independently though devised and led by individuals with similar philosophies, and there is now a deepened synergy to collaboration between them at the conceptual and application levels. The four projects are:

Child Health Monitoring Indicators – a European Commission funded project to seek a composite set of indicators measuring all aspects of child health at the level of Member States.

KIDSCREEN – A project funded by a different European Commission programme, to devise a tool to obtain the views of children on their own health and wellbeing, particularly focussed on younger children.

Teenage Internet Health Sites – two linked projects seeking to make relevant 'evidence based' health information easily available and culturally accessible to teenagers.

Best Health for Children – an initiative of the Chief Executives of the Irish Health Boards to influence policy and service provision in health and social care.

All these projects focus on improving the health of children, taking that in the widest sense of well-being and function as well as absence of disease or incapacity. All are based on sound use of information, and in turn are seeking to generate information for use by individuals or by policy makers.

Child health indicators of life and development (CHILD)

The Child Health Indicators of Life and Development (CHILD) project was funded by the Health Monitoring Programme of the Health and Consumer Protection Directorate of the European Commission. The parent Health Monitoring Programme (HMP) is charged with developing a suite of indicators, which will monitor the health of the population of Europe, selecting indicators applicable at the member state level. The CHILD project is a third wave project within that, which reported back to the Commission in September 2002 (Rigby and Köhler, 2002).

Health monitoring (including health service monitoring) requires robust data sources, which are comprehensive and reliable, and are independent of any internal bias. The indicators must relate to topics and measurements which are comparable across the range of the countries concerned – in this case European Community Member States and those within the European Economic Area (Iceland, Liechtenstein, and Norway). The CHILD project comprised one expert from each of the 17 participating countries (Liechtenstein not having taken part), supported by targeted input by others, as defined in the final report.

A systematic approach

The CHILD project team recognised the importance of developing the concept of child public health as earlier expounded by Köhler (1998), and at the same time saw this as an opportunity to promote understanding of the population view amongst child health practitioners, whilst concurrently projecting evidence about the state of child health and its determinants to a wider audience including the political one.

The CHILD project took a systematic approach by initially considering and defining the principle areas of child health and its determinants. The resulting list is shown below:
- Demography
- Socio-economic Status and Inequity
- Social Cohesion/Capital
- Migrants
- Marginalised Children
- Family Cohesion
- Mental Health
- Quality of Life
- Well-being
- Lifestyles
- Health Promoting Policies
- Nutrition and Physical Growth
- Development (including Intellectual and Social)

▶ Mortality, Morbidity, Injuries
▶ Environment
▶ Access and Utilisation of Services

Following on from this, individual members of the project assumed responsibility for specific topics, and studied the literature on these to identify firstly the key issues in this aspect of child health, and then secondly the possible measures which might exist and be applicable across Europe for each of these.

The project took cognisance of the wide range of determinants of child health, as well as the number of aspects of health status and illness, which ideally ought to be measured. Drawing on previous work in Sweden (Socialstyrelsen, 1998), these can be mapped into a set of dynamics as shown in Figure 1.

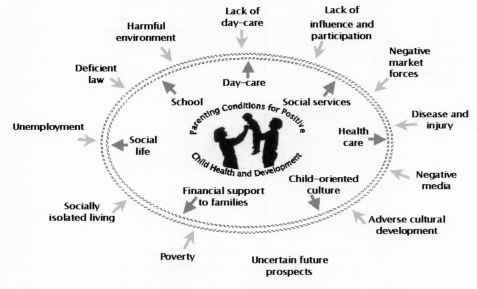

Adapted by Gunnlaugsson G and Rigby M from
Skolhälsovården 1998. Underlag för egen kontroll och
tillsyn. Stockholm: Socialstyrelsen, 1998.

Fig. 1. Determinants of the Child Health and Development Context

Criterion-based selection

The project then embarked on a three-stage process of moving from a long list of potential indicators, through a medium list of the more promising items which appeared to have adequate and comparable definitions and reasonable data availability, down to a final short-list for which evidence, definitions, and data sources could be defined. At the same time, it was seen as important to have a good spread of indicators, both by age group and by field.

Indicators needed to be technically sound, otherwise they did not pass the first filter. The key criteria applied were:

- Validity
  - Face validity
  - Content validity
  - Construct validity
- Consistency
- Sensitivity
- Feasibility

From those that passed through this scrutiny, a prioritising mechanism led to the short list. The criteria used at this stage were:
- **Evidence-based**, underpinned by research
- Significant **Burden to Society**
- Significant **Burden to Family**
- Significant **Burden to Individual**
- **Representative** of **Significant Population Groups**
- **Regularity** and **Repeatability**, to enable trend analysis
- Data **Availability**
- Topic amenable to **Effective Action**
- **Understandable** to broad audience.

Drawing on a preceding Health Monitoring Programme Project, the CHILD project identified four broad types of topic for measurement, namely:
A Demographic and Social Economic (Upstream Health Determinants)
B Health Status and Wellbeing
C Determinants of Health, Risk and Protective Factors
D Health Systems and Policy

In practice, the project experts found difficulty in defining proven and validated comparable indicators for some of the important issues in contemporary child health. These challenging areas included child abuse and child mental health, and therefore the project has included in its report recommendations for further research in a number of defined areas – a resonance with the underlying theme of this chapter.

The full report gives the detailed definition of each of the 38 indicators recommended, and an outline and justification for each of the 17 areas for which further research is believed desirable. It is noteworthy that nine of the aspects where it was felt that adequate indicators with comparable and reliable data flows did not exist were in the domain of Child Health Systems and Policy. This must be of concern, as it indicates that there is not adequate accepted means of monitoring the relevance and quality of services to meet children's health needs. It also reflects earlier concerns that stated priorities for child health care did not manifest as committed policy application (Aynesly-Green, 2000).

Figure 2 shows the topics of the indicators proposed – the full report (Rigby and Köhler, 2002) also contains a detailed template for each recommended indicator, comprising evidence, definition, and potential data sources. The report also explains the reason why further research to identify robust indicators is needed in the following areas:
- Child Abuse
- Childhood Behaviour Disorders
- Learning Disorders/Intellectual Disability
- Educational Development
- Perceived Well-being, Quality of Life and Positive Mental Health
- Children with permanent or severe disability
- Family Cohesion and Social Cohesion

Aspects

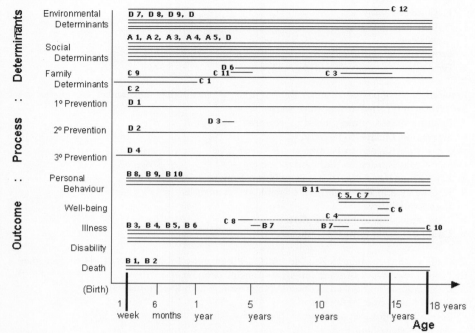

Determinants
- Environmental Determinants
- Social Determinants
- Family Determinants

Process
- 1° Prevention
- 2° Prevention
- 3° Prevention

Outcome
- Personal Behaviour
- Well-being
- Illness
- Disability
- Death
- (Birth)

ABBREVIATED KEY TO INDICATORS

A. Demographic & Socio-Economic
A 1 Socio-economic Circumstances
A 2 Children in Poverty
A 3 Parental Educational Attainment
A 4 Child in Single Parent Households
A 5 Asylum Seekers

B. Child Health Status, Well-being
Child Mortality
B 1 Child Mortality Rates
B 2 Selected Cause-specific Mortality

Child Morbidity
B 3 Cancer
B 4 Diabetes
B 5 Asthma
B 6 Infectious Diseases
B 7 Dental Morbidity

Injuries to Children
B 8 Burns Necessitating Admission
B 9 Poisoning Necessitating Admission
B 10 Fracture of Long-bones

Mental Health of Children
B 11 Attempted Suicide

C. Health Determinants, Risk, and Protective Factors
Parental Determinants
C 1 Breastfeeding
C 2 Household Environmental Tobacco
C 3 Parental Support

Child Lifestyle Determinants
C 4 Physical Activity
C 5 Tobacco Smoking
C 6 Alcohol Abuse
C 7 Substance Misuse

Other Factors
C 8 Overweight and Obesity
C 9 Children in Care
C 10 Early School Leavers

C 11 Educational Enrolment
C 12 Air Pollution Exposure

D. Child Health Systems & Policy
Health Systems Policy
D 1 Marginalised Children's Health Care
D 2 Parental Inpatient Accompaniment

Health System Quality
D 3 Immunisation Coverage
D 4 Leukaemia 5-year Survival

Social Policy Indicators
D 5 Physical Punishment
D 6 Anti-bullying policies in schools

Physical Protection Policy
D 7 Child Transportation Safety
D 8 Exposure to Lead
D 9 Exposure to Hazardous Noise
D 10 Environmental Tobacco Smok

Fig. 2. Spread of CHILD Project Proposed Health Indicators

- Nutritional Habits
- Healthcare Access
- Inpatient Service Quality
- Health Service Access for Socially Restricted Children
- Medication
- Play and Leisure
- Assessment of Children with Special Needs
- Integration of Children with Special Needs
- Health Parenting
- Mental Health Education

In a research and developmental context, the CHILD project sought to be modestly progressive. It has identified indicators where the raw data are potentially available in each case in the majority of Member States, either from current data sets such as hospital discharge data or from civil registration data, or could be obtained from surveys. At the same time, it has been progressive not only in the sense that for each item some countries will need to develop either their routine data flows or the analysis and presentation of the item, but also because it is recommended that the data be broken down by both gender and socio-economic group in order to identify differential biases within population groups, and these sub-groupings are not likely to be available currently (though the information will be available at case level).

In conclusion, therefore, the CHILD project seeks to bring child health monitoring into the overall Health Monitoring Programme commissioned by the European Parliament Health and Consumer Protection Directorate General. Its recommendations are firmly based on published research, and it has the defined those areas where further research is believed to be needed in order to yield necessary indicator definitions.

KIDSCREEN

As stated in the World Health Organization (WHO) definition of health, health should be viewed as a subjective representation of function and well-being (WHO, 1948). The WHO definition holds an important expansion of the view of health, which is not only understood by somatic indicators, but also comprises how a person feels, psychologically and physically, and how she or he manages with other persons and copes with every day life (Rosser, 1988; Spilker, 1990). This perceived health is known as health related quality of life (HRQoL), and this is one of the major descriptors and outcome criteria that has been discussed in the health care systems in recent years.

Quality of life of children and especially children at risk however is yet an under-researched area. To fill this gap, the development of a generic HRQoL measure is warranted. It should meet a European standard in which the children's self report and parental perception of their children's health is included. The importance of subjective measures of well being and function (i.e. subjective health) has increased over the past decade (Stewart et al., 1992; WHOQOL Group, 1996). Especially for children and adolescents it is important to know how they view their lives and how they rate their function and well-being. Including HRQOL instruments in public health surveys allows researchers to monitor population health status over time, to detect sub-groups within the general population who might be at risk for poor HRQOL, and to assess the impact of public health interventions within a given population.

While several European countries have recently included health-related quality of life in representative surveys of the adult population, surveys including children and adolescents are relatively rare in the European community and often do not include self perceived health. Cross-cultural aspects of health related quality of life in children have so far not been addressed. An appropriate way of ensuring that measures on subjective health perception are appropriate for use in cross-cultural research is to develop the measure simultaneously in several countries. This is the approach taken by members of the KIDSCREEN project, a collaborative effort between researchers in Europe.

The project "Screening for and promotion of Health Related Quality of Life in Children and Adolescents – a European Public Health Perspective" (Acronym: KIDSCREEN) is part of to the program "Research and Technological Development Activities of the Generic Nature" in the Area Public Health as described in the EC work program within the 5th Framework Program 'Quality of Life and Management of Living Resources' and is funded by the European Commission for three years (Ravens-Sieberer et al., 2001). It started in February 2001 and involves ten European countries: Austria, France, Germany, Netherlands, Spain, Switzerland, United Kingdom and the newly associated states Czech Republic, Hungary and Poland.

The project aims at a co-operative European development of a standardised screening instrument for children's quality of life, which will be used in representative national and European health surveys. It also aims at identifying children at risk at terms of their subjective health to suggest early intervention possibilities by including the instrument in health services research and health reporting.

The project consists of three main phases: (1) instrument development, (2) instrument application in public health surveys, and (3) an implementation phase in which the possibility of using the instrument in different settings will be tested. The study centre is located at the Robert Koch Institute (RKI), a central institution of the Federal Ministry of Health, in Berlin, Germany. All partners have experience both in conducting public health surveys as well as in HRQoL research in children and adolescents.

Initial development

The **first phase**, the development of the questionnaire, was based on a literature review, expert consultations (Delphi method), and children's focus groups in all participating countries, to identify dimensions and items of HRQoL, which were suitable for inclusion in the new instrument and relevant to respondents in all countries. The systematic literature review concerned the development and use of generic quality of life measures for children and adolescents in public health settings. Relevant studies were reviewed by all participating centres according to Cochrane review criteria using a standardised evaluation sheet and the collected data were recorded in a KIDSCREEN data bank. This literature review provided an initial identification of relevant dimensions and available assessment methods for the project.

A *Delphi method* was used to determine the degree of consensus among experts regarding the conceptualisation and operationalisation of HRQoL in children and adolescents, and to identify preliminary content for the new measure at the dimension level (Herdman et al., 2002). The Delphi process in the KIDSCREEN project consisted of three rounds of questionnaires administered to a multidisciplinary group of experts from the participating European countries. High agreement was reached on the following KIDSCREEN QoL working definition: "Health Related Quality of Life (HRQoL) in children and adolescents is a multidimensional construct with the broader domains: social well-being, physical well-being, psychological well-being (including cognitive & emotional facets) and perception of personal environment. It includes aspects of functioning as well as satisfaction from the child's and adolescent's perspective, taking into account the context of developmental, personal, social and cultural goals and expectations. If self-report cannot be obtained from the children and adolescents, parents as proxies are asked to report their perspective on the child's/adolescent's quality of life". The Delphi results also emphasised that a distinction between HRQoL itself and determinants of HRQoL (e.g. socio-demographic variables, health services utilisation, morbidity) had to be made for further analysis and explanation of the variance of HRQoL and that the measure had to ensure equivalent measurement across different languages.

The results of the literature review and the Delphi process provided a preliminary structure for the *focus groups* with children and adolescents (Bruil et al., 2002; Detmar et al. 2002). Focus groups were chosen because they are an important tool for cross-national qualitative work. They were conducted in each of the participating countries aiming at the generation of potential questions for domains and dimensions from the family perspective. The selection of participants to be recruited was described in a focus group manual. Within the KIDSCREEN project in summary 146 children and adolescents as well as 83 parents participated in the group interviews. In addition relevance ratings for different aspects of HRQoL were provided. The focus group sessions were audio-taped, transcribed and analysed. The natural setting, the flexibility and the semi-structured nature yielded rich data from widely different populations using the standardised protocols. The conducting of the focus groups provided an important methodological safeguard against idiosyncratic dimensions, questions and items.

Resulting items from the literature, Delphi procedure and focus groups were now based on the suggestions of experts and lay-people. They used simple language, avoided ambiguity in terms of either wording or phraseology and were short. Items also avoided double negatives, were amenable to rating scales, asked about a single issue, were applicable to individuals with a broad range of health status and were phrased as questions. The resulting KIDSCREEN item list reflected the following aspects of HRQoL: Physical-Well-being, Social Support and Peer Relation, Cognitive and School-functioning, Parent Relation and Home Life, Psychological Well-being (Negative Emotions, Positive Emotions and Life Satisfaction), Self-Perception (Body-Image and Self-Esteem) and Autonomy.

Items were thereafter translated according to international standards (The WHOQoL Group, 1998; Bullinger et al., 1998) to achieve an optimal conceptual equivalence amongst all language versions rather than only linguistic and literal equivalence. The degree of conceptual equivalence amongst the respective national translations was checked on an international basis in two cross-cultural harmonisation sessions. Results of subsequent national cognitive interviews with children, adolescents and parents provided additional information about the suitability of the national versions. Thereafter all participating countries wrote national reports including detailed descriptions of the translation processes as well as of the outcomes of the respective cognitive interviews.

Instrument application in surveys

Within the **second phase**, the application of the questionnaire, primarily a testing of the national translations, was conducted in a pilot study in seven countries (Ravens-Sieberer et al., 2002). A total of 3952 children and adolescents between 8 to 18 years of age and their parents from different regions (urban vs. rural) and different socio-economic environments were included. Beside the new generated KIDSCREEN items additional determinants (e.g. Socio-demographic variables, Health status, and Health care utilisation variables) were applied. The pilot questionnaire was administered to perform statistical testing of validity of the KIDSCREEN questionnaire.

Once all the data were nationally collected, entered and checked, the national data pools were merged to build an international data base. Item response theory and structural equation modelling were used to determine the optimal item and scale characteristics of the questionnaire in addition to common psychometric analysis. Analysis also involved European cross cultural comparison of the instrument. After item reduction the questionnaire consisted of less than 50 five point Likert scaled items; the dimensions represented social, physical, and psychological well-being (including cognitive & emotional aspects) and perception of personal environment.

The generic HRQoL measure is now available in English, German, Dutch, French, Spanish, Italian, Czech, Hungarian, Polish as well as Swedish and will be used in representative mail and telephone surveys on HRQoL in the respective countries for further validation and to obtain norm data. At least 2000 interviews with both parents and children in each participating country are to be realized. Families in all ten participating countries will be asked via telephone interview to participate in the study, to give their written informed consent and to respond to a mailed survey. The potential cross cultural implementation of the instrument tool in health services and health monitoring will be planned, tested and evaluated.

Implementation

Modes of implementation of the new measure are going to be discussed among all national partners in the **third phase**, the implementation of the KIDSCREEN project. On the basis of the survey data collected, round table discussions with health services officials will be initiated in order to tailor possibilities for each nation to implement the instrument in health promotion programs on the basis of the identified children at risk. The implementation phase will include preparation of user friendly guidelines and user manuals in order to facilitate practical use of the instrument. These will be made available via modern communication technologies.

The project contributes to European policies by providing information about the types and distribution of quality of life impairments (nationally as well as Europe wide). By giving each country and centre the possibility to be involved already at the item construction phase of the current project, a truly international collaborative effort is made. European added value consists in having at hand a cross-cultural comparable and usable instrument, which will be easy to use and to apply. To devise an instrument to assess quality of life for children and adolescents in major European languages makes it easier on a national and international level to communicate the approaches to and experiences with monitoring representative populations, with health promotion as well as with communication about improvement possibilities.

Providing a quality of life assessment measure, the KIDSCREEN project adds an important indicator for health assessment and health monitoring. A cross-cultural screening instrument may also serve as a prototype for further application of quality of life health surveys in other countries. In sum the contribution to public health research of the KIDSCREEN project exists on several levels:
1. the provision of a standardized instrument available in several languages for European countries to monitor routinely subjective health and well-being of the children in the European Union;
2. to screen for and early detect possible impairments in well-being and function in children, which can be the basis of early interventions;

3. to identify social and behavioural determinants of health (e.g. socio-economic factors and health behaviours, acute and chronic health conditions); and
4. the assessment of the relative impact of such quality of life assessment on monitoring the health of children and adolescents in the European region.

It is expected that the KIDSCREEN project will contribute to a better understanding of perceived health in children and adolescents in Europe and will contribute to planning, carrying out and evaluating innovations in the health care field.

Teenage health websites

At the individual level, the older child as an autonomous agent is a very important concept. Whilst on the one hand children's views and behaviours are not well-enough captured in population-level data, equally the importance of getting reliable information to older children in formats which are attractive and accessible, and which they both understand and respect, are inadequate considered. Macfarlane and McPherson have been working to redress this balance, with the aim of improving the provision of 'evidence based' health information to young people in an appropriate confidential, interactive, form that can be accessed by young people 24 hours a day, 365 days a year, and which helps young people decide on appropriate health related behaviours.

Rationale

Health promotion to young people is considered important because there is evidence that certain health related behaviours laid down during adolescence are continued into adulthood. This is most obvious in the area of smoking, where 80% of those young people smoking by the age of 20 began smoking before the age of 16. (Thomas et al., 1998). In other areas of adolescent behaviours such as their diet, the evidence is more complicated. For instance, although we know that two out of three obese children will go on to being obese adults, the majority of obese adults were not obese as children. Further, there is evidence that those obese adults who were obese as children are more likely to suffer health consequences than those who were not obese as children (Vanhala et al., 1998).

The actual delivery of health promotion to adolescents is based around two main areas of intervention. The first concerns general social interventions via manipulation of young people's environment, such as increasing the price of cigarettes, making appropriate play areas available for young people, using traffic calming methods for improving road safety for young people cycling to school. The second method involves health promotionalists and others trying to influence young people's health related behaviour by individual direct exhortation to behave in health responsible ways, for instance by telling them that they should not smoke, that they should use contraceptives, that they should brush their teeth everyday, that they should eat less fatty foods etc.

Evidence from present research indicates that the first method is very much more successful than the second method when trying to influence the health related behaviours of young people (Jepson, 2000). However, there is a third way, which, at the present time, has been under researched. The method involves the provision of 'evidence based' health information for young people in a format that they find useful and that they can access when they, as individuals, need it and want to use it. An initial attempt at doing this was carried out by the authors by publishing a series of 'faction' (a mixture of fact and fiction) books (Macfarlane and McPherson, 2002 a–c) in which 'evidence based' health related information was provided to young people in a format which young people appeared to accept. The success of this format can only be assessed by the fact that these books have sold around a million copies to young people in the UK and have been translated into 22 other languages.

Unfortunately, at the present time there are no specific scientific research methodologies which allow us to examine the direct 'impact' of this information presented in this format on health related behaviours of young people. However, as a result of the success of the books, it was decided to set up a website for teenagers based around the same concept as the books, but allowing easier and quicker access 365 days a year, 24 hours a day to those teenagers with connection with internet facilities (3.6 million young people in the U.K)

Design of the websites

Two linked websites www.teenagehealthfreak.org and www.doctorann.org were designed and set up in consultation with groups of young people (mainly using the internet itself a consultation facility). The first site includes the daily diary of a fictional hypochondriacal 15 year old boy. This diary is designed to:
1. show the readers that other young people have similar health worries as themselves, and
2. via hypertexted links, to provide appropriate 'evidence-based' information about these concerns on the second website site.

This second site is a 'virtual doctor's surgery' and consists of an index, a large number of relevant 'evidence based' health facts, along with 'health' quizzes, information about other relevant sources of health information, and an 'interactive Agony Aunt' where young people can e-mail in their concerns and receive answers.

Throughout the second site, as far as is possible, the information provided is 'evidence based'. In order to do this, the authors rely heavily on two sources of information (BMJ, 2002; www.cochrane.org/cochrane/revabstr/mainindex.htm). Where clear evidence for an intervention does not exist, this is often stated in the website text.

Assessing the website use

In order to assess the use of the website by young people, information is collected about the number of visitors and the number of hits recorded on the websites. This varies from week to week according to (1) whether the week is a 'school term' week or a 'holiday week' as the site is heavily promoted by Physical and Social Health Education teachers to young people within schools who then access via the school computers, and (2) whether there has been any recent media publicity about the site. At present the number of visitors per week varies between 20000 and 30000, and the number of hits recorded in a week varies between 200000 and 300000. Analysis of the sex of the young people answering the quizzes on the site indicates that the gender ratio of those using the site is 6 girls to 4 boys, and that the modal age group of the users is 14–17 years.

Assessing young people's concerns

An e-mail link on the website also allows young people to e-mail comments about the site itself, and again these allow for the authors to change aspects of the site accordingly. Most of these comments have, to date, been positive. A further use of the site is that analysis of e-mail questions from young people (29 000 received in the last 36 months) also allows identification of the major concerns of adolescents.

Assessing the ability of the site to change young people's health related behaviours

Research on the evidence for the effectiveness of health promotion for young people presently indicates that the most effective forms of intervention are related to social interventions, such as raising the price of cigarettes, banning cigarette advertising, or using road traffic calming methods. The method demonstrated here of providing young people with the most up to date 'evidence based' information about health 'facts' is designed, not so much to change young people's behaviours, but rather to provide suitable information in a suitable format for young people to access when they need it and to use according to their own individual needs. The only method of assessing this at the present time is presented above – e.g. the number of young people actually accessing the information and (assessed via the e-mailed comments) finding it useful.

Further directions

The teenage website has been highly successful in terms of the number of young people accessing the sites. The information on the website is, as much as is feasible, 'evidence based' and this information is then presented in a format which teenagers find appropriate. Experience from this website will now be used to develop a further website www.dipex.org in the field of teenage illnesses. This site will not only use teenage patients' own experiences of illnesses but also use links to the Cochrane database to provide young people with further information concerning 'evidence based' treatments in such areas as 'cancer', 'diabetes' and epilepsy.

Best Health for Children (Ireland)

The fourth complementary component to this chapter reports on an initiative in the Republic of Ireland, which seeks in an organisational yet flexible and innovative way to have a positive influence on services for children – using services in the widest sense. Importantly, it is organisationally owned by the Health Boards within Ireland. Also significantly, it has an evaluation element built into its funding and structure.

Background

There are over 50 000 births per annum in the Republic of Ireland. Approximately one third of the population is under 18 years. Concerns regarding the health of children in the country include the following:
- One third of deaths in the 0–14 age group are due to unintentional injury
- Uptake rates of childhood immunisation are unacceptably low
- The same is true of initiation and maintenance rates for breastfeeding

Child Health Services

Child Health services in the Republic of Ireland have, in the recent past, been under-resourced, lacked a research base or have failed to apply what evidence exists. They have also lacked flexibility and have not been consumer friendly. Training for staff has not been available, while Information systems to support quality service delivery have been poorly developed. The resulting lack of standardisation has led to major inequities in child health service experience throughout the country.

The report *"Best Health for Children – Developing a Partnership with Families"* (Denyer et al., 1999), suggested a new model for delivery of child health services in the Republic of Ireland in an attempt to address these issues. Its major themes are:
- ▶ Promotion of an evidence based culture
- ▶ Developing a child centred, health promotion approach
- ▶ Creating a partnership between parents and professionals
- ▶ Quality assurance
- ▶ A standardised and co-ordinated approach to child health service delivery.

Best Health for Children

The Best Health for children (BHFC) initiative was established in 1999 by the Chief Executive Officers of the ten Health Boards in the country, to drive the implementation of the report. The vision statement of BHFC is that "The health and well-being of all children is valued and sufficiently provided for to enable each child to reach his/her full potential".

Its objectives are:
1. To develop policy and strategy on behalf of the health boards in relation to child and adolescent health.
2. To disseminate research and good practice in relation to child and adolescent health.
3. To develop partnerships with relevant government departments, including the Department of Health and Children, and voluntary organisations.
4. To facilitate joint working by the health boards.
5. To monitor implementation of policies in relation to child and adolescent health.
6. To carry out projects and reviews in relation to child and adolescent health as determined by the CEOs.

Translating research into practice

Culture shift

Traditionally, each of the health boards developed its own programme for delivery of child health services. The fact that the Chief Executive Officers of the ten health boards agreed to support this work in a conjoint fashion represented a major cultural shift in work practice.

Structures

- ▶ Two Assistant Directors with complementary skills (backgrounds in Public Health Medicine and Education respectively) were employed in 1999 to drive the initiative.
- ▶ Reflecting the National thrust of the initiative, team members are located at three sites.

- A National Conjoint Child Health Committee was formed to act as a scientific advisory group to the initiative. This committee includes representatives from the ten health boards, the Departments of Health and Children, and Education and Science, professional bodies and representatives from the National Parents Council.
- Multidisciplinary committees are established to address specific topics identified in the original report. They consist of "Key Players" and reflect a geographical spread. They disband upon production of a report.
- Steering committees have been set up in each health board to drive the implementation of the report.

Communication

BHFC works with the Health Boards Child Health Steering Committee to:
- Co-ordinate implementation of the initiative at health board level
- Share best practice
- Achieve standardisation throughout the country.

Taking on board the need to consider the broad determinants of child health, BHFC has forged links with EU and Australian child health initiatives, a wide range of government departments, voluntary organisations and interest groups, academic institutions and all the health boards. BHFC has hosted three national conferences to showcase child health initiatives and to facilitate networking among health professionals. BHFC publishes and disseminates an annual report. A website www.besthealthforchildren.com has been set up as a further resource.

Demonstration projects

In order to avoid duplication and to promote a cost-effective use of resources, each health board has agreed to select a certain aspect of the report as a demonstration project. Upon evaluation and refinement national roll-out is planned.

Policy development

Building on the original report "Best Health for Children – Developing a Partnership with Parents", BHFC has produced further reports to provide a framework for child and adolescent health service provision, namely.
- The adolescent health strategy, "Get Connected – Developing an adolescent friendly health service" (National Conjoint Child Health Committee, 2001a).
- The supporting parents strategy, "Investing in Parenthood to achieve best health for children" (National Conjoint Child Health Committee, 2002).
- Documents addressing specific topics such as performance indicators and training for staff in child health surveillance have also been produced.
- Focused work is currently ongoing regarding Neonatal Metabolic Screening, and planning for the introduction of National Universal Hearing Screening.
- BHFC has also been requested by the Department of Health and Children to consider issues around the implementation of a Neonatal Cystic Fibrosis Screening Programme.

All are available on the website.

Endorsement

The BHFC initiative has been endorsed in:
► The National Health Strategy, "Quality and Fairness" (2001). ["Best Health for Children represents a co-ordinated approach to protect and promote children's health in partnership with parents and health professionals and this approach is fully endorsed in the health strategy."]
► The National Childrens' Strategy, "Our Children – Their Lives". (National Children's Office, 2000)
► The report of the Chief Medical Officer on child health, "The Health of our Children". (Department of Health and Children, 2000)
► The National Anti-Poverty Strategy (2002).

BHFC submitted a report, "Use of H.I.P.E. Data in development of Child Health Indicators" to the CEOs (National Conjoint Child Health Committee, 2001b). This work has lead to the suggested indicators being included in a suite of nationally accepted performance indicators.

Outcomes to date

Heightened awareness

BHFC has put child health on the agenda of many relevant organisations and government departments. This is evidenced by the inclusion of child health in key strategies. Furthermore, these organisations have been actively involved in conferences and working groups arranged by BHFC.

Funding

To date, BHFC has succeeded in acquiring a total of 2.8 m Euro from the Department of Health and Children on behalf of ten health boards in order to commence implementation of the initiative.

Framework

An effective communication network has facilitated co-ordination and lack of duplication. Two strategy documents and a number of minor reports have been published. The initiative has been endorsed in four major national strategies.

Concluding overview

This chapter draws together four very different but research-based practical activities to further the availability and use of information to illustrate the current pressing issues of child health in Europe and its member states, and the way in which the span from research to policy can and must be bridged. None of these projects is at the position of standing still, or considering its work to be finished, yet at the same time each is sufficiently firmly grounded to be a foundation stone upon which further practical progress can be made in child health service delivery and development. The pivotal role of sound and reliable information is clear throughout the four examples, as is the dependence upon research in order to identify and define the necessary information and its data sources.

Children are particularly dependent upon the use of reliable and comparable data, turned into structured information systems, to act as their advocate, and this is particularly important for children who fall into disadvantaged groups who are likely to have no natural advocate. These projects indicate the affinity between different research approaches and action initiatives within public health, but also the synergy which can be obtained by very different projects coming together and sharing experiences within the European context.

What stands out clearly is the exciting potential of linking together better information, achieved through research into method and use as well as subject, and better application to enable individuals and policy makers to make better decisions. If that can be achieved, then important gains in child health will result, to the benefit of current children and present and future society.

Acknowledgements. *The CHILD Project was part funded under the European Commission Community Health Indicators Programme as Project 2000 IND 2049, Grant Agreement S12.289740 (2000CVG3-505). The KIDSCREEN Project is funded by the European Commission Quality of Life Research Programme, contract number: QLG-CT-2000-00751. Both projects comprise teams of contributors as listed in project documents, whose input has been pivotal to the work.*

References

Aynesly-Green A, *et al* (2000). Who is Speaking for Children and Adolescents and for their Health at Policy Level? British Medical Journal, 321:229–232.

BMJ (2002) Clinical Evidence; a compendium of best available evidence for effective health care, 6th Edition. BMJ Publishing Group.

Bruil J, Detmar S, Phillips K, Bisegger C, Herdman M, Rajmil L, Duer W, Boltzmann L, Auquier P. Gosch A. Ravens-Sieberer U & the European KIDSCREEN Group (2002). Itemdevelopment in the European Kidscreen Project. HRQOL in healthy children, from focusgroups to pilot questionnaire. Quality of Life Research, 11, 7:638.

Bullinger M, Alonso J, Apolone G, Leplège A, Sullivan M, Wood-Dauphinee S, Gandek B, Wagner A, Aaronson N, Bech P, Fukuhara S, Kaasa S, Ware J (1998). Translating health status questionnaires and evaluating their quality: The International Quality of Life Assessment Project approach. J Clin. Epidem. 51, 11:913–924.

Department of Health and Children (2000). "The Health of our Children". Stationery Office, Dublin.

Department of Health and Children (2001). The National Health Strategy "Quality and Fairness". Stationery Office, Dublin.

Department of Social Community and Family Affairs (2002). National Anti-Poverty Strategy. Stationery Office, Dublin.

Detmar S, Bruil J, Bisegger C, Phillips K, Herdman M, Auquier P, Ravens-Sieberer U & the European KIDSREEN Group (2002). Using Focus groups to determine what constitutes the quality of life of healthy children. Quality of Life Research; 11, 7:631.

Denyer S, Thornton L, Pelly H (1999) Best. Health for Children – Developing a Partnership with Families. Conjoint Body of Chief Executive Officers, Republic of Ireland.

Herdman M, Rajmil L, Ravens-Sieberer U, Bullinger M, Power M, Alonso J, and the European Kidscreen and Disabkids groups (2002). Expert consensus in the development of a European health-related quality of life measure for children and adolescents: a Delphi study. Acta Paediatrica; 91:1–6.

Jepson R (2000). The Effectiveness of Interventions to change Health Related Behaviours: a review of reviews. MRC Social and Public Health Sciences Unit. Occaisonal Paper No 3.

Köhler L (1998). Child Public Health – A New Basis for Child Health Workers. European Journal of Public Health, 8:253–255.

Macfarlane A, McPherson A (2002a). The Diary of a Teenage Health Freak (3rd Ed) Oxford University Press, Oxford.

Macfarlane A, McPherson A (2002b). The Diary of the Other Health Freak (3rd Ed) Oxford University Press, Oxford.

Macfarlane A, McPherson A (2002c). RU A Teenage Health Freak? Oxford University Press, Oxford.

National Children's Office (2000). The National Children's Strategy, Our Children – Their Lives. Stationery Office, Dublin.

National Conjoint Child Health Committee (2001a). Get Connected – Developing an Adolescent Friendly Health Service. Best Health for Children, Dublin.

National Conjoint Child Health Committee (2001b). Use of Hospital Inpatient Enquiry data in development of Child Health Indicators. Report presented to the Conjoint Body of Chief Executive Officers. Best Health for Children, Dublin

National Conjoint Child Health Committee (2002). Investing in Parenthood – to achieve best health for children. Best Health for Children, Dublin.

Ravens-Sieberer U, Gosch A, Abel T, Auquier P, Bellach B-M, Dür W, Rajmil L & the European KIDSCREEN Group (2001). Quality of life in children and adolescents: a European public health perspective. Social and Preventive Medicine 46:297–302.

Ravens-Sieberer U, von Rueden U, Power M, Rajmil L, Cloetta B, Erhart M, & the European KIDSCREEN Group (2002) the KIDSCREEN Project: results from the Pilot test in seven European countries. Quality of Life Research; 11, 7:637.

Rigby M (1998). Information in Child Health Management. In Rigby M, Ross EM, Begg NT (eds). Management for Child Health Services, Chapman and Hall, London.

Rigby M (1999). Realising the Fundamental Role of Information in Health Care Delivery and Management (Reducing the Zone of Confusion). Nuffield Trust, London.

Rigby M, Köhler L (2002). Child Health Indicators of Life and Development (CHILD) – Report to the European Commission. Centre for Health Planning and Management and Health and Consumer Protection Directorate, European Commission, Keele, UK.

Roberts R (1999). Information for Evidence-based Care (Harnessing Health Information Series No. 1); Radcliffe Medical Press, Abingdon.

Rosser RM (1988). Quality of Life: consensus, controversy and concern, in Quality of Life: assessment and application. In Walker SR and Rosser RM (eds). 1988, MTP Press: Lancaster.

Sackett et al (1996). Evidence Based Medicine: what it is and what it isn't. British Medical Journal, 312:71–72.

Socialstyrelsen (1998). Skolhälsovården 1998: Underlag för egen kontroll och tillsyn. Stockholm. Socialstyrelsen, Stockholm.

Spilker B (1990). Quality of life assessment in clinical trials. Raven Press, New York.

Stewart AL and Ware J (1992), Measuring function and well-being. Duke University Press, Durham NC.

Thomas M, Walker A, Wilmot A, Bennet N (1998). Living in Britain. Results from the 1996 General Household Survey. The Stationary Office, London.

United Nations (1989). Convention on the Rights of the Child. United Nations, New York.

Vanhala M, Vanhala P, Kumpusalo E, Halonen P, and Takala J (1998). Relation between obesity from childhood to adulthood and the metabolic syndrome: population based study. Brit Med Journal, 317:319–320.

World Health Organisation (1948). Constitution of the World Health Organization. 1948, World Health Organisation, Geneva.

WHOQOL-Group (1996). What is quality of life? The WHOQOL Group. World Health Organization Quality of Life Assessment. World Health Forum, 14 (4):354–356.

WHOQOL Group (1998). The World Health Organisation Quality of Life Assessment (WHOQOL): Development and general psychometric properties. Social Sci Med. 46:1569–1585.

Hospital patient migration: analysis using a utility index

Nicola Nante · Gualtiero Ricchiardi · Oussama al Farraj · Sergio Morgagni
Roberta Siliquini · Fulvio Moirana · Gabriele G. Messina · Franco Sassi

Introduction

Patient migration as an effect of patients being able to choose where they wish to be treated (or of following the advice of their general practitioner as an "agent") has always been a decisive factor for the financial equilibrium of private health facilities and now, since Italian Decree Law 502/92 came into force, it has also become equally decisive for public facilities.

The term "patient migration" is used to describe the fact of people residing in a particular area (e.g. a Local Health Organisation or Region) travelling to health facilities in other areas for treatment (Ministero della Sanità, 1996).

In fact it has been calculated that one patient in ten in Italy is hospitalised in Regions other than their own (Biscella 1998); this means approx. 1 000 000 transfers out of approx. 10 000 000 annual admissions (Ministero della Sanità, 2000).

The study of the mechanisms at the basis of this widespread phenomenon is even more important for healthcare planning than it is for its financial implications.

There are two kinds of transfers:

▶ one is caused by objective considerations linked to an actual lack in the patients' local health facilities. In this case the transfers are necessary and are caused by factors other than the patients' own preferences;

▶ the other is derived from subjective reasons. This takes place when patients "emigrate" either because they think they will be taken care of better in other facilities, or for various other reasons which do not necessarily imply negative judgements on the facilities linked to their own residential area (Tessier 1985).

In order to enable accurate forecasts, overcoming the uncertainty caused by the subjective nature of such evaluations and by the consumer's profiting by the freedom of choice, it is a good rule to focus one's attention on the multiple aspects of the complicated chain of provider – producer – consumer of the service. In the field of healthcare, moreover, one needs to remember that the demand for welfare is normally induced, as mentioned above, by the prescriptions of general practitioners or specialists trusted by their patients (Hodgkin 1996; Rozenberg 2001).

Much research has shown that there is a connection between the quality of hospital service and patient migration (Skinner 1977; Egunjobi 1983; Luft 1990; Phibbs 1993; Hansen 1994; Hodgkin 1996; Chernew 1998).

The quality of a service is perceived according to how its characteristics are evaluated. This takes place on a basis of individual judgements, a hospital service thus acting as a set of stimuli on which the person's evaluation is founded.

Many authors have studied the phenomenon of hospital patients migrating (Addari 1995; Degli Esposti 1996; Fabbri 1996; Ugolini 1998; and Baccarani 1998); little research, however, has left the main track of administrative data analysis to investigate directly with the deciders what motivates them to give expression to their preference and actually choose one particular facility instead of another (Skinner 1977; Egunjobi 1983; Luft 1990; Mahon 1993; Phibbs 1993; Mapelli 1993; Hodgkin 1996; Fiorentini 1997; Rozenberg 2001).

The aim of this study is to propose a statistic model for analysing the phenomenon of patient migration capable of explaining and forecasting the deciders' (patients' and general practitioners') choices and providing elements for evaluating the perceived quality of the hospital service by means of a measurement of utility.

Materials and methods

Within the sphere of studies on sanitary economics several methods have been identified for measuring utility as linked to the state of health: Standard Gamble – SG (McNeil 1978, 1981), Visual Analogue – VA (Nord 1991), Time Trade Off – TTO (Torrance 1972), Willingness to Pay – WTP (Donaldson 1993), Conjoint Analysis – CA (Ryan 1997).

A further development of CA, the technique Discrete Choice – DC, has also been used to measure utility as perceived in relation to the use of health services (Mor 1985; Rozenberg 2001). This technique has been referred to in this study.

Assumption terminology

The general structure of a DC model can be represented by a set of assumptions (Ben-Akiva 1985), which concern the decider, the alternatives, the attributes and the decisional rules:

▶ **Decider:** this is the specific entity (e.g. an individual, family, group of people or organisation), which makes a choice. One can ignore all the internal interactions of the group and consider only the decisions in their entirety. In order to explain the variety of the deciders' preferences it will be necessary to include their characteristics, i.e. the socio-economical variables of age, gender, education, profession, income, etc.

▶ **Alternatives:** these are the options open to the decider; the set of alternatives taken into consideration is called the *set of choices*. If such a set is *discrete*, i.e. it contains a limited number of alternatives, which can be listed clearly, it can be analysed with the technique we chose (DC). The preferences among the possible alternatives can be measured using the methods Ranking, Rating Scale or Discrete Choice Exercises (Green 1978). The latter method was chosen for this investigation.

▶ **Attributes:** these are the elements taken into account by deciders when making their decisions. An attribute is not necessarily a directly measurable quantity. The DC technique enables both the attribute itself and its logarithmic transformation to be considered, so that the most suitable one can be identified.

▶ **Decisional rules:** these describe the process followed by the decider to come to his/her decision. Economic theory assumes that the decider's preference for an alternative is determined by a value (called the Utility Index) and that the decider chooses the alternative, which supplies him with the highest level of utility.

The Discrete Choice technique

The Discrete Choice – DC technique makes it possible to evaluate preferences (in the specific case of the patient or doctor) with respect to some of the characteristics of a particular service.

In order to prepare the economic model we hypothesised that when the patient or his/her doctor acting as "agent" needs to select a hospital facility they evaluate the utility of the combination of attributes (see the next paragraph) according to the degree of importance they have themselves allotted to each one.

Let us consider a general decider "i" (doctor or patient) who needs to choose between two alternatives: the hospital belonging to the Local Health Organisation – LHO where he resides (from now on referred to as the "Origin-O") and a hospital outside the circuit of this LHO (from now on referred to as "Destination-D").

If we assume that "i" attributes a certain level of utility to each alternative, the choice will be the one with the highest level. More specifically speaking, "i" will choose "D" if he decides to be transferred (alternative 1), or "O" if he decides to stay in his own area (alternative 0).

For every "i" decider only one possibility (Yi *dummy*) chosen between two possible alternatives can be observed.

$$Y_i = \begin{cases} 1 \text{ if the decider } "i" \text{ moves to Destination } "D" \\ 0 \text{ if the decider } "i" \text{ does not move and prefers to remain in Origin } "O" . \end{cases}$$

$$(2\text{-}1)$$

Let us assume that:
U_{i1} (A_D, C) utility for the decider "i" deriving from alternative 1
U_{i0} (A_O, C) utility for the decider "i" deriving from alternative 0

Then the decisional rule would be:

$$Y_i = \begin{cases} 1 & \text{If } U_{i1}(A_D, C_i) > U_{i0}(A_O, C_i) \\ 0 & \text{If } U_{i0}(A_O, C_i) \geq U_{i1}(A_D, C_i) \end{cases}$$

$$(2\text{-}2)$$

Where A_D represents the attributes characterising the destination facility "D", A_O – represents the attributes characterising the structure of origin "O", and C_i indicates the characteristics of the decider "i".

Since the role of our research in this context is to explain the variation in Y_i and to forecast the choices made by the deciders on the basis of the attributes considered (see next paragraph), we needed to create an economic utility model derived from the choice of each decider.

Generally speaking we can assume that the utility derived from the choice of an alternative "J" ($j = 1$ or 0) made by the decider "I" ($i = 1, 2, ..., T$) is a function of the pre-selected attributes (e.g. reputation of the facility, waiting times, distance, etc.) and of the decider's characteristics (e.g. gender, age, education, profession, income, etc.).

When one chooses between two alternatives (1,0) the key utility factor is the difference between them.

The difference relating to the decider ith, indicated as ΔX_i, would be:

$\Delta x_i = (\text{Attribute "1"}) - (\text{Attribute "0"})$

If $\Delta X_i > 0$ the decider "i" will choose 1 depending on the attribute considered.
If, on the other hand, $\Delta X_i = 0$ the attribute will play no role in his/her choice.

Determining the variables and preparing the questionnaires

We used the Focus Group technique (Corrau 2000) to collect information and indications about the attributes, which can create the patient migration phenomenon and the relative levels of quantitative expression. Two groups were investigated separately:
► patients (5 males and 5 females over 18, recently discharged from Sienna hospital where they had been admitted for certain Diagnosis Related Groups – DRGs (see sampling)
► 6 general practitioners (some Siennese and some from other parts of Italy, in Sienna for training) and 4 privately employed out-patient specialists.

Each group was given an information sheet on the extension of the patient migration phenomenon in Italy and on the work programme planned. Before asking the key question it was thought advisable to prepare each group with an initial warming-up phase of approx. 15 minutes to start the participants interacting with each other, suggesting free associations on patient migration. After this initial phase came the key questions for our research:
► for the first group (patients): "What are the reasons (attributes) for a patient deciding on hospitalisation far from home?"
► for the second group (general practitioners): "What are the criteria (attributes) a doctor follows when advising a patient's admittance (in non-urgent cases) to one hospital rather than another?"

Each participant's opinions were written on a chart.
After this phase the participants were asked to determine the attributes considered most important among those emerging from the discussion.
In this way the main factors concerning the demand (deciders) and the supply (hospital services) emerged, i.e. those connected to the perception of quality and to the decisional process being studied (activation or non-activation of the patient mobility phenomenon):
► demographic factors (such as gender and age);
► socio-economic factors (education, profession, income). It can be intuited that high income levels can facilitate transfers, since, besides treatment costs, the indirect expenses (travel, family members' board and lodging, night nurse, etc.) also play a strong role;
► type (urgent, planned) and causes of admission (seriousness, complexity);
► factors linked to the hospital network's structure, which can be evaluated in terms of presence or absence of the service on the spot, and of the distance between home and hospital. It was agreed to measure this distance in travelling time;
► quality of the facility (judgement of the capability of the hospital facility to solve the health problems in question);
► waiting times for admission;
► communication and co-operation between the hospital and the patient's GP.

The two groups were then asked to suggest the possible levels of expression for each attribute. The information thus obtained was used to prepare two questionnaires: one for the patients and one for the GPs. They were designed to collect general data needed for the use of the "DC" technique (gender, age, education, income, type of admission, etc.) and information on reputation, distance, waiting times, co-operation (for the doctor) on the "Origin" and "Destination" hospitals. (These coincide where patients residing in a Local Health Organisation area are admitted to the hospital belonging to that area or referring to it.) The first section of each questionnaire was aimed at establishing the logic behind the patient's/doctor's choice (*Why did you decide to enter this hospital? Who advised you to enter this hospital? What weight did the reputation of this facility, the waiting time, the distance from your home have in your decision to be admitted here? According to your opin-ion, what is a hospital's good reputation based on? etc.).* The questionnaire for the doctors covers the activity of the previous 30 days and is divided into two sections: the first for the most recent recovery they prescribed for a patient residing in Sienna and admitted to Sienna hospital; the second for their latest patient residing in Sienna and sent to a hospital outside the province of Sienna. The two questionnaires were then perfected by a pilot study covering ten doctors and ten patients.

Samples and methods

Since it was not possible to define which population the investigation on the patients should be referred to, we followed the fundamental indications given in the literature for a statistical study of this kind (Champion 1970; D'Ascani 1987; Bailey 1995) and decided to acquire at least 100 questionnaires correctly filled in by patients and 30 by doctors. The criteria for selecting patients for the study were:

► a random sample of adult patients admitted to Sienna Hospital in March 2001;
► In order to describe the seriousness and complexity of the cases and render them more homogenous the DRG system, as adopted by all Italian hospitals (Bonoldi 1998), was used. The DRGs to be examined were identified on the basis of the following criteria:
  – The DRGs were selected from those with many documented cases (normal recovery in public hospitals);
  – Above all DRGs where recovery could be postponed for a medium or long period were considered, since DRGs of emergency cases do not normally allow the patient any choice. In order to allow comparisons, a few typical, urgent case DRGs were in-cluded (DRGs 127 and 87);
  – Relative importance (in the sample there must be DRGs of various degrees of relative importance); in fact, for some authors this importance is a variable positively corre-lated to the migration level (Fabbri 1996);
  – Low Coefficient of Variation – CV (DRGs with little variation in the inter-group aver-age stay in hospital, i. e. more homogeneous than the others). The average hospitali-sation CV measures the relative inter-group dispersion and can thus be used to com-pare the relative dispersions of two or more DRG distributions. It is known that each DRG represents cases of hospitalised patients with a similar consumption of re-sources (days in hospital); therefore, DRGs with $CV < 1$ are considered homogeneous, whereas a $CV \geq 1$ expresses an excessive dispersion, higher than the group's mean hospital stay. The CV of the length of the stay is influenced by the homogeneity of the cases and by the efficiency of the facility where they are being treated. While it can be hypothesised that in-house efficiency does not change, the seriousness can or cannot change whether or not a selection of pathologies exists. A low CV should be proof of a scarce selection, whether active or passive;
  – Pathologies not belonging to very high specialities (treatment supply not monopo-lised);
  – Inclusion of both surgical and medical pathologies.
► The departments with more frequent admissions due to the above-described DRGs were identified first of all and the investigation was performed there (Table 1).

The survey on the patients was carried out in the Sienna Hospital within 20 days, from 8th March to 1st April, 2001. 151 questionnaires were distributed personally to the patients. The doctors were surveyed by mailing the questionnaires to 50 GPs operating in the Sien-

Table 1. Selection criteria and characteristics of the sample of patients studied

Diagnosis Related Group – DRG	Criteria					Departments						Cases studied		
	Frequency	Relative weight	Possib. of deferment	Variation Coefficients	Non monopolised treatment	General surgery	General medicine	Obstetrics Gynaecology	Ortho-paedics	Urology	Haema-tology	Male	Female	Total
87 Pulmonary oedema and respiratory failure		1.263	X		X		X					2	3	5
127 Heart failure and shock.	X	1.260	X	X	X		X					0	7	7
134 Hypertension	X	0.775	X	X	X		X					1	3	4
162 Operations for inguinal and femoral hernia in people over 17, w/o complications	X	0.75	X	X	X	X						2	3	5
167 Appendectomy with uncomplicated main diagnosis, w/o complications	X	0.68	X	X	X	X						4	1	5
206 Liver diseases except malignant neoplasm, cirrhosis, alcoholic hepatitis w/o complications	X	0.80	X		X		X					4	3	7
209 Major operations on the articulations, arms and legs	X	3.31	X						X			7	11	18
243 Medical disorders of the back	X	0.770	X	X	X		X					2	2	4
245 Bone diseases and specific arthropathies, w/o complications	X	0.759	X	X	X		X					5	2	7
294 Diabetes in people over 35	X	1.008	X	X	X		X					1	3	4
324 Urinary calculosis, w/o complications	X	0.53	X	X	X	X				X		1	4	5
359 Operations on the womb and adnexa, not for malignant neoplasm and w/o complications	X	1.043	X	X	X	X		X				0	9	9
373 Vaginal birth with diagnosed risk of complications	X	0.64	X	X	X			X				0	11	11
391 Normal birth	X	0.20	X	X	X			X				0	9	9
473 Acute leukaemia w/o operation in people over 17		6.82									X	1	2	3
Total												30	73	103

na Commune. Our surveyors then visited each patient and doctor personally to collect the filled-out questionnaires, helping to complete the forms in case of doubt.

Factorial analysis

In the questionnaires given to the patients and doctors the set of input variables which can create patient migration, such as "Reputation of the hospital" (HOSPREP), "Reputation of the department" (DEPTREP), "Reputation of the Chief Physician" (CHIEFREP), "Distance from home" (DIST), "Short waiting list" (SHORTLIST), "Doctor's advice" (DOC-ADV), "Direct acquaintance of a doctor at the hospital/dept." (DIRKNOW), "Direct co-operation with the hospital/dept." (DIRCOOP), etc. Factorial analysis was used to reduce the number of these variables. Factorial Analysis (FA) is a statistical technique for investigating the correlation between the variables/items being considered with regard to a certain phenomenon. FA also identifies any factors explaining such correlation (Royce 1963, Morizet-Mahoudeaux 1983). The SPSS software automatically performed *the analysis of the main components* (Hotelling 1933) and the *Scree Test* (Cattell 1978), identifying three factors, which were named I, II and III. It was seen that these factors were not correlated to each other and were therefore independent. Then the values of these factors were calculated automatically using the method *Direct Oblimin* (Gorsuch 1983) and the *Varimax* normalisation (Kaiser 1958). The correlation values were estimated in terms of factorial correlations (between the variables and the factors) and factorial configuration (weights applied to the variables) (Kline 1997). At this point it was necessary to determine the factor and optimum reading scale for weighing up the single variables. Where the doctors' survey is concerned, as already mentioned, the minimum amount of 100 cases, considered as optimum (Kline 1997) could not be achieved. However, in agreement with a substantial amount of literature, we believe that an item, which reaches the value of 0.2 at least, independently of its positive or negative sign, can be considered as sufficiently correlated to a factor (Cattell 1978; Bailey 1995; Kline 1997; Comrey 1995).

Structuring of the model

The DC model we hypothesised is intended to investigate the reasons behind patient migration on a basis of the differences between the utility values of the attributes of the "Destination" hospital and those of the "Origin" hospital. The Focus Groups, Pilot Studies (and the first data processing phases later on) directed us to those attributes and characteristics of the deciders, which could be adopted in the final structure of the DC model, and to the relating levels of expression (Table 2). When the relationship between the variables is not linear, or when the independent variable is not of the quantitative kind (Dominick 1985; Kazmier 1986), as happened for some cases we took into consideration, we can apply multiple linear regression models, such as the Linear Probability Model – LPM, and multiple logistics regression models such as Logit and Probit, used by Discrete Choice. Analysis with these models offers the advantage of being useful for forecasting and estimating too, instead of only verifying the significance of the relationships existing between the variables. As we have already mentioned, where the relationship between the variables is not linear, it is, in any case, possible to transform the function which expresses this non-linearity into a linear function using a logarithm.

This makes it possible to apply coefficient estimation methods (Ordinary Least Squares) for the LPM and Log Likelihood for models Logit and Probit. The LPM model's parameters

Table 2. Factors studied determining the choice of hospital

Attributes	Levels
Considered in the preparation of the patients' model:	Excellent, Good, Medium, Poor[a]
Reputation of the hospital facility (Rep)	Up to 1, 7, 14, 21, 28, 42, 56, 70, 84 and beyond (days)
Waiting times (Times)	8, 24, 38, 53, 68, 83, 106, 136, 166[c] (minutes)
Distance (Dist)	1 = Male, 2 = Female
Gender[b]	
Considered in the preparation of the doctors' model:	Excellent, Good, Medium, Poor[a]
Reputation of the hospital facility (Rep)	Up to 1, 7, 14, 21, 28, 42, 56, 70, 84 and beyond (days)
Waiting times (Times)	8, 24, 38, 53, 68, 83, 106, 136, 166[c] (minutes)
Distance (Dist)	Constant, Sufficient, Sporadic, None[a]
Co-operation (Co-op)	

[a] In the statistical processing these levels were categorised as follows: ("Excellent, Good = 1", "Medium, Poor = 0") and ("Constant, Sufficient = 1", "Sporadic, None = 0").
[b] It was seen that other characteristics of the patient (age, income, profession, level of education) initially included in the model did not improve it, probably because of the criterion adopted for selecting the sample.
[c] Average values considered as representative of the intervals proposed (e.g. 8 = from 1 to 15 minutes, 24 = from 16 a 30 minutes; ... 166 = from 151 to 180 minutes, the rare excess values were also considered in this last level.

are linear and when the explanatory variables vary there is no guarantee that the probability (in our case the migration) will be included between 0 and 1.

For this reason it is preferable to substitute this linear probability model, or back it up, with statistic models such as Probit and Logit which, not having linear parameters, allow measurement of the relationship between the dependent variable (expressed in terms of probability) and a set of independent variables, and whose interval of probability always lies between 0 and 1 (Aldrich 1984; Griffiths 1993).

The fact that the relationship between the probability that Y will assume value 1 (he/she migrates) and every explanatory variable X_i (reputation of the facility, waiting times, distance, co-operation) is non-linear means that the effect of X_i on the probability of Pr $(Y=1)$ is less evident than in the linear probability model. Therefore, in the model we adopted the utility the deciders "i" perceived of migrating from "O" to "D" is described (estimated) by the following linear functions U (.):

$$\Delta U_i = \beta_0 + \beta_1 C_i + \beta_2 \Delta\text{Rep} + \beta_3 \Delta\text{Temp} + \beta_4 \Delta\text{Dist} + e_i \text{ (Patients' model)} \quad (2\text{-}3)$$

$$\Delta U_i = a_0 + a_1 \Delta\text{Rep} + a_2 \Delta\text{Temp} + a_3 \Delta\text{Dist} + a_4 \Delta\text{Coll} + e_i \text{ (Doctors' model)} \quad (2\text{-}4)$$

where:

▶ ΔU_i indicates the difference between the level of utility the decider "i" attributes to "D" and "O";

▶ ΔRep, ΔTimes, ΔDist and ΔCo-op refer, respectively, to the difference in level of reputation, waiting times, distance/travelling times in minutes and that of the co-operation between the GP and the hospital facility where the patient is admitted. The natural logarithm Ln of the variable distance "$Dist$" was considered in the statistic processing;

▶ the parameters β_0 and a_0 are the constant terms or intercepts of the regression and give the estimated value of ΔU_i when the independent variables ΔRep, ΔTimes, ΔDist and ΔCo-op (for the GP) = 0;

▶ C_i indicates the characteristics of the decider "i" and refers to his/her parameter with β_1;

▶ The parameters β_k ($k = 2, 3, 4$), a_w ($w = 1, 2, 3, 4$) measure the variation of ΔU_i for every unit variation of the independent variable when the other independent variables are kept constant; the parameters β and α are coefficients of the partial regression, since they correspond to the partial derivative of ΔU_i with respect to the independent variable;

▶ Finally, e_i represents the imponderable factors in the utility function of the decider "i".

During the course of the processing phases on the basis of the interactions encountered amongst the variables for the estimation of the ΔUi utility index the following equations were found to be the best:

$$\Delta U_i = \beta_0 + \beta_1 \text{Sesso} + \beta_2 \Delta \text{Rep} + \beta_3 \Delta \text{Temp} + \beta_4 \Delta \text{Dist} + \beta_5 \Delta \text{Dist}^2 +$$
$$+ \beta_6 (\Delta \text{Dist} * \Delta \text{Rep}) + e_i \quad \text{(Patients)} \tag{2-5}$$

$$\Delta U_i = \alpha_0 + \alpha_1 \Delta \text{Rep} + \alpha_2 \Delta \text{Temp} + \alpha_3 \Delta \text{Dist} + \alpha_4 (\Delta \text{Dist} \times \Delta \text{Rep}) +$$
$$+ \alpha_5 \Delta \text{Coll} + \alpha_6 (\Delta \text{Rep} \times \Delta \text{Dist}^2) + e_i \quad \text{(Doctors)} \tag{2-6}$$

The marginal effects of each independent variable on the probability $P(Y = 1)$ in the Probit and Logit models are identified with the mark β_k, α_w, which determines the direction of each effect, which tends to grow as β_k, α_w increases, while the relative size varies together with the variation of the independent variable ΔX_i. The data were processed with statistics software SAS version 6.00 and SPSS version 10.

Results and considerations

Table 2 as mentioned in the "Materials and Methods" (Structuring of the model), contains the attributes and deciders' characteristics (factors determining the choice of hospital), and the relating levels of expression adopted according to the results of the Focus Groups and pilot studies. The following tables and figures refer to the outcomes of the sample investigations performed on hospitalised patients and GPs.

Of the 151 questionnaires distributed to the patients, 27 (17.9%) were refused; 17 patients (11.3%) were discharged straight after the distribution and were, therefore, non longer available; in 4 cases (2.7%) the name and address were not filled in and so they were not included in the processing. 103 questionnaires (68.2%) were completely filled in and processed; (Table 1) refers to these.

Of the 50 questionnaires sent to the doctors 30 (60%) were sent back correctly completed, while in 20 cases (40%) there was no co-operation. 8 of the 30 doctors who co-operated (26.6%) had sent all their patients needing hospitalisation to different hospitals than those belonging to their LHO in the 30 days prior to the interview. 8 (26.6%) turned to both local facilities and other structures, while the remaining 14 (46.6%) had patients hospitalised within their own LHO. In all, the 30 doctors co-operating prescribed 38 admissions in the thirty days preceding the interview. The following results refer to these cases. From an examination of Table 3 one can see that the patients felt that all the attributes included in the study were important (reputation 80.6%, waiting times 64%, distance 55.4%). On the other hand it was clear that the doctors were insensitive to the distance from the patient's home to the hospital prescribed (reputation 81%, waiting times 73.7%, distance 31.6%, co-operation 86.8%). In general, distance seems to be the least important attribute amongst those considered, for both patients and doctors. Reputation and (for the doctors) co-operation appear to be the most important attributes.

Table 4 analyses the motives supplied by those interviewed for their deciding on admission to Sienna Hospital, whether the patients belonged to Sienna LHO no. 7 (not migrating) or not (migrating).

Table 3. Judgement of the importance of the variables considered

Attributes	Patients' judgement (n = 103)				Doctors' judgement (n = 38)			
	Unimport.	Not very Important.	Import.	Very Import.	Unimport.	Not very Important.	Import.	Very Import.
Reputation	10.7%	8.7%	49.5%	31.1%	5.3%	13.2%	36.8%	44.7%
Waiting times	23.3%	12.6%	31.1%	33%	5.3%	21.1%	52.6%	21.1%
Distance	26.2%	18.5%	28.2%	27.2%	47.4%	21.1%	15.8%	15.8%
Co-operation	–	–	–	–	5.3%	7.9%	34.2%	52.6%

Table 4. Percentage distribution of the Deciders according to the criteria adopted for their choice of hospital for admittance

Criteria for choice and/or migration	Patients (n = 103)		Doctors (n = 38 patients)	
	No migration	Migration	No migration	Migration
Hospital's reputation (HOSPREP)	19.4	8.7	0	0
Department's reputation (DEPTREP)	20.4	6.8	30	26.7
Chief physician's reputation (HEADREP)	12.6	9.7	0	0
Nearness to own home (DIST)	33	9.7	0	0
Short waiting list (SHORTLIST)	3.9	1.9	3.3	6.7
Doctor's advice (DOCADV)	11.7	11.7	–	–
Direct acquaintance with a hosp./dept. doctor. (DIRACQ)	14.6	16.5	6.7	10
Direct co-operation with the hospital/departm. (CO-OP)	–	–	6,7	10

It is noticeable that the doctors and patients use different criteria when making their decisions: while reputation, especially that of the department for the recovery, is important for both categories, the distance of the hospital is important only for the patients and does not affect the doctor, and the waiting times influence the doctor, and also the patient, but much less.

Table 5 carries the results of the factorial analysis (analysis of the main components, Scree Test, Direct Oblimin, Kaiser Varimax normalisation) of the relations between the variables listed in the previous table corresponding to the patients interviewed. The correlations between the variables and their linking factors are thus determined.

Where the doctors' model is concerned no statistics were calculated since the variances of the items (HOSPREP, CHIEFREP, DIST) equal zero; moreover, the sample is not large enough for this analysis to achieve any statistical significance.

One can see that the average of all the items lies between 0.22 and 0.34, and the standard deviation between 0.42 and 0.47, except for item SHORTLIST with an average of 0.05 and standard deviation of 0.24. These results show that the above variables are almost equally important as reasons for migration, while the "Waiting Times" variable differs from the others.

The items over 0.2, considered the significance threshold, are shown in bold. It can be seen that:

▶ the first factor is significant for items HOSPREP ($r = 0.74$), DIRKNOW, ($r = 0.71$), DEP-TREP ($r = 0.48$) and DIST ($r = -0.25$); this suggests that a hospital's reputation is linked to the fact that when doctors working in a particular department are known directly, they attract patients even from far-off areas.

Table 5. Results of the factorial analysis (analysis of main components, Scree Test, Direct Oblimin, Kaiser Normalisation) on the observations reported by the 103 patients interviewed

	Item		Factorial Correlations			Factorial Configuration		
	Average	S.D.	Factor I	Factor II	Factor III	Scale I	Scale II	Scale III
HOSPREP	0.28	0.45	0.736	0.042	−0.014	0.547	0.020	−0.090
DIRACQ	0.31	0.47	0.712	0.044	0.121	0.516	0.019	0.022
DIST	0.34	0.48	−0.245	0.737	−0.211	−0.170	0.593	−0.160
SHORTLIST	0.05	0.24	0.095	0.586	0.094	0.054	0.461	0.058
DOCADV	0.23	0.42	−0.172	−0.583	−0.157	−0.105	−0.455	−0.098
HEADREP	0.22	0.42	−0.138	−0.0003	0.865	−0.186	−0.108	0.718
DEPTREP	0.27	0.45	0.479	0.196	0.662	0.290	0.131	0.484
Total variation percentage explained			21.45	17.93	16.14			
Kaiser Meyer Olkin Test			TKMO=0.458					
Barlett Test		$\chi^2=35.49$	DF=21	P<0.025				

Table 6. What does a hospital's "good reputation" mean for patients? (values per cent)

Reputation Indicators	Patients (n = 103)	Doctors (n = 38)
No judgement	1.0	0.0
Presence of valid and well-known specialists	53.4	44.7
Availability of sophisticated, modern equipment	11.7	2.6
Large number of cases treated	4.9	10.5
Recovery rates	7.8	21.1
Percentage of satisfied patients	10.7	13.2
Percentage of patients of other regions/provinces	1.0	0.0
Polite, willing staff	7.8	2.6
Modern facility	1.9	5.3

▶ the second factor is significant for items DIST ($r=0.74$), SHORTLIST ($r=0.59$), DOCADV ($r=-0.58$) and DEPTREP ($r=0.20$); this factor suggests that where there is no advice from doctor lack of co-operation? "do-it-yourself" patients?) the distance and short waiting times come to the fore; i.e. accessibility conditions the patient's choice;

▶ the third factor is significant for items CHIEFREP ($r=0.87$), DEPTREP ($r=0.66$) and DIST ($r=-0.21$); this factor shows that the reputation of a department is founded on that of its chief physician and both attract patients from afar.

The same table shows the loads of each item according to its actual contribution to a particular scale. According to the Kaiser Meyer Olkin test (KMO) the sample is sufficient (KMO index = 0.458). The correspondence (i.e. how far the data foreseen by the model correspond to those actually measured) evaluated by the Barlett test ($\chi^2=35.49$ with 21 degrees of freedom-DF and $p<0.025$) was significant. The table contains the percentages of the explained variance attributable to the single factors; it would obviously be best to identify all the factors so as to explain the variance totally. It is not normally considered advisable to go so far ahead with the investigation. Justifying the 55.52% of the variance with only a few factors (Factor I = 21.45%, Factor II = 17.93%, Factor III = 16.14%) is a result we can consider more than satisfying (Kline 1997) and we decided not to proceed further. Table 6 shows the significance of a hospital's reputation (the main selection criterion according to the results) for the 103 patients and 30 doctors interviewed.

It is noticeable that the highest percentages are generally expressed by the *presence of excellent, well-known specialists* (53.4% for the patients and 44.7% for the doctors). Then come:

▶ for the patients, the technical equipment (11.7%), the satisfaction reported by acquaintances and relations (10.7%) and the courtesy, availability and willingness of the staff (7.8%);

▶ for the doctors, clinical efficacy (21.1%), the amount of pathologies treated (10.5%), the satisfaction reported by previous patients (13.2%).

Table 7 shows the results obtained using the DC technique.

Among the decider's various characteristics only gender was seen to be important, although it was not statistically significant, as we shall see. Age, income, profession and education, initially included in the model as explanatory variables, were then removed because they brought no improvement and do not clarify the variation in Y_i.

▶ age: most of the patients interviewed were more than 75 years old;

▶ income: the majority stated they had a low annual income of less than 10 000 000 Lit.;

▶ profession: given their age, the patients were retired;

▶ education: most were blue-collar workers and housewives.

For conciseness the table only contains the results obtained by logistic regression (model Logit – main effects) since both models, Logit and Probit, have proved, also in our investigation, to correspond to each other where the interpretation of the results is concerned (Liao 1994). Several authors have found that it is possible to obtain approximately the coefficients of the Probit model starting with the values obtained with Logit, dividing the parameters estimated calculated by the factor 1.814 according to Aldrich (1984) or by the factor 1.6 according to Amemiya (1981).

From a first reading of Table 7 emerges a very high significance for both models (patients $p[X^2(6) > 13.232] = 0.0001$ or doctors $p[\chi^2(6) > 34.406] = 0.008$): i.e. the Likelihood Ratio shows that at least one coefficient relating to the independent variables is other than zero. Therefore, the models explain the variability of the phenomenon studied. An analysis of the table shows that:

▶ the intercept in both models has a negative sign (*Patients: –7.48, t = 2.24, p < 0.13; Doctors: –1.86, t = 6.72, p < 0.01*); this means that, when all the characteristics of the two facilities Origin and Destination are the same, the decider is not willing to move away from his own area.

▶ The "gender" parameter in the patients' model was negative (*+6.08, t = 2.39, p < 0.12*); although the "gender" variable has a low significance level, its inclusion is justified by the improvement it brings to the model's adaptation.

▶ The ΔRep parameter was positive in both models (*Patients 6.79, t = 3.81, p < 0.05; Doctors 6.51, t = 0.93, p < 0.33*); when the level of reputation of the Destination facility grows with respect to the Origin, the utility for the decider also grows, and with it the probability of migration.

▶ The ΔTimes parameter was negative in both models (*Patients –0.03, t = 0.39, p < 0.53; Doctors –0.37, t = –7.11, p < 0.007*); this shows that the increase in the waiting times of a nearby facility with respect to the one further away increases the utility and consequent probability of migration.

▶ The ΔDist parameter is, paradoxically, positive in both models (*Patients 0.15, t = 3.88, p < 0.049; Doctors 0.31, t = 8.91, p < 0.003*). Logically speaking, one would expect a negative sign: if the distance increases, the probability of migration should be less. It seems that distance has an effect on reputation (the patient who has no faith in his local hospital prefers to go to a distant one which he presumably knows less about).

Table 7. Comparison of the estimators (Logit – Main Effects of the two models)

Estimation of	Patients	Doctors
Intercept	−7.4847	−1.862
Standard Error	4.9964	0.719
T-ratio	2.24	6.715
Significance	0.1341	0.010
Gender	6.0845	–
Standard Error	3.9349	
T-ratio	2.39	
Significance	0.1220	
Rep	6.7933	6.516
Standard Error	3.4864	6.746
T-ratio	3.81	0.933
Significance	0.0514	0.334
Times	−0.0318	−0.369
Standard Error	0.0512	0.140
T-ratio	0.39	6.960
Significance	0.5340	0.008
Dist(*)	0.1519	0.305
Standard Error	0.0770	0.102
T-ratio	3.88	8.908
Significance	0.0486	0.003
Dist*Dist	0.0011	–
Standard Error	0.0005	
T-ratio	4.83	
Significance	0.0280	
Rep*Dist	0.0435	−0.209
Standard Error	0.0454	0.295
T-ratio	0.92	0.499
Significance	0.3372	0.480
Co-op	–	−5.339
Standard Error		2.597
T-ratio		4.227
Significance		0.040
Rep*Dist2	–	0.0003
Standard Error		0.003
T-ratio		0.007
Significance		0.932
−2LLR	13.232	34.406
DF	6	6
Overall significance	p < 0.0001	0.008

* Was considered the natural logarithm of the distance Ln (Dist) in the regression analysis

▶ All the squares of the various attributes were examined and only the square of the distance in the patients' model was found to be significant and to improve the model (*0.0011, t = 4.83, p < 0.03*);

▶ The par ameter of the *Δ*Coop variable has a negative sign (*–5.34, t = 0.0001,n.s.*), a condition which leads one to think that there is little communication and co-operation between the doctor and the hospitals, both of Origin and of Destination. It is likely that the negative sign is determined above all by the poor co-operation between the GP and the local hospital, which encourages patient migration.

▶ In our endeavours to improve the model, we examined the square effects of the various attributes: only the distance square of the patients' model was significant, with an improvement of (*0.0011, t = 4.83, p < 0.03*); it was thus included in Table 6;.

▶ If we associate the Distance (or square distance for the doctors' model) to the reputation, we get a positive sign for the parameter (*Patients 0.041, t = 0.92, p < 0.34; Doctors 0.0003, t = 0.007, p < 0.93*);

▶ We interpret this datum in the sense that when the level of reputation increases, there is an increase in the probability of migration independently of the fact that the hospital is far from home. The negative sign obtained for the Rep * Dist parameter with the doctors' model is not so easy to interpret.

Figure 1, structured fundamentally with the application of the DC models described above (see Appendix) illustrates the dynamics resulting from increases or reductions of some variables (waiting times, reputation, reputation associated with distance, co-operation). It can be seen that:

▶ a reduction of the waiting times in favour of the hospital of Destination causes an increase in the probability of migration, both of "do-it-yourself" patients (A) and of patients sent by their GP (a);

▶ the interaction of Reputation and Distance improves the significance of the values, as explained above, but it does not alter the behaviour profile already noted for Reputation alone;

▶ the lower the level of co-operation between GP and local hospital, the greater the tendency to hospitalise patients in distant facilities;

▶ there are different profiles in the curves referring to the decisional models of both patients and doctors.

Conclusions

This study was aimed at finding a statistical model capable of explaining (and forecasting) patients' and GPs' choices of hospitals for admission.

By means of Focus Groups and interviews conducted on samples of GPs and patients we discovered the main principles determining their choice of hospital for treatment:

▶ the reputation of the hospital, waiting times and distance were the most important factors for the patients;

▶ co-operation with the hospital, its reputation and the waiting times were the most important for the doctors.

Logically, doctors and patients seem to use different decisional criteria: while reputation, especially that of the department for admission, is important for both categories, the distance from home is important only for the patients and does not affect the doctors' judgement; waiting times affect the doctor's choice but are not nearly so important for of the patient.

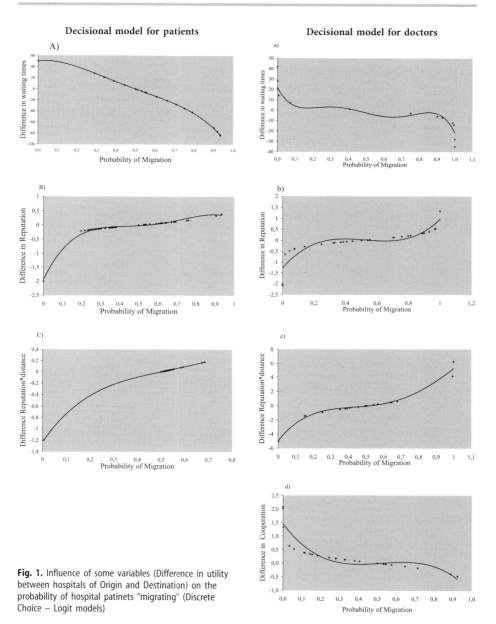

Fig. 1. Influence of some variables (Difference in utility between hospitals of Origin and Destination) on the probability of hospital patinets "migrating" (Discrete Choice – Logit models)

The asymmetry existing between the information possessed by doctors and patients is the most natural explanation of this phenomenon: e.g. whether it is advisable to solving the clinical problem as soon as possible or how long the waiting times are for other hospitals. Mahon (1993) has observed that most GPs are well informed about the hospital waiting times in their area, while the information is not normally readily available for patients. We shall come back to this subject later.

Using Factorial Analysis on the patients' answers, we investigated the links between the above-mentioned decisional criteria. This technique proved it could clarify the nature of the variables examined and we determined the weights for each variable. The main indications emerging from this analysis are:

▶ the reputation of the hospital chosen is often linked to the patient's direct knowledge of a doctor working in a certain department, even though he may be far away (Factor I). This leads us to emphasise the importance of the promotional role held by hospital doctors' activities (mostly freelance) in different out-patients' clinics/surgeries from where they are employed;

▶ when the GP does not advise a department/hospital for admission (and only then) the importance of ease of access (first distance and second a short waiting list) emerges (Factor II);

▶ the department's reputation derives mainly from that of its chief physician. (Factor III).

Special attention was paid to investigating the genesis of the main selection criterion, the hospital's reputation, and the results showed that the reputation of a department or hospital is, in fact, unequivocally due to the presence of excellent, well-known specialists. Doctors and patients thus agree on human resources being prevalent in determining quality. Although technical equipment is also important, it is subordinate for how utility is perceived.

In creating the reputation of a hospital/department, humanity and relationships were decisive for the patients (e.g. satisfaction reported by acquaintances and relations, polite, kind and willing staff), while the doctors considered "objective" knowledge (clinical efficiency and efficacy, a wide range of pathologies treated) but also the satisfaction reported by previous patients as more relevant.

The DC model we prepared investigated the differences between the values of the variables-attributes (the motives we studied determining patients migration) concerning the hospitals of Destination and Origin. (Skinner 1977; Egunjobi 1983; Luft 1990; Mahon 1993; Phibbs 1993; Hodgkin 1996; Rozenberg 2001). The main results achieved were:

▶ the deciders are willing to sacrifice the benefits of a hospital facility near their home for one with a better reputation;

▶ when the level of the Destination hospital's reputation increases with respect to the hospital of Origin, the utility for the decider, and consequently the probability of migrating, also increases, and the latter pursues the good reputation independently of the distance involved. The probability of the patient migrating does not lessen with the increase in distance. On the contrary, a paradoxical "effect of reputation" was observed (the patient who does not trust his own hospital of reference prefers to be admitted to another he knows less about).

▶ Shorter waiting times for the hospital of Destination mean that both "do-it-yourself" patients and those sent by their GPs will probably migrate. Long waiting times in the nearby hospital with respect to the distant one naturally increase the probability of transfer. Shorter waiting times locally can limit hospital patients' migration, so it is excellent that the strategic aims of the Italian National Health Programme 2002/2004 include "adapting the waiting times and ease of access to the consumers' requirements" (Ministero della Salute, 2002).

▶ The lower the level of co-operation is between the GP and the hospital of reference, the greater the tendency to admit patients to distant hospitals. Co-operation and communication are, therefore, important for motivating a GP to send a patient to a particular hospital and, once more, this study has highlighted the insufficiency in this field.

▶ Various different profiles can be seen in the curves referring to the decisional models of the patients and doctors.

This latest discovery, already emerging with the comment to Table 4 and Figure 1, is a function of the asymmetry in information, which justifies the GP's role of agent.

It can be hypothesised that the differences between these profiles increase or decrease according to the era and the social/cultural contexts, and that they become less substantial where information is readily available and the patient trusts in his doctor.

In fact, for a GP to become an Agent, a foundation of mutual trust should be there: he acts on behalf and in the interest of the patient and interprets his needs, taking his place in choosing the health care providers necessary for satisfying them. The decisional incidence of the GP's role is decisive in all phases of the process of converting the need for health into a request for treatment and in the choice of the quality and substance of the health services capable of satisfying the request (Rozenberg 2001). On the other hand, besides being the patient's intermediary for the request, the GP normally takes part in actually producing health care, so he may be conditioned by factors of an economic-professional nature. For this reason he could be an "imperfect agent" (Rossi 1994; Brenna 1999).

Correcting the lack of access to information, which conditions the patient's freedom of choice, or developing the role of the GP as an agent and his trustful relationship with the patient are two potential alternatives for future strategic action to be taken by the Italian National Health Service.

The Italian National Health Programme 2002/2004 appears to be indicative here, since, besides aiming to reduce the time required for diagnosis and treatment, it provides for monitoring of the relative data and their sharing via a computer system dedicated to structures and professional people (hospitals, LHCs, regional councils, central administrational bodies, doctors). However, this system is not meant to be directly accessible by citizens/patients (Ministero della Salute, 2002).

Phibbs (1993) used the Logit Conditional model, inserting control variables (quality, prices for services and road distance between hospitals) to demonstrate that the choice of a hospital depends on how long the treatment of the pathology can be deferred.

For our research we considered above all DRGs with a medium and high possibility of deferment; those cases with possibility of deferment zero (emergencies, accident victims) do not normally allow any choice and are directed to the nearest hospital (Hansen 1994).

A patient with cancer, perceived as the most worrying problem, is intuitively more willing to move to distant facilities (naturally where there is no clinical emergency) than a patient needing selective interventions for solving other pathologies.

There is no doubt that more analytical studies on patient migration in relation to specific pathologies could lead to more useful indications on the determinants of the migration flows.

The fact that, in the absence of other input, and also for pathologies where treatment can be postponed, patients in general tend to apply for admission to the nearest hospital has been ascertained (Chernew 1998).

Hansen (1994) found that patients residing on the border between different hospital consumer areas considered the technical quality of the treatment, comfort and humanity, previous experiences (Gooding 1996) and easy access (e.g. public transport) to be most important when selecting a hospital.

Payment terms or insurance constitute another well-known determinant, which we did not study since they do not affect the Italian National Health Service (Chernew 1998).

The possibility of making choices without having to worry about the financial side is in itself a sign of the quality of our health system.

The programme for the hospital networks proposes to eliminate the less quantifiable financial conditioning deriving from the distance of the hospital.

However, it is becoming clearer and clearer that emphasising the patients' freedom of choice, keeping up the network and developing the quality of the assistance (e.g. through competitive mechanisms) are goals reconcilable only with the availability of substantial financial means and the capability of attentive evaluation.

Where there is the same level of coverage, and patients have received objective information about it (e.g. post-hospitalisation mortality with specific causes, availability of advanced technology), the technical quality of the treatment provided appears to be the main determinant for patients transferring and, therefore, the main thing the hospitals are asked for (Hodgkin 1996; Chernew 1998).

We leave our observations on this determinant to other studies, including our own (Nante 1999; Nante 2000a; Nante 2000b; Nante 2001).

The model we created enables calculation of a "utility index". On the one side the utility index can help the patient to make the right choice and, on the other, it is actually a perceived quality evaluator. In fact, this instrument transcends the function of the techniques for measuring the consumer's satisfaction *a posteriori* (Nante 2002; Pellegrino 2002), which are useful for management, and assumes an important planning role. The model enables:

▶ the identification of the possible transfers of a patient/group of patients, while improving the weak spots;

▶ the establishment, on a simulation basis, of the features that a hospital/department already existing, or being built, should have in order to overcome competition in the vicinity.

We believe this second use could be even more helpful than the first.

To give an example, Table 8 compares two hospitals: one of Origin "O" and one of Destination "D"; in both there is an identical level of reputation 0 (1(D)-1(o)=0), but different waiting lists (5(D)-10(O)=-5 days) and a different distance from the patient's home (20(D)-6(O)=14 minutes) in "O" with respect to "D".

The result is a utility level (index) of approx. -0,817 equal to a likelihood of 0,31, for (male) patients to migrate towards the Destination hospital.

The example given in Table 8, with vector of the explanatory variables [1 0 -5 14], compares 2 hospitals; however, it is possible to hypothesise uses for improving a single hospital, starting from the actual data and, on the basis of viable planning choices, simulate the changes these factors would cause in that hospital.

Furthermore, one can obtain the marginal effects of each single independent variable on the probability (PrY = 1), as shown in Table 8; if the if the ΔTime (Difference in waiting times) increases by one unit, the probability diminishes by approx. 0.01, while, if ΔDist (Difference between the distances) increases by one unit, the probability grows by approx. 0.03. Finally, if the increase in ΔDist is accompanied by an increase in ΔRep (Difference in reputation), we will obtain a probability increase of approx. 0.01.

Table 8. Results obtained with the patients' Logit using simulation

Coefficients	β_0	β_1	β_2	β_3	β_4	β_5	β_6	Utility Index	Prob.
Patients' Logit model estimators	−7.48	6.08	6.79	−0.03	0.15	0.001	0.043		
Hypothesised vector of the explanatory variables (ΔX_i)	1	1 (Maschi)	0	−5	2.6391**	6.965	0		
Results	−7.45	6.08	0	0.15	0.396	0.007	0	−0.82	0.31
Marginal effects		*	*	−0.01	0.03	0.0002	0.01		

* The marginal effects of the categorised variables are not calculated (Liao Tim 1994); ** Ln (14) = 2.6391

Our study was limited by the fact that we began with real decisions already taken (hospitalisations in course or over) and went back to the characteristics, as perceived by the decider (doctor or patient), which motivated their choice.

This represents an inverted route with respect to the traditional DC path, which starts with a predefined set of characteristics and asks the subject to imagine which choices he would make on that basis. This led us to analyse a limited number of possible observations (levels of the variables studied in different combinations) for each subject, while with the traditional approach many hypothetical scenarios can be proposed to the subjects being interviewed. However, the methodology we adopted achieves more realistic results.

The importance of our research does not lie so much in our having discovered new reasons for patient migration, the determinants of which have been known for some time (Hansen 1994; Hodgkin 1996; Chernew 1998), as in the fact that we have attributed specific decisional weights to them and have identified forecasting models based on the values taken on step by step by the determinants.

In the near future we propose to apply these weights to actual data and situations in order to see how the model presented here works in practice.

There is another possible interesting development of our findings, i.e. the application of the game theory to the strategic interaction (competition?) between the Local Health Companies or Hospitals. The function we found to measure the utilities is used to discover which is the best strategy (improving the reputation, reducing the waiting times, reducing the distances between the hospital facilities and their potential consumers) to adopt in order to achieve the equilibrium of the game, i.e. the equilibrium which provides the maximum utility for the players-competitors.

Summary

The aim of this study is to determine a statistical model capable of explaining (and forecasting) the choices of patients and their doctors (GPs) regarding hospitals for admission:

Using focus groups and interviews carried out on samples of patients and doctors (GPs), we found that the main determinants for the choices of a place for treatment made by the above deciders are:

▶ for the patients – **reputation** of the hospital, **waiting times** and **distance** (most important determinants for the patients;

▶ for the doctors – **co-operation** with the hospital, its **reputation** and the **waiting times.**

By performing a factorial analysis on the replies given by a sample of patients we investigated the connections between the decisional criteria shown above and their relative weights. By means of a Discrete Choice model (a development of the Conjoint Analysis technique) we investigated the differences between the value of the variables-attributes (the above-mentioned motivations determining patient migration) we studied in the hospitals of Destination and Origin, observing that:

▶ the deciders are willing to sacrifice the benefits of a hospital facility near home for one with a better **reputation**;

▶ as the level of **reputation** of the Destination hospital grows with respect to the one of Origin, the decider's utility also grows and with it the probability of migration. The deciders follow a good **reputation**, independently of **how far away** the hospital is. The probability of the patient migrating does not diminish as the distance involved increases;

▶ an improvement in the waiting times in favour of the Destination hospital causes an increase in the probability of migration on the part of both "do-it-yourself" patients and of those sent by their GPs. Long waiting times in the nearby facility with respect to the distant one increase, rather obviously, the probability of the patient migrating. The reduction in the waiting times can limit this migration.

▶ The less co-operation there is between the GP and the reference hospital, the greater is the tendency to admit patients to far-off facilities.

▶ Different profiles can be seen in the curves referring to the patients' and doctors' decisional models.

Appendix

When the random variable is discrete, such as Y_i in equation (2-1), we can obtain all the possible values with their respective probabilities by means of a probability density function, which is the basis of a DC statistical model:

(P_i) shall be the probability that the ith decider chooses alternative 1 (he transfers) and ($1 - P_i$) the probability of his choosing alternative 0 (he does not transfer).

In this case the probability density function of Y_i is:

$$g(y_i) = p_i^{y_i}(1 - p_i)^{1-y_i}; \; y_i = 1, 0$$

Therefore, the probability that the decider "i" transfers is:

$$g(1) = p[y_i = 1] = p_i$$

On the other hand, the probability that the same decider "i" does not transfer is:

$$g(0) = p[y_i = 0] = 1 - p_i$$

The mean and variance of the discrete probability distribution of a discrete casual variable Y_i are respectively:

$$E[y_i] = p_i$$
$$Var[y_i] = p_i(1 - p_i)$$

The probability distribution of Y_i is, therefore, completely determined by P_i which expresses both the probability of choosing alternative 1, and the expected value of Y_i.

The random utility model

Since the random utility function is not known with certainty (Aldrich 1984), it is expressed as the sum of an observable component and an idiosyncratic component (random errors):

$$U_{ij} = \bar{U}_{ij} + \varepsilon_{ij}$$

where U_{ij} is the random utility of alternative "J" ($j = 1$ o 0) chosen by the decider "I" ($i = 1, 2, \ldots, T$).

If we wish to express utility U_{ij} as a function of the attributes (Rep, Time, Dist, Co-op) of the alternative preferred and of the decider's characteristics (Gender, Age, Education, Income, Profession), we can write the systematic component, which represents the indirect utility, as

$$\bar{U}_{ij} = A_{ij}\beta + C_i a_j \tag{2}$$

where,

A_{ij} is the vector of the attributes of the alternative "J" of the decider "I" (A_{ij} = Rep, Time, Dist, Co-op);

C_i is the vector of the characteristics of the decider "I" (C_i = Gender, Age, Education, Income, Profession);

β, a_j are vectors of the known parameters.

Combining (1) with (2) we obtain:

$$U_{ij} = A_{ij}\beta + C_i a_j + \varepsilon_{ij} \qquad (3)$$

assuming that the errors are independent for each decider and alternative and that they are distributed normally with a mean of zero and a variance of $\sigma_j^2 2$; ($j = 0, 1$). These hypotheses imply that the utility a decider attributes to an alternative is not correlated with the utility attributed by another decider.

Since we are not sure of being able to find out which alternative will be chosen, but we can foresee the probability of one of the possible alternatives being chosen, specifically, we represent the probability of the decider "i" choosing each alternative as:

$$p_i = p_r[y_i = 1] = p_r[U_{i1} \rangle U_{i0}]$$
$$1 - p_i = p_r[y_i = 0] = p_r[U_{i1} \leq U_{i0}]$$

Given the random utility model in equation (3) we can write:

$$p_i = p_r(U_{i1} \rangle U_{i0})$$
$$p_i = p_r(\bar{U}_{i1} + \varepsilon_{i1} \rangle \bar{U}_{i0} + \varepsilon_{i0})$$
$$p_i = p_r(\varepsilon_{i0} - \varepsilon_{i1} \langle \bar{U}_{i1} - \bar{U}_{i0}) \qquad (4)$$

On this basis we can identify a DC statistical model by substituting (3) with (4) and specifying the distribution of the probabilities of the difference in the random utility errors, $\varepsilon_{i0} - \varepsilon_{i1}$.

First of all, let "I_i" be the utility index representing the difference of utility in the systematic component in the right-hand part of equation (4):

$$I_i = \bar{U}_{i1} - \bar{U}_{i0} = (A_{i1} - A_{i0})\beta + C_i(a_1 - a_0) \qquad (5)$$

$$I_i = [(A_{i1} - A_{i0})C_i]\begin{bmatrix} \beta \\ a_1 - a_0 \end{bmatrix}$$

$$I_i = X_i \eta \qquad (6)$$

We point out that, if the parameters (a_1, a_0), were originally equal, the different characteristics of the individual would not then contribute to the difference in utility. Therefore, the utility index "I_i" is the difference between the systematic component of alternative (1) and that of alternative (0); the bigger "I_i" is, the bigger the systematic component of the alternative (1) is with respect to (0). Consequently, the higher "I_i" is, the higher the probability that alternative (1) will be preferred to (0).

By substituting (4) with (6) we obtain:

$$p_i = p_r[\varepsilon_{i0} - \varepsilon_{i1} \leq X_i \eta] = p_r[e_i \leq X_i \eta] \qquad (7)$$

Equation (7) highlights the fact that the probability that alternative 1 will be chosen is the probability that the difference in the random errors e_i will be less than or equal to the utility index.

Given that the errors ε_{ij} are independent random variables, with a mean of zero and variance σ_j^2, their difference is $e_i \sim N(0, \sigma^2 = \sigma_0^2 + \sigma_1^2)$:

$$p_i = p_r[e_i \leq X_i \eta]$$

$$p_i = p_r\left[\frac{e_i}{\sigma} \leq \frac{X_i \eta}{\sigma}\right] \tag{8}$$

$$p_i = p_r[\kappa_i \leq X_i \beta]$$

where

$$\kappa_i = \frac{e_i}{\sigma}, \quad \beta = \frac{\eta}{\sigma}$$

The random variable κ_i is distributed normally with a mean of zero and a variance of one: $N(0, 1)$.

The probability that the random variable κ_i is "less than" or "equal to", is provided by the cumulative distribution function of the random variable. Consequently, the probability that alternative 1 will be chosen is:

$$p_{i1} = p_r[\kappa_i \leq X_i \beta] = \phi(X_i \beta)$$

where

$\phi(X_i \beta)$ is the value of the cumulative distribution function of the standardised variable and is calculated by means of the following formula, called the "Probit Model":

$$p_i = \phi(X_i \beta) = \phi(I_i) \tag{9}$$

where $\phi(.)$ is the cumulative distribution function of the standardised random variable.

Generally we can write:

$$\phi(I_i] = \phi X_i \beta = \int_{-\infty}^{X_i \beta} 2\pi^{-\frac{1}{2}} \cdot e^{-\frac{\kappa^2}{2}} \cdot d\kappa \tag{10}$$

When the random errors e_i assume a logistic instead of a standardised normal distribution, another formula called the "Logit Model" and its expression is:

$$\phi(I_i) = \frac{1}{1 + e^{-1}}$$

In order to measure the marginal effect of every independent variable on the probability $P(Y=1)$, in the models of the Probit e Logit type, we can apply the following formulas respectively in which the sign β_i determines the direction of such effect, which tends to grow as β_i increases, while the relative size varies together with the variation of the exogenous variable X_i.

$$\frac{\partial P(Y=1)}{\partial X_i} = \frac{1}{\sqrt{2\pi}} \cdot e^{-\frac{I^2}{I^2}} \cdot \beta_i \equiv \phi(I)\beta_i \tag{11}$$

$$\frac{\partial P(Y=1)}{\partial X_i} = \frac{e^I}{1+e^1} \cdot \frac{1}{1+e^1} \cdot \beta_i \tag{12}$$

These considerations lead us to formula (13) in which the relationship between the probability $P(Y=1)$ and the variation in X_i will be visible.

$$\frac{\partial P(Y=1)}{\partial X_i} = \frac{e^{\beta_i(X_{1i}-X_{0i})}}{1 + e^{\beta_i(X_{1i}-X_{0i})}} \tag{13}$$

References

Addari P, Nante N, Giannuzzi P, Ngoyi Ngongo K, De Bedin C, Mara E (1995) Studio della mobilità sanitaria relativa al bacino di utenza del policlinico senese. Atti Sez. Toscana S.It.I.; VII: 51–59

Aldrich JH, Nelson FD (1984) Linear Probability, Logit, and Probit models. SAGE; 45

Baccarani C (1998) La qualità delle prestazioni e la libera scelta dell'utente. In Economia e direzione delle aziende sanitarie, Achard PO (ed), Fontana, Roma: RIREA, Quaderno di ricerca no. 8

Bailey KD (1995) Metodi della ricerca sociale. Il Mulino, Bologna

Ben-Akiva M, Lerman SR (1985) Discrete choice analysis: Theory and application to travel demand. MIT Press, Cambridge

Biscella M, Deponti F (1998) Il Nord attira i malati in trasferta. Il Sole 24 ore, 23 Feb.

Bonoldi P (1998), Sistema DRG e finanziamento degli Ospedali: un'opportunità per programmare la qualità dell'assistenza. Centro Scientifico Editore, Turin

Brenna A (1999) Manuale di economia sanitaria per una gestione razionale delle risorse; CIS Editore, Milan

Cattell RB (1978) The scientific use of Factor Analysis. Plenum, New York

Champion, Dean J (1970) Basic statistics for social research. Scaranton PA: Chandler

Chernew M, Scanlon D, Hayward R (1998) Insurance type and choice of hospital for coronary artery bypass graft surgery. Health Services Research; 33:447–466

Comrey LA (1995) Introduzione all'analisi fattoriale. Zanichelli, Bologna

Corrau S (2000) Il focus group, Franco Angeli, Milano

D'Ascani G, Candida-De Matteo G (1987) La conjoint analysis fornisce al progettista di hardware/software le specifiche informazioni di mercato richieste nella fase creativa dell'innovazione. In Innovazione tecnologica, discipline economiche e organizzative e indirizzi di ricerca, Pagliarani G, Gottardi G (eds), Atti workshop Bressanone, 3–4 ottobre; Padova

Degli Esposti G, Rimondi M, Virgilio G, Ugolini C (1996) Matrici di mobilità per DRG's: analisi descrittiva ed applicazioni per la programmazione e le politiche sanitarie regionali. Management ed Economia Sanitaria (MECOSAN); 19: 53–62

Dominick S (1985) Statistica ed econometria, Collana Schaum teoria e problemi, ETAS Libri

Donaldson C (1993) Theory and practice of willingness to pay for health care. Health Economic Research Unit Discussion Paper No. 01/93. Aberdeen: University of Aberdeen

Egunjobi L (1983) Factors influencing choice of hospitals: a case study of the northern part of Oyo State, Nigeria, Social Science & Medicine, vol 17, Issue 9, pp 585–589

Fabbri D, Fiorentini G (1996) Mobilità e consumo sanitario: metodi per la valutazione di benessere. Management ed Economia Sanitaria (MECOSAN); 19: 37–52

Fiorentini G, Rebba V, Daniele F (1997) La regolamentazione della qualità delle prestazioni ospedaliere mediante tariffe: un'analisi dei sistemi di pagamento prospettico. In Economia della Sanità, Petretto A (ed), il Mulino, Bologna 201–219

Gooding SK (1996) The relative importance of information sources in consumers' choice of hospitals. Journal of Ambulatory Care Marketing, vol 6, Issue 1, pp 99–108

Gorsuch RL (1983) Factor Analysis, 2nd edn, Erlbaum, Hillsdale

Green P, Srinivasan V (1978), Conjoint analysis in consumer research. Issues and outlook. Journal of Consumer Research, vol 5: 103–123

Griffiths WE, Carter Hill R, Judge GG (1993) Learning and practising econometrics. John Wiley & Sons: 736–760

Hansen TB (1994) What factors affect choice of hospital in cases of trauma? A study of conditions in the county of Ringkøbing, Ugeskrift for Laeger, vol 156, Issue 5, January 31, pp 652–655

Hodgkin D (1996) Specialized service offerings and patients' choice of hospital: the case of cardiac catheterization. In Journal of Health Economics, vol 15, Issue 3, pp 305–332

Hotelling H (1933) Analysis of a complex of statistical variables into principal components, Journal of Educational Psychology, 24, pp. 417–441

Kaiser HF (1958) The varimax criterion for analytic rotation in factor analysis, Psychometrika, 23, pp. 187–200

Kazmier LJ (1986) Statistica aziendale, Schaum Teoria e Problemi Series, ETAS Libri

Kline P (1997) Guida facile all'analisi fattoriale, Astrolabio-Ubaldini Editore, Rome

Liao Tim F (1994) Interpreting probability models Logit, Probit, and other generalized linear models. SAGE, 101

Luft HS, Garnick DW, Mark DH, Peltzman DJ, Phibbs CS, Lichtenberg E, McPhee SJ (1990) Does quality influence choice of hospital?, JAMA, the Journal of the American Medical Association, vol 263, Issue 21, pp 2899–2906

Mahon A, Whitehouse C, Wilkin D, Nocon A (1993) Factors that influence general practitioners' choice of hospital when referring patients for elective surgery. The British Journal of General Practice: the Journal of the Royal College of General Practitioners, vol 43, Issue 372, pp 272–276

Mapelli V (1993) Libertà di scelta ed equità nel sistema sanitario italiano: un'indagine campionaria. In Economia Sanitaria, France G, Attanasio E, Milan (eds): Giufrè A: 345–361

McNeil B, Weichselbaum R, Pauker S (1978) Fallacy of five year survival in lung cancer. The New England Journal of Medicine; 299: 1397–1401

McNeil B, Weichselbaum R, Stephen G, Pauker S (1981) Speech and survival. The New England Journal of Medicine; 305: 982–987

Ministero della Sanità (1996) Relazione sullo stato sanitario del Paese. Servizio Studi e Documentazione

Ministero della Sanità (2000) Relazione sullo stato sanitario del Paese. Servizio Studi e Documentazione

Ministero della Salute (2002) Schema di Piano Sanitario Nazionale 2002–2004, Servizio Studi e Documentazione

Mor V, Wachtel TJ, Kidder D (1985) Patient predictors of hospice choice. Hospital versus home care programs, Medical Care, vol 23, Issue 9, pp 1115–1119

Morizet-Mahoudeaux P, Dubuisson B (1983) Analysis of the criteria of choice of hospital materials and technologies, International Journal of Bio-Medical Computing, vol 14, Issue 1, pp 53–63

Nante N, Moirano F, Giusti E, Galanti C, Giuliano G, Taddei M, Marenco C, Savioli V, Isoardi MA, La Ferlita G, Autieri G, Addari P (1999) Mortalità intraospedaliera DRG specifica in alcuni nosocomi italiani, Organizzazione Sanitaria, XXIII, 4, pp 78–91

Nante N, De Marco MF, Balzi D, Addari P, Buiatti E (2000a) Prediction of mortality for congestive heart failure patients: results from different wards of an Italian teaching hospital, European Journal of Epidemiology, XVI, pp 1017–1021

Nante N, Siliquini E, Morgagni S, Moirano F, Renga G (2000b) In-hospital mortality DRG related in Piemonte, Italy. J Prev Med Hyg 41:91–99

Nante N, Brandini S, Autieri G, Isoardi MA, Piazza A, Furfaro V, Panella M, Di Stanislao F (2001) Uno strumento per la valutazione del processo assistenziale ospedaliero: la qualità redazionale della cartella clinica, Difesa Sociale, 5, 143–155

Nante N, Fattorini A, Groth N, D'Ostuni R, Quercioli C, Moirano F (2002), Qualità assistenziale percepita dai ricoverati in ospedale: messa a punto di uno strumento valutativo, Annuale d'Igiene XIV, 51–72

Nord E (1991) The validity of a visual analogue scale in determining social utility weight for health states. International Journal of Health Planning and Management; 6: 234–242

Pellegrino P, Groth N, Cento G, Beodogni C, Moirano F, Nante N (2002), Esperienze di analisi partecipata della qualità in un'azienda ospedaliera, Annali d'Igiene XIV, 37–50

Phibbs CS, Mark DH, Luft HS, Peltzman-Rennie DJ, Garnick DW, Lichtenberg E, McPhee SJ (1993) Choice of hospital for delivery: a comparison of high-risk and low-risk women, Health Services Research, vol 28, issue 2, pp 201–222

Rossi G (1994) Mercato e non mercato in sanità: l'efficienza dei sistemi sanitari e la razionalizzazione dei consumi delle risorse, Edizioni Copinfax, Siena

Royce JR (1963) Factors as theoretical constructs in Jackson DN, Messick S (eds), Problems in Human Assessment, McGraw-Hill, New York

Rozenberg S, Ham H (2001) Effect of physician's opinion on patients' choice of treatment, European Journal of Obstetrics, Gynecology, and Reproductive Biology, vol 96, issue 2, pp 215–217

Ryan M, Hughes J (1997) Using conjoint analysis to assess women's preferences for miscarriage management. Health Economics vol 6: 261–273

Skinner TJ, Price BS, Scott DW, Gorry GA (1977) Factors affecting the choice of hospital-based ambulatory care by the urban poor, American Journal of Public Health, vol 67, issue 5, pp 439–445

Tessier G, Contandriopoulos AP, Dionne G (1985) Patient mobility for elective surgical interventions, Social Science & Medicine, vol 20, Issue 12, pp 1307–1312

Torrance G, Thomas W, Sackett D (1972) A utility maximization model for evaluation of health care programs. Health Service Research, 7: 118–133

Ugolini C, Fabbri D (1998) Mobilità sanitaria ed indici di entropia. Management ed Economia Sanitaria (MECOSAN); 26: 9–24

The impact of disasters: long term effects on health

Joris Yzermans · Gé Donker · Peter Vasterman

Introduction

Disasters occur more often since the world gets overpopulated, air traffic is busier, terrorists are operating worldwide and therefore, risks are increasing. According to the Federal Emergency Management Agency major disasters in the USA have been increasing in frequency, from fewer than 25 per year in the 1980s to more than 40 per year in the 90s (Washington, 1998).

Disasters have happened throughout history. But the reaction to these events has varied according to the mood that prevailed in society at the time. As Frank Furedi stated (2002): "Many of our fears are *not* based on personal experiences. Despite an unprecedented level of personal security, fear has become an ever-expanding part of our life. Western societies are increasingly dominated by a culture of fear". Characteristic of trauma after a disaster is a perceived loss of control. The accustomed sense of security has vanished; the victim fears being struck by a new calamity.

Especially after 9–11 there is a lot of attention to the aftermath of disasters, to post-traumatic stress (disorders), medically unexplained physical symptoms (MUPS) and functional somatic syndromes (FSS). However, there is not much long-term research on this phenomena (with a few exceptions like Three Mile Island (Cleary & Houts, 1984; Prince-Embury & Rooney, 1989; Dew & Bromet, 1993), which was only a disaster because residents thought it was, and the Gulf war (Rook & Zumla 1997; Straus, 1999; Unwin et al., 1999; Ismail et al., 1999; Haley, 1997; Haley & Kurt, 1997; Haley et al., 1997; Wegman et al., 1997; Holmes et al., 1998; The Iowa Persian Gulf Study group, 1997; Southwick et al. 1993 and 1995)). For that reason we use in this chapter the Amsterdam air disaster as a 'casus belli'. For public health and for the authorities there are lessons to be learned, in the absence of a protocol for dealing with disasters, and in the lack of experience in dealing with man-made disasters.

We pay attention to the role of the media in the aftermath of disaster as well: "The ironic thing about the seemingly endless coverage of the 1986 Chernobyl accident – and the relatively harmless, because much diluted, radiation that then blew around the world-, is that, with few exceptions, the media have done more injury to the truth than was ever done by cover-up or whitewash. Television is the worst offender because the visual impact is unforgettable and any reasonable sense of proportion goes out of the window..." (Brewin, 1994). Earlier research showed the impact of media on consultation frequency in general practice (Elie, 1992; Foets et al., 1993).

The narrative of the Amsterdam air disaster

On the evening of the 4th of October 1992, two engines of an El Al Boeing 747-cargo broke from a wing. The Israeli crew tried to return to Schiphol Airport, mistakenly flying over a densely populated part of Amsterdam. The plane crashed onto two apartment buildings in the multicultural 'Bijlmermeer'. Thirty-nine residents and the 4 crewmembers died in the inferno of burning buildings, plane, cargo and fuel. Remarkably enough, very few persons suffered immediate physical injuries, except for some people with burns and fractures. Several hundreds of rescue workers were soon on the spot. A campaign was launched in the media to inform people and caregivers about possible psychological after effects; the slogan "a normal reaction to an abnormal event" was used. Initially the health effects were typical stress reactions and several hundreds of adults and children received some form of trauma intervention.

According to the authorities, the cargo of the plane was not toxic: flowers, perfume and PCs. This initial information soon appeared to be incomplete. Suspicion rose about nearly everything and one year after the crash rumors were confirmed that depleted uranium was in the plane's tail as a counterweight. Dutch and Israeli authorities were not able to retrieve full cargo specifications. A chain of events started ("a disaster after the disaster") in which people attributed their somatic symptoms to their presence at the disaster scene. Similar concerns arose among employees of the hangar at Schiphol Airport where the plane's wreckage had been stored and among rescue workers. Local authorities responded slowly and disconnectedly to the rising fears. Suspicions were fuelled by private investigations, lawyers, members of parliament and the media (often generalizing from individual cases).

Five years after the crash the Ministry of Health, Welfare and Sports commissioned us to conduct an exploratory study into possible health problems. At the same time the National Institute for Public Health and the Environment (RIVM) concluded that no additional negative health effects were to be expected as a result of the known agents in the cargo or the fire.

Six years after the crash the Dutch parliament decided to conduct a 'parliamentary inquiry' to determine the causes and consequences of the plane crash and its possible health effects. Individuals were heard under oath and the hearings were broadcasted live on national television. Finally, the complete list of the cargo was published: no dangerous toxic substances were aboard the plane. Nevertheless, the authorities started a comprehensive medical examination at the end of 1999 to which more than 6400 persons should take part. Finally 75% of them showed up for this examination, with, strangely enough, a large majority of rescue workers.

Literature review

Introduction

Almost daily disaster (natural or 'man-made') strikes somewhere in the world (Noij, 1997) and large proportions of the general population are exposed to some traumatic event in their lifetime (Green, 1994). The stress that is associated with disasters and other traumatic events has short-term health effects, and an increasing amount of studies suggests that disasters and other traumatic events may have long-term health consequences as well (Dew and Bromet, 1993; Ismail et al., 1999; Green et al., 1990; Bland, 1996; Winje, 1996; Marmar, 1999; Donker et al., 2002, Yzermans, 2003). These health effects may be reflected in an increased prevalence of psychiatric disorders like posttraumatic stress disorder (PTSD), major depression, generalized anxiety and substance abuse or in increased rates of domestic violence or functional disabilities (Noij, 1997; Kleber, Figley & Gersons, 1995; Rubonis & Bickmann, 1991). Health effects (on shorter and longer notice) are furthermore reflected in raised scores on questionnaires measuring psychological distress (Winje, 1996; Marmar, 1999; Ursano, Fullerton, Tzu-Cheg-Kao & Bhartiya, 1995).

Increased self-reports of non-specific psychological and general physical symptoms (fatigue, headaches, difficulty concentrating, sleeping problems, joint/muscle pains, etc.) are seen long after civil traumatic events, like for instance the Three Mile Island incidence (Dew & Bromet, 1993), the Buffalo Creek disaster (Green et al., 1990) and the Amsterdam air disaster (Yzermans, et al., 1999; Donker et al., 2002; see table 1). The same symptoms are also reported by veterans, long after military traumatic events, like for instance the Gulf War (Hyams, Wignall & Roswell, 1996; Ismail et al., 1999).

This chapter on literature concerning short- and long-term impact of disasters focuses on the type and persistence of symptoms reported after traumatic events. Special attention is given to the Amsterdam air disaster, a disaster studied by the authors of this chapter.

Studies were identified through a search of the MEDLINE database. The bibliographies of the retrieved articles were then searched for additional publications. The emphasis was on recent studies of 'man-made' (technological) traumatic events. Instead or besides psychiatric diagnosis (like posttraumatic stress disorder or depression) and/or standardized questionnaires, self-reported symptoms had to be presented in the overviewed studies. This because self-reported non-specific symptoms were the major concern after the Amsterdam air disaster.

Symptoms reported after traumatic events

Post-traumatic stress disorder (PTSD). Characteristic of PTSD is a perceived loss of control. The accustomed sense of security has vanished. The victim fears being struck by a new calamity. PTSD is characterized by symptoms such as re-experiencing, hypervigilance and poor concentration. Victims are sharply alert to danger but have trouble focusing on more trivial matters. This leads to sleep disturbances and intense fatigue. Presumably such symptoms are perpetuated by feelings of rage about what has happened and by feelings of grief – not only at the loss of loved ones, but at the destruction of a life perspective and fundamental sense of security (Yzermans & Gersons, 2002).

In literature concerning people undergoing a disaster or an individually significant trauma, a percentage of 10% developing PTSD is reported (Bromet & Dew, 1995; Palinkas et al., 1993; Breslau et al., 1991). Although symptoms may decrease in course of time, even years after a disaster part of the victims may show a full-blown PTSD (Breslau & Dew, 1995; Noij, 1997; Rubonis & Bickmann, 1991). In the National Comorbidity Survey an average lifetime prevalence of PTSD of 8% was reported with a higher prevalence among women and divorced persons. A high comorbidity of depression addiction and personality disorders was reported as well (Skodol et al., 1996). Studies concerning airplane disasters, like Lockerbie (1988), reported high prevalence's of PTSD in the years following the disaster (Brooks & McKinlay, 1992; Livingston et al., 1992). Type of symptoms and impact on life appeared to be the same in all age groups (Livingston et al., 1992). Earlier research concerning the Amsterdam air disaster also revealed a high incidence of PTSD during the first year after the disaster; 26% complete PTSD and 44% partial PTSD among eye witnesses and others involved, six months after the disaster (Meijer JS, 1992; Carlier & Gersons, 1997). A direct comparison to the 5% found in the study of the Amsterdam air disaster, six years after the crash, is not valid as the study population is not comparable. Neverthe-less, the high rate of depression and PTSD in the latter study even years after the crash is consistent with literature (Yzermans et al., 1999; Donker et al., 2002).

Air- and other transportation disasters. Given the nature of the event in Amsterdam, the re-ported symptoms were initially compared to symptoms reported after other air disasters. Air disasters are a particular kind of traumatic experience in which not only crew, passen-gers and rescue workers are involved but also people residing on the site of the crash may be victimized. Crashing of planes may be sudden (explosion, collision) – like in the Am-sterdam air disaster and the Lockerbie and New York terrorist attacks –, less explosive (turbulence, lightning) or gradual (broken engine, open door) (Eckert, 1990; Yzermans et al., 1999; Brooks and Mc Kinlay, 1992; Schuster et al., 2001).
In 1984 a basketball team and supportive personnel crash-landed at an airport in Alabama. There were no serious injuries but the sight of smoke and fire while being on flight and the desperate escape after landing when the plane was destroyed by fire was a very trau-matic experience. Initially (12 days after the crash) the survivors presented high levels of stress which decreased rapidly and gradually levelled-off over one year. The symptoms re-ported 12 days after the crash were mostly psychological and general physical: loss of con-centration or memory (initially 79%), intrusive thoughts (71%), hyper-irritability (71%), sleep problems (68%), physical pain symptoms (65%), dreams of the event (50%) (Sloan, 1988).
    Intimates of people exposed to a traumatic event are exposed indirectly as well. By hearing about the event and by identification with the victims they may develop so called 'secondary posttraumatic stress symptoms' (Figley & Kleber, 1995). This was demonstrated when an Army jetliner crashed shortly after taking off in 1985 from Gander International Airport in Newfoundland. Assistance workers were assigned to care for the families of the killed soldiers. These assistance workers were exposed to extreme emotional reactions. Six months after starting their support activities they reported many symptoms and one year after twice as many. Most commonly reported symptoms one year after the crash were: headache (40–63%), feeling nervous/tense (33–52%), sleeping problems (31–49%), general pain (29–56%), common cold (25–59%), feeling depressed (21–40%), tiredness (20–51%), concentration problems (49%), gastrointestinal problems (40%) (Bartone et al., 1989).
    The findings of the above-mentioned studies are summarized in Table 1. It is shown that the symptoms that are reported after air disasters are all among the most frequently reported symptoms after the Amsterdam air disaster. The same applies for the other trans-portation disasters, like train accidents and disasters at sea (Lundin, 1995) that are pre-sented in the table.

Fire, smoke and collapsed buildings. A huge fire, a lot of smoke, and the collapse of two apartment buildings accompanied the Amsterdam air disaster. Therefore, symptoms reported after traumatic events with comparable characteristics were also addressed (Table 1). After a fire in a Norwegian hotel building rescue workers reported anxiety, irri-tation and dizziness (Hytten & Hasle, 1989). In another study, survivors of fires were assessed for posttraumatic symptoms after discharge from hospital. Reported symptoms were, among others, sleeping problems, nightmares, irritation and difficulty concentrating (Roca et al., 1992). After a bushfire in Australia fire fighters reported respiratory, gastroin-testinal, musculoskeletal and neurological (mainly headaches) symptoms (McFarlane et al., 1994).
    Destroyed buildings characterized the collapse of the Hyatt Regency Hotel skywalks in 1981 like the Amsterdam air disaster. Symptoms reported after this disaster by victims, guests and rescue workers were fatigue, sleeping problems and nightmares, concentration

Table 1. Self-reported symptoms after air and other transportation disasters, fire disasters, collapsed buildings and (supposed) exposure to toxic agents

Reported symptoms	Air disasters			Other transportation disasters				Fire disasters			Collapsed building	(Supposed) exposure toxic agents	
	Bijlmer*	Newfoundland	Alabama	Gothenburg	California	Zeebrugge	Norway	Norway	Burn survivors	Australia	Kansas City	Three mile Island	Bhopal
Fatigue/weakness	1	x										x	x	x
Headache	2	x				x					x	x	x	x
Shortness of breath	3					x					x			
Sleeping problems	4	x	x	x	x	x				x		x	x	x
Complaints skin	5	x			x									
Difficulty concentrating	6	x	x		x	x			x		x	x	x
Memory problems	7	x	x								x		x
Anxiety/nervousness	8	x			x	x	x				x	x	x
General pain muscles/joints	11–12	x	x							x			
Depressive feelings	14	x		x	x	x		x			x	x	
Irritation/anger	17		x			x		x	x		x	x	
Dizziness	18				x			x	x		x		x
Nightmares	25	x	x	x									x
Gastrointestinal	29	x			x					x	x		

* The figures correspond with the list of thirty most frequently mentioned symptoms after the Amsterdam air disaster (Yzermans et al., 1999). Frequent mentioned symptoms that are not presented are: complaints of the back (9), coughing (10), itching (13), complaints of the shoulders (15) and transient situational disturbance (16).

problems, loss of memory, feelings of anxiety and depression, anger and psychosomatic symptoms (Wilkinson, 1983).

Supposed exposure to toxic agents. After the nearly nuclear incident on Three Mile Island controversy and uncertainty existed – for a long period – about whether people had been exposed to radiation; if so, how much exposure and for how long (Cleary & Houts, 1984; Prince-Embury & Rooney, 1989; Dew & Bromet, 1993). Ultimate study results showed no raised exposure to radiation at all. However, the immediate response by government and by the media was so confusing and contradictory that it led to reduced trust, and as a consequence, people were far less receptive for accurate information that corrected conflicting earlier reports. Until ten years after this near-disaster psychological symptoms like sleeping problems, concentration problems, anxiety, depressive feelings and anger were reported (Table 1).

The nuclear accident in 1986 in Chernobyl was also surrounded by many uncertainties (Havenaar et al., 1997; Havenaar et al., 1996). A long-term impact on psychological well-being was found after this accident in the Gomel region. No serious effects on physical health were found, although health authorities, journalists and politicians persistently claimed alarming increases in the incidence on cancers, birth defects and other ailments.

After the chemical disaster in Bhopal exposed people reported headache, dizziness, fever and weakness, symptoms that were related to the gas exposure. Emotional effects were reported as well: symptoms of anxiety, depression, nightmares, loss of concentration and memory, sleeping problems (Gerson, 1986). The railroad chemical spill, in California, that was classified earlier as a transportation disaster could also be classified as a chemical disaster. Exposed persons showed psychological and medically unexplained physical symptoms (MUPS) (Bowler et al. 1994).

War and possible exposure to toxic agents. Serving in a war is another traumatic experience in which (supposed) exposure to toxic agents may result in psychological distress. Gulf War veterans for instance have been exposed to a broad scale of known and potential dangers for health. Besides clearly war related symptoms, many veterans have reported MUPS (Table 2). The most commonly reported symptoms are fatigue, dyspnea, headache, muscle- and joint pain, loss of concentration and/or memory, sleeping problems and digestive symptoms (The Iowa Persian Gulf Study Group, 1997; Hyams et al., 1996; Hyams, 1998; Unwin et al., 1999; Ismail et al., 1999). Depleted uranium (Miller et al., 1998; Jamal, 1998), multiple vaccinations (Rook & Zumla 1997; Jamal, 1998) and mycoplasma-fermentas-incognitus (Gray et al., 1999; Nicolson & Nicolson, 1998) were – among others – discussed as possible cause of the reported symptoms. Despite systematic clinical examination of more than 100 000 Gulf War veterans and despite many studies in the USA and in England no distinctive clinical sign or laboratory abnormality has been identified (Rook & Zumla 1997; Straus, 1999; Unwin et al., 1999; Ismail et al., 1999; Haley, 1997; Haley & Kurt, 1997; Haley et al., 1997; Wegman et al., 1997; Holmes et al., 1998; The Iowa Persian Gulf Study group, 1997; Southwick et al. 1993 and 1995). Although there is still much controversy, the broadly supported assumption is that in some cases the symptoms may have been associated with an (un) identified toxin but that in most cases the symptoms are caused by psychological stress associated with being in a combat area far away from home (Hyams, 1998; Hyams et al., 1996; Rook & Zumla 1997; Straus, 1999; Unwin, 1999; Ismail, 1999). This hypothesis, although controversial among veterans, is supported by a study in which symptoms are compared that were reported after five wars in different eras (between 1860–1980), in which the USA took part (Hyams et al. 1996). In these wars, veterans were exposed to different toxic substances and yet they reported comparable psychological and general physical symptoms (Table 2). The similarity in symptoms despite the exposure to

Table 2. Self reported symptoms after participation in war

Reported symptoms	Traumatic (U.S.) war experiences						Dutch war traumas		Functional somatic syndromes
	Bijlmer*	Civil War	World War I	World War II	Vietnam War	Gulf war	Cambodia	Bosnia	
Fatigue/weakness	1	x	x	x	x	x	x	x	x
Headache	2	x	x	x	x	x	x	x	x
Shortness of breath	3	x	x	x	x	x	x	x	x
Sleeping problems	4	x	x	x	x		x	x	x
Complaints skin	5					x	x	x	x
Difficulty concentrating	6	x	x	x	x	x	x	x	x
Memory problems	7	x	x	x	x	x	x	x	x
Anxiety/nervousness	8						x		x
General pain muscles/joints	11–12				x	x	x		x
Depressive feelings	14					x	x	x	x
Irritation/anger	17								x
Dizziness	18	x	x	x	x	x	x		x
Palpitations	22	x	x	x	x	x			x
Nightmares	25					x	x		x
Gastrointestinal	29	x		x	x	x	x	x	x

* The figures correspond with the list of thirty most frequently mentioned symptoms after the Amsterdam air disaster (Yzermans et al., 1999). Frequent mentioned symptoms that are not presented are: complaints of the back (9), coughing (10), itching (13), complaints shoulder (15) and transient situational disturbance (16). Figures US experiences (Hyams, 1996).

different toxic substances suggests a relation of the symptoms with psychological stress. This hypothesis was also supported by two studies on health problems reported by Dutch veterans who served in Bosnia and in Cambodia (Mulder & Reijneveld, 1999; DeVries, Soetekouw, Bleijenberg & VanderMeer, 1998). These veterans were exposed to different toxic substances as well but they shared the psychological stress that is associated with the combat area. The reported symptoms by these Dutch veterans are highly comparable with the reported symptoms in the American veterans (Table 2).

Medically unexplained physical symptoms (MUPS). MUPS, frequently reported after traumatic events (Tables 1 and 2), are symptoms with high incidences in the general population as well, characteristic of so called 'functional somatic syndromes' (FSS) (Table 2) (Barsky & Borus, 1999; Wessely et al., 1999; Wyke, 1998; Sharpe et al., 1992; Kroenke & Mangelsdorff, 1989; Verbrugge & Ascione, 1987; Speckens et al., 1996; Robbins et al., 1997). According to Kellner (1987) between 60–80% of healthy individuals experience MUPS in any one week, and for a substantial proportion of these symptoms no organic cause can be found. Among new referrals to a general medical outpatient clinic the proportion of patients with MUPS was 52% (VanHemert et al., 1993), and 34% of women and 27% of men consulted a general practitioner for 'vague' common symptoms (Wyke et al., 1998). These MUPS mostly fall within the symptom-repertoire, characteristic for traumatic events, presented in this overview. Barsky and Borus (1999) classify the "Gulf War syndrome" as a FSS. Other FSS's are, for instance, chronic fatigue syndrome, fibromyalgia, multiple chemical sensitivity, the sick building syndrome, repetitive stress injury, chronic whiplash, the side effects of silicone breast implants and hypersensitivity (Barsky & Borus, 1999; Wessely et al., 1999). These syndromes share similar phenomenology's, high rates of co-occurrence, similar epidemiological characteristics and higher than expected prevalence of (psychiatric) co-morbidity. They are more characterized by comparable non-specific, diffuse symptoms than by disease-specific, demonstrable abnormalities of structure or function.

We would like to assess the hypothesis expressed in this paragraph in the view of the Amsterdam air disaster. The symptoms attributed to the crash by patients six years after the crash will be compared to symptoms and diagnoses noted in their GP's medical records and to a standard Dutch population.

Symptom attribution after a plane crash: comparison between self-reported symptoms and GP-records

[Another version of this material was published in: Donker GA, Yzermans CJ, Spreeuwenberg P & Zee J van der. (2002) Symptom attribution after a plane crash: comparison between self-reported symptoms and GP records. *Brit J Gen Pract*, 52, 917–922]

Introduction

Six years after the Amsterdam air disaster (see narrative), the Dutch parliament decided to conduct a 'parliamentary inquiry' to determine the causes and consequences of the plane crash and its possible health effects. One year earlier (1997) the Ministry of Health had decided to enhance an exploratory study of the health of all those who considered themselves as victims of the crash. This study was carried out in 1998 and 1999 (Yzermans et al., 1999). Victims were invited to report their symptoms by telephone and were asked informed consent to study their medical records. Although literature about health effects in the aftermath of disasters was growing, little was known about doctor-patient interaction in general practice in the years following a crash. The subject of this study was a comparison between patient's symptoms attributed to the crash, the consistency with symptoms and diagnoses as noted in their medical records in general practice, and GPs' perception of a possible association with the crash. This investigation was possible as in the Dutch Health Care System each person is (obligatory) registered on the list of only one GP, who functions as a gatekeeper (consultation of a medical specialist is not possible without being referred by the GP). Medical specialists report final results of their examination to the patient's GP.

The following questions were answered:
1. How many and which symptoms reported to the call centre were also reported to the GP?
2. Were the reported symptoms and diagnoses caused by the disaster according to the GP?

Methods

Respondents and GPs

A toll-free call centre, staffed by 25 professional multilingual interviewers, was established to which people could present the health problems they attributed to the plane crash. During two months (June and July 1998) ten telephone lines were open between eight a.m. and ten p.m. The interviews lasted on average 45 minutes. People were requested to call in themselves, unless if they were too young (younger than 14 years, i. e. 8 years at the time of the crash), too ill, or had a serious language barrier. In those cases a proxy was allowed to present the health problems in his or her place. At the end of the telephone interview objectives were explained and consent was requested to the respondent to inquire his or her GP about symptoms in their medical records. Data entry of the telephone interview in a computerized database took place immediately after each call.

Data on the GP records were collected by sending questionnaires to patients' GPs after receiving signed informed consent forms from their patients who contacted the call centre. Most GPs (90%) only had one or two of such patients in their practice. All GPs with three or more patients (maximum 22) were offered to be assisted in examining the medical records. In case additional information was considered appropriate, GPs' forms were accompanied by copies of specialists' letters, laboratory results etc. About 50% of GPs provided such extra documents.

The questionnaire, sent to the GP, reported symptoms and diagnoses as presented by the patient during the telephone interview and included the following questions: 'Did this patient consult you with the reported symptoms and if so, when?' 'Do you relate the symptoms to the disaster?' 'Why (not)?'; 'Were the symptoms converted into a diagnosis?'; 'Can you confirm this diagnosis?'; 'When was this diagnosis made?'; 'Was the diagnosis related to the disaster?'; 'Why (not)?'

Measurement and measures

Telephone interviews: Trained interviewers used an adapted version of the International Classification of Primary Care (ICPC) to classify the symptoms (IJzermans et al., 1999; Lamberts and Woods, 1987).

GP-questionnaires: Four time frames were distinguished retrospectively, i. e. before the disaster took place (before October 1992), and three periods after the disaster took place

(October 1992–'94; 1995–'97; and 1998/'99). The time of the first presentation to the GP of symptoms attributed to the crash by patients was assessed.

The GP was requested to indicate on a three-point scale whether a relationship between symptoms (and/or diagnoses) and disaster was considered realistic (1 = unrealistic; 2 = possible; 3 = (very) realistic). The contents of the plane cargo had not yet been disclosed at the time of data collection.

Results

Were the reported symptoms noted in GP's medical records? Finally, 553 questionnaires (89% of those who gave informed consent) were received from 345 GPs scattered all over the country with a concentration in Amsterdam. Comparison of baseline variables between respondents whose medical records were examined and those who were not, revealed no difference in distribution of sex, age and country of origin. Responders (48%) were more frequently rescue workers than non-responders (37%, p < 0.05) and less often lived in the destroyed apartments (35% versus 43%, p < 0.05). Responders (42%) more often reported psychological problems and problems of the nervous system (25%) than non-responders (34% and 14% respectively, p < 0.05 for both comparisons).

The 553 respondents reported in total 2358 signs and symptoms (average 4.3 symptoms per respondent). Of these, 2211 (94%) could be used for statistical analysis. In the other 6% analysis was not possible due to incomplete information of the GP. The majority of signs and symptoms (N=1636, 74%) had been reported to the GP (Table 3). Fatigue, skin symptoms, feeling anxious or nervous, dyspnea and backache were most frequently reported (80% had been reported to the GP). From the top-10 symptoms reported to the call centre memory disorder was least known to the GP (53% of cases reported to the GP, Table 3). Of all symptoms reported to the call centre: hyperventilation, digestive symptoms and neurasthenia were most frequently reported to the GP. Contrary, instability of weight (gain

Table 3. Ten most reported symptoms to the call centre, the percentage of respondents who reported these symptoms to the GP (N = 553 respondents), and the percentage probably related to the disaster as judged by the GP (N = 2211 reported symptoms)

Symptom	Percentage of respondents (N=553) reporting symptom to call centre*	Percentage of respondents with this symptom who reported to their GP	Percentage of symptoms probably related to disaster according to GP**
Tiredness, fatigue	45%	80%	3%
Headache	18%	73%	6%
Sleeping problems	16%	70%	23%
Dyspnea	15%	79%	3%
Concentration disorder	14%	83%	3%
Dry skin	13%	81%	15%
Memory disorder	13%	53%	16%
Feeling anxious, nervous	12%	81%	18%
Cough	9%	75%	0%
Backache	9%	80%	3%

* It was possible to mention more than one symptom, the average symptom score was 4.3; ** Scored as '(very) realistic' on a 3-point scale indicating the assumed association between diagnosis and disaster (1 = unrealistic, 2 = possible, 3 = (very) realistic).

or loss), hoarseness, frequent fever and common cold were least frequently presented to the GP (Donker et al., 2002).

Since when have these symptoms been known to the GP? The time of onset was known in 1456 (89%) out of 1636 symptoms reported to the GP. One out of nine symptoms, attributed to the disaster by the patients, was reported to the GP before the disaster took place (especially cardiovascular symptoms, anxiety and nervousness). Most symptoms (74%) were reported between October 1992 and 1998, while 15% were reported to the GP in 1998/'99 mainly symptoms of the cardiovascular and musculoskeletal system.

GP's translation from reported symptoms to diagnoses. In 553 patients GPs interpreted 2211 presented symptoms to 862 diagnoses. Analysis made clear that a symptom can be associated to several diagnoses, but frequently the diagnosis could not be specified (MUPS). Fatigue could besides being unspecified in most cases, lead to diverse diagnoses such as depression in 5% of cases, upper respiratory tract infection and diabetes mellitus in 1% of cases. Headache was presented as a symptom of stress as well as of sinusitis. Dyspnea was related to asthma/COPD (18%) and allergy (2%), but also to hyperventilation (6%).

One third of the patients (33.8%) showed one or more of the top-ten of diagnoses (not in Table). Depression (6.7%) and PTSD (5.2%) were most frequently diagnosed. Neurasthenia (4.7%), muscle pain (3.1%), hyperventilation (3.1%) and tension headache (2.9%) appear in the top-ten diagnoses in this study (not in Table), while usually less frequently diagnosed in general practice.

Did the GP relate reported symptoms and diagnoses to the disaster? Only 6% of all 2211 reported symptoms were related to the disaster by the GP. Although fatigue was expressed by 45% of the patients, the GP related this in only 3% of cases to the disaster (Table 3). Coughing reported by 9% of respondents was never related to the disaster. For sleeping problems, reported by 16% of the patients, the percentage related to the disaster was much higher (23%). Only a few diagnoses were frequently related to the disaster (Table 4); not surprisingly PTSD and acute stress most frequently. Highly incident diagnoses of the musculoskeletal system and skin were rarely related to the disaster.

Table 4. Ten diagnoses (from disorders diagnosed > 4 times) most suspect of relationship to the disaster according to GP's perception (as scored on a 3-point scale indicating the assumed association between diagnosis and disaster: 1 = unrealistic; 2 = possible; 3 = (very) realistic)

Most suspect relationship between diagnosis and disaster			
Diagnosis	% (Very) Realistic	% Possible	N
PTSD	72.4	20.7	29
Acute stress	28.6	35.7	14
Disease of esophagus	20.0	20.0	5
Anxiety disorder	16.7	33.3	6
Depression	16.7	27.8	36
Tension headache	13.3	40.0	15
Other social problems	12.5	25.0	8
Other skin problems	11.1	33.3	9
Emphysema/COPD	9.1	63.6	11
Problems with working conditions	7.7	15.4	13

What were reasons for GPs to relate symptoms or diagnoses to the disaster? In case GPs related a symptom or diagnosis to the disaster, the time of diagnosis was the most important reason to do so (Yzermans et al., 1999). Especially when the symptoms were presented before the disaster took place or with a long delay after it took place (at the time of high media attention during the Parliamentary Inquiry) a direct relationship with the disaster was thought to be highly unrealistic. When the GP did not relate a diagnosis to the disaster, he was questioned about other specific causes. In 46% of cases the GP mentioned other psychosocial causes, in 13% an existing somatic disease, in 30% no clear cause and in 8% a personality trait (Yzermans et al., 1999).

Conclusions

Three quarter of symptoms reported to the call centre was also found in GPs' medical records. A quarter of these were reported before the disaster took place, or six or more years after, co-incident with a lot of media attention at the time of the Parliamentary Inquiry. Symptoms existing before the disaster took place, may have been aggravated by the disaster. A direct relationship with the disaster seems unlikely, however. Most symptoms did not fit in a clear diagnosis and could be classified as MUPS. By GPs PTSD was frequently related to the disaster, but in general there was a high discrepancy between patients and GPs in attributing symptoms and diagnoses to the disaster.

Comparison of symptoms attributed to the Amsterdam air disaster with symptoms collected in the Dutch National Survey

Introduction

The study took place six years after the disaster, and the neighbourhood concerned was a multicultural one with a majority born abroad. It was impossible to create a control group for an epidemiological study, but nevertheless, we compared the group who contacted the call centre and their symptoms with data from the Dutch National Survey performed by the Netherlands Institute for Health Services Research (NIVEL) in 1988 (Foets et al., 1992). The Dutch National Survey is a stratified random sample of 103 GP-practices (162 GPs) and their registered patients (Van der Velden, 1999). Large differences exist between the two datasets: a period of six years after a disaster for a selection of people who contacted (self reported) the call centre because they attributed their symptoms to the disaster, versus a selection of patients who presented their symptoms to their GP during a period of three months. This comparison was performed to assess how much and in which aspects the population attributing symptoms to the Amsterdam air disaster was different from a standard Dutch population.

Method

The Dutch National Survey is the most important national reference. During three months contact registration data concerning 335000 persons was collected in the practices of 162 GPs. Like in the study on the health effects of the Amsterdam air disaster, the International Classification of Primary Care (ICPC) was used. In this system it is possible to register the reason for encounter (in the words of the patient) as well as the diagnosis (as reported by the GP). The under mentioned attempts were undertaken to make it possible to compare the two datasets:

▶ In order to exclude seasonal influences: from the Dutch National Survey only those practices wre selected where data were collected during the same period of the year (three months registration period), when symptoms were reported to the call centre; 95 000 persons remained for analysis.

▶ In three ways the dataset of the Dutch National Survey was 'weighed':

 a For the people from Amsterdam the reference group consisted of persons from one of the four biggest cities in The Netherlands (more than 400 000 residents). For the persons living outside Amsterdam, persons not living in the four biggest cities,

 b Persons from the two groups were equalized after weighing for gender, age and country of origin,

 c Policemen and fire fighters were compared with colleagues from the Dutch National Survey dataset.

Obviously, chances of presenting a symptom during the period studied, were 20 times greater for the Amsterdam air disaster population (nearly 6 years vs 3 months). The mean symptom score of the Amsterdam air disaster study population was 4,3 compared to 0.8 in the National Survey. Therefore, it should be possible to standardize on the number of symptoms. *Advantage*: the chance of a symptom among the victims should be twice as high. Differences between the two groups should be larger than factor two to be statistically significant. *Disadvantage*: it is well possible that the Amsterdam air disaster population experienced and presented more symptoms than they mentioned to the call centre. Moreover we counted persons only in case they presented one or more symptoms in a certain cluster. Above, we presented non-standardized results. In case we would have standardized the differences in the cluster 'Psychological symptoms' remained. Analysis of the individual symptoms is decisive for the necessity to standardize.

Results

Clusters of symptoms. Eight clusters of symptoms were made using correspondence analysis (Yzermans et al., 1999). The proportions between the two groups for six of these clusters were:

	Amsterdam Air Disaster	Dutch National Survey
General, non-specific symptoms	1,75	1
Psychological problems	3,3	1
Respiratory symptoms	1,4	1
Skin symptoms	2	1
Musculoskeletal symptoms	1	1,7
Problems of eyes and metabolism	2	1

Comparing specific symptoms. Per cluster we looked for scores of difference between the two datasets for more than 1% and a statistical significance level of at least 5%. The two most important groups were analysed: residents of Amsterdam and persons living elsewhere (in majority rescue workers) at the time of the disaster. We weighed for gender, age and country of origin (Table 5).

Table 5. Top 15 symptoms for victims living in Amsterdam or elsewhere compared to patients from the National Survey, weighed for gender, age and country of origin

Rank	Symptom	Cluster	Amsterdam		Elsewhere	
			Vict	NS	Vict	NS
1	Tiredness	General	40,8	7,8	49,9	6,7
2	Dyspnea	Respiratory	20,0	3,1	11,7	3,1
3	Problems sleeping	Psychol.	18,6	2,3	10,2	2,2
4	Disturbance Memory	Psychol.	13,8	0,5	10,2	0,4
5	Dist. Concentration	Psychol.	13,3	0,5	13,9	0,4
6	Anxious, nervous	Psychol.	16,6	3,5	4,1	3,5
7	Headache	General	19,8	7,4	12,4	7,7
8	Nightmares	Psychol.	7,9	–	0,5	–
9	Dry skin	Skin	11,4	4,2	14,4	3,9
10	Joints (> 1)	General	7,9	0,9	7,3	0,6
11	Anger, irritation	Psychol.	7,0	0,1	3,6	0,2
12	Down, depressive	Psychol.	8,2	1,9	3,6	0,2
13	Aching muscles	General	6,8	1,1	6,6	1,2
14	Hair loss	Skin	6,1	0,5	1,5	0,2
15	Stress (ac + chronic)	Psychol.	7,5	2,4	0,9	1,3

The differences are large, especially among symptoms, which are relatively frequently presented to GPs, such as tiredness, headache, nervousness and dyspnea. People from Amsterdam presented some symptoms more frequently when compared to those living elsewhere (dyspnea, anxiousness, nightmares). On the other side rescue workers (living elsewhere) presented more tiredness, disturbances in concentration and dry skin. The analysis per specific symptom provides some extra information, although in general the standardization procedure is more useful for clusters of symptoms. Both comparisons together show that although the Amsterdam air disaster population is not homogeneous (more stress-related symptoms among those living in Amsterdam compared to those living outside Amsterdam at the time of the study), the population as a whole differs very much from a standard Dutch population with comparable degrees of urbanization in type and number of symptoms presented to their GP. A limitation of the Amsterdam air disaster study is the self-selection of patients. Everybody who considered him- or herself a victim of the crash, who experienced symptoms and attributed these to the crash, was allowed to call and was accepted for the study. No respondents without symptoms were participating in the study. By study design the study population was one with symptoms, which limits comparison to other primary care surveys. The comparison to the Dutch National Survey confirms the high rate of psychosocial symptoms in the Amsterdam air disaster population. Depression, PTSD, hyperventilation and tension headache, all in the top-ten diagnoses of the Amsterdam air disaster population, are not in the top-ten of prevalent diagnoses of the National Survey (Foets et al., 1986).

Media-hypes and risk amplification

Media coverage of risk issues can play an important role in the social amplification of risk, especially when media-hypes occur. Media-hypes can be defined as massive news waves, generated by self-reinforcing processes within the media.

In post-modern society, coined by sociologists as the 'risk society', people feel threatened by invisible risks like air pollution, contaminated food or radiation. These risks only exist in terms of knowledge (Beck, 1992), which means that all depends on the social construction of that risk. In that respect the social definition of a specific risk can be manipulated, magnified or minimized, depending on the activities of social actors involved (industries, health departments).

The mass media fulfil a key role in the way society deals with risk issues. Their function is not limited to just 'reporting the news that is happening'; media are also involved in 'making news' and 'making sense of the news'. The media can pursue a topic by selectively digging for 'new' facts, exposing other angles or interviewing social actors. By doing so the media can 'frame' a topic, which means that news coverage shapes and promotes a specific problem definition, causal interpretation, moral evaluation and problem solving recommendations (Entman, 1993). The role of the media is often described as 'agenda setting', but the 'frame setting' role is in many cases much more important for the way society defines problems. Especially in situations, like in the aftermath of the Amsterdam airplane disaster, where new risk issues come to the surface, 'uncertainty' reigns, and the public has to rely on the messages communicated to them by the media.

The Amsterdam airplane disaster proved the vulnerability of complex technological systems and the magnitude of risks for society. However, in the aftermath it was not the risk of a busy airport in a densely populated area that became the number one issue, but the health risks for rescue workers and residents during the disaster. Over the years more and more people began to attribute their health problems to some kind of intoxication related to the explosion of the (alleged) toxic cargo (chemicals and military equipment) and parts of the depleted uranium (used as counterweight in the tail of the 747). For many years this became the most important topic for the media in the coverage of the aftermath. The media were actively pursuing the topic and by doing so they contributed to a process that is described as the 'social amplification of risk' (Kasperson et al., 1988). A chain of events develops in which a specific risk is magnified, causing in turn all kinds of secondary social, political and economic consequences. The media, the government, the experts, the interest groups, the 'victims'; each 'social actor' will be dragged along in this seemingly uncontrollable avalanche of incidents, actions and reactions. While the authorities try to develop a 'de-escalating' strategy, the media, as their natural enemy, will probably hunt for scoops, scandals and cover-ups. The result is that the rational assessment of the actual risks involved can be completely over clouded by all the social outrage about who is to blame.

This amplification process gets a boost each time a media-hype occurs. A media-hype is defined as a news wave in which the media are 'leading' and not as usual the (independent) events. During a hype news coverage seems to develop a life of its own, pushed forward mainly by self-reinforcing processes within the news production itself. The metaphor of 'hyperventilating media' seems appropriate: fear and stress can create intensive breathing, but this hyperventilation will reinforce fears, resulting in a spiral of growing anxiety.

Media-hypes are triggered by the intensive news making activities of the media en then reinforced again and again by the extensive coverage of the social actors' reactions, responding to the massive media attention for a topic. News selection is based on criteria for newsworthiness, but what is newsworthy is to some extent a tautology: once a topic gains a certain level of attention in the media, it attracts more, and because it attracts more attention, it becomes more newsworthy (Kitzinger, Reilly, 1997). This self-referential system creates positive feedback loops, expanding the news wave. During the hype the media will generate more news on the topic by reporting comparable incidents, by reinterpreting incidents in the past, by digging into backgrounds, by (morally or ideologically) evaluating events and performances, and by paying attention to reactions in society, triggered by the previous news wave (Kepplinger, Habermeier, 1995).

It is important to notice that during a media-hype a specific frame, a specific definition of the issue, structures newsgathering and news making. Reporters are looking for confirmation of this frame and tend to focus on all the events and statements that do so. This selective perception and selective reporting reinforces the original frame and seems to prove its tenability. During a hype the media act as amplifiers of one voice, weakening others. These alternative voices can still be aired, but their frames do not structure the news making process and the pursuance of 'newer' news. That is why media-hypes can push forward the process of risk amplification and thereby elicit new social developments.

During the long aftermath of the Amsterdam airplane disaster, media-hypes played a decisive role in the governments' decision to keep a Parliamentary Enquiry in 1999 to investigate the role of the different state departments, the air controllers, the firefighters and the rescue services. Also during the Enquiry in February and March of 1999 media coverage produced several media-hypes with huge social outrage.

In 1998 two media-hypes strongly reinforced a specific frame that stated that 'there must be a cover-up about an unknown toxic agent causing all health symptoms'. The first one in April 1998 was triggered by the publication of a controversial research, which claimed to have found traces of uranium in the blood and faeces of rescue workers. A newspaper scoop ignited a second media-hype in September 1998, revealing that the Boeing carried components of the nerve gas Sarin on board. Although in itself harmless, the presence of these components was defined as confirmation of the cover-up and the link between the explosion and the health symptoms. During the Parliamentary Enquiry, February 1999, another media-hype was triggered by the discovery of a tape, which seemed to prove that an air traffic controller gave in to the request of an El Al employee to keep information over the dangerous cargo confidential. Although this turned out very quickly misinterpretation of the conversation in which the wrong cargo list was used.

During these media-hypes the same dynamic reoccurred in the news coverage. Although the newly revealed 'facts' were quite dubious (or controversial to say the least), the media created a flow of news on the basis of the 'toxic agent cover-up' frame. They would follow up on the numerous health symptoms, the feelings of betrayal among the Bijlmer residents and rescue workers, the other 'mysteries' linked to the El Al crash (involvement of the Israeli Mossad, unknown men in white suits on the disaster site, etc.), and of course on political responsibility. Who was to blame and would this minister retain her position in this 'scandal-in-the-making'? The domination of the 'toxic agent' frame was supported by the abundant attention some of the sources (victims, lawyers, advocacy groups) received from the media. Spokespersons from the other side (departments, experts) were forced to respond within the dominant framework, thereby unwillingly reinforcing that frame. The same applied to all the governments' efforts to respond, it did fan the flames of the media-hype. In contrast, the revelation of new facts that contradicted the central frame did not lead to a comparable hype. This news was reported once, but the media would not create the same follow-up as in the case of the 'confirming' facts. The news on November 6 1998 that the risk of cancer due to the inhalation of depleted uranium after the crash was 'negligibly small', did not create any news dynamic at all.

This kind of coverage, dominated by media-hypes, contributes to the social amplification of risk by setting the agenda and framing the risk. Risk perception in general is to a large extent shaped by media coverage, but in this specific case the media have had more specific effects. The number of people claiming to have developed health problems due to the disaster increased over the years between 1993 and 1999 from a few dozen to more than 6000. This group involved at first only Bijlmer residents and rescue workers, but later other groups joined like the employees who removed the debris from the site and the people who worked in the hangar at the airport where the wreckage of the Boeing was stored.

By 1999 even people with hardly any connection to the disaster itself, but still living in the area, reported health problems linked to the crash.

The health problems of these groups were very diverse and diffuse, although in some rare cases identifiable diseases were diagnosed like autoimmune diseases. Most people reported symptoms like skin rashes, respiratory problems, sleeplessness, concentration and memory problems and (chronic) fatigue, for which no physical cause was found after extensive medical investigation. Research (Yzermans et al., 1999) showed that some of these health problems were linked to posttraumatic stress disorders, while most symptoms were classified as MUPS that could be found in any 'normal' population, although usually in a lower frequency. Sometimes these general and stress related symptoms are clustered and labelled as a new 'disease'. These so called 'functional somatic syndromes' are "characterized more by symptoms, suffering, and disability than by disease-specific, demonstrable abnormalities of structure or function (Barsky & Borus 1999)". The 'Bijlmer syndrome' meets the criteria of a functional somatic syndrome: stress related and medically unexplained physical symptoms are clustered together and defined as caused by a specific toxic agent.

In this longstanding attribution process between 1992 en 1999 the media seem to have played a decisive role with their repetition of media-hypes based on the 'cover-up/toxic agent' frame. An important indication for this is the fact that each time after a media-hype new groups of people reported to be suffering from 'Bijlmer-related' health problems (Fig. 1).

After the first hype in the spring of 1998 more than 600 people registered for the first general health survey, followed by another 500 in the slipstream of the Sarin hype. The media-hype in February 1999 about the 'keep secret' audiotape generated another 2000 and by the end of the Parliamentary Enquiry 6460 was registered for a medical check-up. Under normal circumstances one would expect a reverse relationship: more media coverage because more people apparently developed health symptoms. In this case there is reason to believe that the intensive media-hypes contributed to the development of a FSS. In

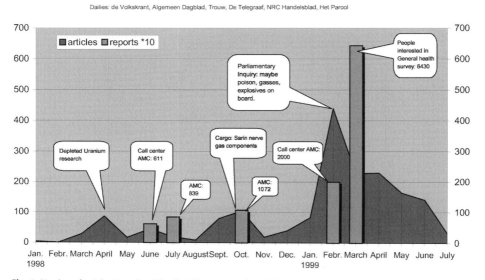

Fig. 1. Number of articles in national Dutch dailies per month and the number of people reporting health problems

other words, the media contributed to the development of stress related symptoms, which were defined as being symptoms of a new syndrome. Another indication for this conclusion can be found in the reactions of the people reporting to the call centre. In many cases these stories directly referred to the worrying messages in the media about the link between health problems and the disaster.

Discussion

A lot of reported symptoms and diagnoses in the Amsterdam air disaster study would fit in the categories MUPS and/or functional somatic syndrome (FSS) (Barsky & Borus, 1999, Wessely 1999). Muscle pain, hyperventilation, tension headache and irritable bowel syndrome were among the top twenty of GPs' diagnoses. MUPS and FSSs share similar phenomenologies and high rates of co-occurrence. Multi factorial aetiology has been demonstrated (Mumford et al., 1991). The suffering of patients with FSS is exacerbated by a self-perpetuating, self-validating cycle in which common, endemic somatic symptoms are incorrectly attributed to serious abnormality, reinforcing the patient's belief that he or she has a serious disease (Barsky & Borus, 1999). The climate surrounding functional somatic syndromes includes sensationalised media coverage, the mobilization of parties with a vested self-interest in the status of functional somatic syndromes, litigation and a clinical approach that overemphasizes the biomedical and ignores psychosocial factors. All these factors played an increasing role in the Amsterdam air disaster population during the years preceding the study.

Persons who are exposed to traumatic events, report (non-specific) psychological and general physical symptoms that stem from a comparable, restricted symptom 'repertoire'. Similar symptoms are reported following different types of traumatic events, civil and military, among victims and rescue workers (Table 2; Hyams et al., 1996; Yzermans et al, 1999). In our opinion, the common factor across these incidents is an ineffective and/or disconnected response by authorities that leads to chronic stress-related health problems (Yzermans & Gersons, 2002).

People have a need to predict the future and to control events, so in case they are exposed to uncontrollable and unpredictable events they are strongly motivated to explain why the event and/or why their symptoms occurred (Weiner, 1995; Wong & Weiner, 1981). Causal attribution is the central cognitive mechanism involved in the attempt to establish and maintain self-esteem as well as perceptions of the world as predictable and controllable (Joseph et al., 1998). Even if causal attributions are not responsible for the onset of symptoms, they may be responsible for their maintenance. Differences in attributional styles between patients may lead to differences in coping behaviour (Turnquist et al., 1988; Tennen & Affleck, 1990; Joseph et al., 1993). The high rate of psychological distress in the Amsterdam air disaster population has been reported elsewhere (Yzermans et al., 2003). Other studies also confirmed that the level of post-traumatic distress is not directly related to the degree of trauma exposure (Yzermans et al., 1999; Schuster et al., 2001).

Hypothetical explanatory model. Traumatic events like the Amsterdam air disaster, Three Mile Island (nearly) accident and the Gulf War share comparable aftermaths in which uncertainty and controversy are important features. Cultural, social and political forces played important roles in the aftermaths of these events. We propose an explanatory model for the Amsterdam air disaster and events with comparable aftermaths. This model is based on the works of Havenaar & VandenBrink (1997), Baum & Fleming (1993), Bertazzi (1989), Sharpe et al. (1992) and Barsky & Borus (1999). In this model an interaction of *in-*

tra- and *inter*-individual mechanisms leads to the onset, exacerbation and prolongation of symptom reporting. The same kind of mechanisms is also associated to the functional somatic syndromes (Sharpe et al., 1992; Barsky & Borus, 1999).

Intra **individual mechanisms.** Bodily sensations may be caused by a variety of factors like minor physical illness, physiological variations, psychological distress and traumatic events (Baum & Fleming, 1993; Sharpe et al., 1992). People who suppose they have been exposed to a toxic agent (or 'pathogen') may regard these bodily sensations as symptomatic of a disease. The suspicion of disease heightens bodily awareness and symptom perception: people are more conscious of psycho-physiological changes in their body and they will screen their selves more intense on sensations and symptoms. They will also experience more psychological distress, which may cause further bodily sensations. Symptoms will be remembered more easily and people will be more prone to report symptoms (especially those that are mentioned by other 'victims' and in the media). These processes reinforce the belief in the pathological significance of the sensations and these processes may become linked in self-validating and self-perpetuating mechanisms of symptom amplification and disease conviction. The actual interpretation of bodily changes as symptoms caused by the (supposed) toxic agent depends on the individual's character and experiences, and on the responses, the opinions and the expectations of the surrounding society.

Inter **individual mechanisms.** As a consequence of the *intra*-individual mechanisms (more) symptoms will be attributed to the suspect toxic agent (or 'pathogen'). This will initiate a variety of responses by the surrounding society. These responses cause emotional distress like anxiety, fear, arousal, anger and distrust, and eventually this may lead to chronic stress (see for instance, Barsky & Borus, 1999; Baum & Fleming, 1993; Bertazzi, 1989; Havenaar & Vandenbrink, 1997; Bowler et al., 1994; Dew & Bromet, 1993). As a consequence, the intra-individual mechanisms, in persons who already suspected a toxic agent caused their symptoms, are exacerbated and prolonged. Furthermore the responses result in the onset of the same kind of intra-individual mechanisms in other persons, who were exposed to the same toxic agent, but who had not yet related symptoms to it. The perception of people may be altered in such a way that they reattribute existing (medically unexplained physical) symptoms, with another or unknown cause, to the toxic agent. Finally the health effects of real exposure to toxic agents are exacerbated and the same intra-individual mechanisms may be initiated in these sufferers. These processes will all result in an increase in reported symptoms, which will initiate ongoing (and more) responses by the surrounding society.

Influencing responses by the surrounding society. Several responses by the surrounding society can be distinguished that might influence the intra-individual mechanisms (Barsky & Borus, 1999; Baum & Fleming, 1993; Sharpe et al., 1992; Bertazzi, 1989; Havenaar & Vandenbrink, 1997). First, written reports and ventilated opinions in the mass media are sometimes conflicting, ambiguous, preliminary, anecdotal and/or sensational. Different opinions by experts and by politicians, about possible exposure and about possible health consequences that might arise, are debated in the mass media. The available information is sometimes unclear, and ineffective and disparaging statements are made, like "there is nothing going on" and "there is no need to worry". Sometimes there are shifts, over time, in ventilated opinions about factors like whether people and how many people were exposed, to what substances people were exposed, whether negative health consequences could be expected, and so on. Personal accounts of a few sufferers and tentative findings with uncertain scientific and biomedical status were sometimes reported as conclusive medical evidence. Those reports were sometimes alarming and sensational and insinuations were made about cover-ups and denial by societal institutions (the government was often seen as a scapegoat). Such reports and opinions may all have contributed to an increase in emotional distress and convictions to be or become sick.

Furthermore the same effects might result from the actions that were deployed by individuals and organizations, which sometimes had interests themselves in the status of the health problems. Lawsuits were started to seek for liability and fault. Studies were conducted, by (scientific) specialists and institutes, to find out, for instance, whether specific substances might have resulted in the presented symptoms and whether there was a biological base for the symptoms. Advocacy groups, journalists and others, tried to mobilize public opinion and to influence scientific debate.

An overemphasis on a possible biomedical base of the symptoms and resistance against a biopsychosocial explanation is a third type of response that influences the intra-individual mechanisms. This resistance against a biopsychosocial explanation is not only characteristic for the surrounding society. In a climate of uncertainty and contradictions, exposed people become angry and distrustful. When they are told their health problems are psychosocial, they may feel as if they are not taken serious.

Finally, exposed people hear directly from other exposed people, close to them (family, neighbours, friends), about symptoms that are attributed to a suspected toxic agent (or 'pathogen'). This might (further) stimulate people to screen their bodies for these symptoms and/or to (re) attribute symptoms and/or it might reinforce the conviction to be or become sick.

Patients' beliefs about their symptoms are powerful influences on their decision to consult a doctor. It influences the frequency of consultation and the way of presenting the problem. Patients' consulting behaviour in general practice before the plane crash took place, could (by study design) not be analysed. In literature, an increased number of GP-consultations in the fifteen years before development of chronic fatigue syndrome were found, suggesting that behavioural factors have a role in the aetiology (Hamilton et al., 2001). Another study comparing self-reported screening questionnaires and clinical opinion also confirms that in general the greater the number of symptoms a patient reports, the less likely it is that they can all be due to somatic disease (Peveler et al., 1997). Total symptom scores are therefore likely to be associated with somatization for a population.

The challenge for GPs is to recognize patient's attributional style and, while maintaining a good relationship with their patient, to support coping behaviour by switching from continuing the search to the cause of symptoms to concentrating on the impact these symptoms have on patient's life (Kessler et al., 1999; Hemert et al., 2002). The challenge for policymakers is to provide a framework of trust to victims in handling the disaster in an optimal way. Six recommendations to support this process after disasters were developed (Carlier 1993, 1995, 1997. Gersons 1993, 1994, Yzermans 1999, 2002):

1. *Information about the aftercare of victims.* It is important to inform victims about all available services (victim and peer support), for example in a leaflet.
2. *Central information point.* It is very important to have a central advise and information point. All possible victims should be made aware of its existence and it should be operational for several years. It should be outreaching and inform victims about all relevant issues. A small newspaper could be distributed regularly to keep victims informed.
3. *Monitoring.* Long-term monitoring of aftercare provision is essential. It is also important to monitor (developments in) health problems, preferably using existing registration systems and databases.
4. *Mental health care provision following disasters.* A large proportion of the survivors had persistent, chronic PTSD. In most cases, treatment had been too brief and too discontinuous to achieve a satisfactory outcome. Moreover, PTSD often does not stand alone in the diagnosis, but occurs in combination with other disorders. It is important for

both the referring general practitioners and for the care providers at the receiving end, to know that is taking care for medical costs for victims of a disaster. Victims do not always find their way to mental health services (see 1 and 2).

5. *Peer support.* Many victims were offered dwellings outside the area, so they could avoid a daily confrontation with the disaster scene. However, many of them missed the ease of bumping into friends and acquaintances in the well-known 'ethnic subculture' and years later, many of them moved back to the area. Wessely (et al., 2002) added: "Maintaining public confidence is a long, and not just a short, term task. The recent events post September 11 have demonstrated that populations are resilience and may react to assaults with cohesion rather than panic, even if many individuals will experience some psychological distress. Increased communication opportunities, especially those that are initiated by the public themselves, may add further protection against anxiety and distress."

6. *Financial problems.* An emergency fund has to be established for long-term problems, to which people could apply.

Those recommendations formed a blueprint for the aftercare the authorities deployed after the next Dutch disaster eight years later: the explosion of a fireworks depot in the centre of the city of Enschede.

Three final points of consideration:

1. In the aftermath of disasters there is always a threat of a societal conflict, between laymen and authorities and between the general public and authorities (Havenaar, 2002).

2. Disasters tend to happen in neighbourhoods where's a lot of distress beforehand. Moreover, disasters do not happen in a societal vacuum. There are a lot of influences on the course of the aftermaths. If a disaster should happen these days, it is – for instance – in a culture of fear (Furedi, 2002): fear for El Quaida, fear for loss of control and fear for health problems without probable cause(s).

3. Although every disaster is unique or *specific* and strikes in different cultures, there is a need for international planning how to deal with the *generic* aspects of an aftermath, as the abovementioned small repertoire of symptoms disaster victims, war- and peacekeeping veterans experience and present. Two big explosions in Europe within 15 months (Enschede 2000 and Toulouse 2001) and hardly any exchange of approaches took place. It seems that the wheel has to be invented again and again and that is not efficient and potentially harmful for the growing number of disaster victims.

References

Barsky AJ, Borus JF (1999) Functional somatic syndromes. Ann Int Med, 130:910–921.

Bartone PT, Ursano RJ, Wright KM, Ingraham LH (1989). The impact of a military air disaster on the health of assistance workers. Journal of Nervous and Mental Disease, 177, 317–328.

Baum, A. & Fleming, I. (1993). Implications of psychological research on stress and technological accidents. American Psychologist, 48, 665–672.

Beck U (1992) Risk Society, Towards a New Modernity. London: Sage Publications, 1992 [originally publ. 1986].

Bertazzi PA (1989) Industrial disasters and epidemiology. A review of recent experiences. Scandinavian Journal of Work and Environmental Health, 15, 85–100.

Bland SH, O'Leary ES, Farinaro E, Jossa F, Trevisan M (1996) Long-term psychological effects of natural disasters. Psychosomatic Medicine, 58, 18–24.

Bowler RM, Mergler D, Huel G, Cone JE (1994) Psychological, psychosocial, and psychophysiological sequelae in a community affected by a railroad chemical disaster. Journal of Traumatic Stress, 7, 601–624.

Breslau N, Davis GC, Andreski P et al. (1991) Traumatic events and posttraumatic stress disorder in an urban population of young adults. Arch Gen Psychiatry 48:216–222.

Brewin TB (1994) Chernobyl and the media. BMJ 309:208.

Bromet E, Dew MA (1995) Review of psychiatric epidemiologic research on disasters. Epidemiologic Reviews, 17, 113–119.

Brooks N, Mc Kinlay W (1992) Mental health consequences of the Lockerbie disaster. J Traum Stress, 5:527–543.

Bruggen M. van Janssen PC, Kliest JM, Meulenbelt JJG, Smetsers J, UitdeHaag RCGM, DeMik PAM, Elzinga G (1998) Health risks fire El Al–Boeing (in Dutch). Bilthoven: RIVM.

Carlier I'VE, Gersons BPR (1997) Stress reactions in disaster victims following the Bijlmermeer Plane Crash. J Traum Stress, 10:329–335.

Cleary PD, Houts PS (1984) The psychological impact of the Three Mile Incident. Journal of Human Stress, 10, 28–34.

Dew MA, Bromet EJ (1993) Predictors of temporal patterns of psychiatric distress during 10 years following the nuclear accident at Three Mile Island. Social Psychiatry & Psychiatric Epidemiology, 28, 49–55.

Donker GA, Yzermans CJ, Spreeuwenberg P, Zee J van der. (2002) Symptom attribution after a plane crash: comparison between self-reported symptoms and GP records. Brit J Gen Pract, 52, 917–922.

Dooley E, Gunn J (1995) The psychological effects of a disaster at sea. British Journal of Psychiatry, 167, 233–237.

Eckert WG (1990) The Lockerbie disaster and other aircraft breakups in midair. American Journal of Forensic Medical Pathology, 11, 93–101.

Elie I. (1992) Medische berichtgeving in de media en consultatiegedrag bij huisartsen. Afstudeerscriptie. Nijmegen, Katholieke Universiteit.

Emmerik AAP van, Kamphuis JH, Hulsbosch AM, Emmelkamp PMG. 2002 Single session debriefing after psychological trauma: a meta-analysis. The Lancet, 360, 766–771.

Entman RM (1993) Framing: Towards clarification of a fractured paradigm. Journal of Communication, 43:51–58.

Ersland S, Sund LW (1989) The stress upon rescuers involved in an oil rig disaster. "Alexander L Kielland" 1980. Acta Psychiatrica Scandinavica, 80, 38–49.

Figley CR, Kleber RJ (1995) Beyond the "Victim": Secondary Traumatic Stress. In Kleber RJ, Figley CR, Gersons BPR (Eds) Beyond Trauma: cultural and societal dynamics (pp. 75–98). New York: Plenum Press.

Foets M, Velden J van der, van der Zee J (1986) Morbidity and intervention in general practice. A cross-national survey in The Netherlands. Utrecht: NIVEL.

Foets M, Velden J van der, Bakker D de (1992) Dutch National Survey of general practice. A summary of the survey design. Utrecht, NIVEL.

Foets M, Elie I, Rijt G van der (1993) Medische berichtgeving in de media. De invloed op het consultatiegedrag bij huisartsen. Medisch Contact, 48, 617–619.

Furedi F. Culture of fear. Risk-taking and the morality of low expectation. London: Continuum, 2002.

Gerson A (1986) Tragedy can continue in human effects of chemical disaster. Occupational Health and Safety, 55, 20.

Gersons BPR, Carlier I'VE (1993) Plane crash crisis intervention: a preliminary report from the Bijlmermeer, Amsterdam. Crisis, 14:109–116.

Gibbs MS (1989) Factors in the victim that mediate between disaster and psychopathology: a review. Journal of traumatic stress, 2, 489–513.

Gray GC, Kaiser KS, Hawksworth AW, Watson HL (1999) No serologic evidence of an association found between Gulf War and mycoplasma fermentas infection. American Journal of Tropical Medicine & Hygiene, 60, 752–757.

Green BL (1994) Psychological research in traumatic stress: an update. Journal of traumatic stress, 7, 341–362.

Green BL, Lindy JD, Grace MC, Gleser GC, Leonard BA, Korol M, Winget C (1990) Buffalo Creek survivors in the second decade: stability of stress symptoms. American Journal of Orthopsychiatry, 60, 43–54.

Hagström R (1995) The acute psychological impact on survivors following a train accident. Journal of Traumatic Stress, 8, 391–402.

Haley RW (1997) Is Gulf War syndrome due to stress? American Journal of Epidemiology, 146, 695–703.

Haley RW, Kurt TL (1997) Self-reported exposure to neurotoxic chemical combinations in the Gulf War. JAMA, 277, 231–237.

Haley RW, Kurt TL, Hom J (1997) Is there a Gulf War Syndrome? Searching for syndromes by factor analysis of symptoms. JAMA, 277, 215–222.

Hamilton WT, Hall GH, Round AP (2001) Frequency of attendance in general practice and symptoms before development of chronic fatigue syndrome: a case control study. Br J Gen Pract, 51:553–558.

Havenaar JM., VandenBrink W (1997) Psychological factors affecting health after toxicological disasters. Clinical Psychology Review, 17, 359–374.

Havenaar JM, Rumyantzeva GM, VandenBrink W, Poelijoe NW, VandenBout J, VanEngeland H, Koeter MWJ (1997) Long-term mental health effects of the Chernobyl disaster: An epidemiologic survey in two former Soviet regions. American. Journal of Psychiatry, 154, 1605–1607.

Havenaar JM, VandenBrink W, VandenBout J, Kasyanenko AP, Poelijoe NW, Wohlfarth T, Meijler-Iljina LI (1996) Mental health problems in the Gomel region (Belarus): an analysis of risk factors in an area affected by the Chernobyl disaster. Psychological Medicine, 26, 845–855.

Hemert AM van, Hengeveld MW, Bolk JH, Rooijmans HGM, VandenBroucke JP (1993) Psychiatric disorders in relation to medical illness among patients of a general medical outpatient clinic. Psychological Medicine, 23, 167–176.

Hemert AM van, Huijsman-Rubingh RRR, Smeets EC (2002) Rampen en gezondheidsklachten. Essentieel is een goede relatie met de patiënt. Medisch Contact, 57:141–144.

Holmes DT, Tariot PN, Cox C (1998) Preliminanary evidence of psychological distress among reservists in the Persian Gulf war. Journal of Nervous and Mental Disease, 186, 166–173.

Hyams KC (1998) Lessons derived from evaluating Gulf War syndrome: suggested guidelines for investigating possible outbreaks of new diseases.[editorial comment]. Psychosomatic Medicine, 60, 137–139.

Hyams KC, Wignall FS, Roswell R (1996) War syndroms and their evaluation: from the US Civil War to the Persian Gulf War. Annals of Internal Medicine, 125, 398–405.

Hytten K, Hasle A (1989) Fire fighters: a study of stress and coping. Acta Psychiatrica Scandinavica, 80, 50–55.

Inquiry-commission plane crash Bijlmermeer (1999) Final report Bijlmer inquiry (in Dutch). 's-Gravenhage: Sdu Publishers.

Ismail K, Everitt B, Blatchley N, Hull L, Unwin C, David A, Wessely S (1999) Is there a Gulf War syndrome? Lancet, 353, 179–182.

Jamal GA (1998) Gulf War syndrome: a model for the complexity of biological and environmental interaction with human health. Adverse Drug Reactions & Toxicological Reviews, 17, 1–17.

Jones E, Hodgins-Vermaas R, McCartney H, Everitt B, Beech C, Poynter D, Palmer I, Hyams K, Wessely S (2002) Post-combat syndromes from the Boer war to the Gulf war: a cluster analysis of their nature and attribution. BMJ, 324:321–324.

Joseph S, Williams R, Yule W (1998) Understanding post-traumatic stress. A psycho social perspective on PTSD and treatment. Chapter 6.

Joseph S, Yule W, Williams R (1993) Post-traumatic stress: attributional aspects. J of Traumatic Stress, 6:501–513.

Kasperson RE, Renn O, Slovic P et al. (1988) Social amplification of risk: a conceptual framework. Risk Analysis, 8, 177–187.

Kellner R (1987) Hypochondrias and somatization. JAMA, 258, 2718–2722.

Kepplinger HM, Habermeier J (1995) The Impact of Key Events on the Representation of Reality. European Journal of Communication 10, no. 3:271–390.

Kessler D, Lloyd K, Lewis G, Gray DP (1999) Cross sectional study of symptom attribution and recognition of depression and anxiety in primary care. BMJ, 318:436–440.

Kitzinger J, Reilly J (1997) The Rise and Fall of Risk Reporting: Media Coverage of Human Genetics Research, False Memory Syndrome, and Mad Cow Disease. The European Journal of Communication, Vol 12, NO 3.

Kleber RJ, Figley CR, Gersons BPR (1995) Beyond Trauma: cultural and societal dynamics. New York: Plenum Press.

Kroenke K, Mangelsdorff D (1989) Common symptoms in ambulatory care: Incidence, evaluation, therapy, and outcome. American Journal of Medicine, 86, 262–266.

Lamberts H, Woods M (1987) International Classification of Primary Care. Oxford: Oxford University Press.

Livingston HM, Livingston MG, Brooks DN, Mc Kinlay WW (1992) Elderly survivors of the Lockerbie air disaster. Int J Geriatric Psychiatry, 7:725–729.

Lundin TL (1995) Transportation disasters: a review. Journal of traumatic stress, 8, 381–389.

McFarlane AC, Atchison M, Rafalowicz E, Papay E (1994) Physical symptoms in posttraumatic stress disorder. Journal of Psychosomatic Research, 38, 715–726.

Marmar CR, Weiss DS, Metzler TJ, Delucchi KL, Best S, Wentworth KA (1999) Longitudinal course and predictors of continuing distress following critical incident exposure in emergency services personnel. The Journal of Nervous and Mental Disease, 187, 15–22.

Meijer JS (1992) Een jaar na de vliegramp in de Bijlmermeer; posttraumatische reacties in een huisartspraktijk. Ned Tijdschr Geneeskd, 136:2553–2558.

Miller AC, Fuciarelli AF, Jackson WE, Ejnik EJ, Emond C, Strocko S, Hogan J, Page N, Pellmar T (1998) Urinary and serum mutagenicity studies with rats implanted with depleted uranium or tantalum pellets. Mutagenesis, 13, 643–648.

Mulder YM, Reijneveld SA (1999) Health study Unprofor. A study among veterans who served in Lukavac, Santici and Busovaca (Bosnië-Herzegovina) in the period 1994–1995 (in Dutch). Leiden: TNO.

Mumford DB, Devereux TA, Maddy PJ, Johnston JV (1991) Factors leading to the reporting of 'functional' somatic symptoms by general practice attenders. Br J Gen Pract, 41:454–458.

Nakajima T, Ohta S, Morita H, Midorikawa Y, Mimura S, Yanagisawa N (1998) Epidemiological study of sarin poisoning in Matsumoto City, Japan. Journal of Epidemiology, 8, 33–41.

Nicolson GL, Nicolson NL (1998) Gulf War illnesses: complex medical, scientific and political paradox. Medicine, Conflict & Survival, 14, 156–165.

Noij EK (1997) The public health consequences of disasters. New York: Oxford University Press.

Norusis MJ (1990) SPSS/PC+ V2.0 Base Manual. Gorinchem: SPSS International BV.

Palinkas LA, Petterson JS, Russell J et al. (1993) Community patterns of psychiatric disorders after the Exxon Valdez oil spill. Am J Psychiatry, 150:1517–1523.

Peveler R, Kilkenny L, Kinmonth AL (1997) Medically unexplained physical symptoms in primary care: a comparison of self-report screening questionnaires and clinical opinion. J Psychosomatic Research 1997, 42:245–252.

Prince-Embury S, Rooney JF (1989) Psychological symptoms of residents in the aftermath of the Three Mile Island nuclear accident and restart. Journal of Social Psychology, 128, 779–790.

Reijneveld SA (1994) The impact of the Amsterdam aircraft disaster on reported annoyance by noise and on psychiatric disorders. International Journal of Epidemiology, 23, 333–340.

Robbins JM, Kirmayer LJ, Hemami S (1997) Latent variable models of functional somatic distress. The Journal of Nervous and Mental Disease, 185, 606–615.

Roca RR, Spence RJ, Munster AM (1992) Posttraumatic adaptation and distress among adult burn survivors. American Journal of Psychiatry, 149, 1234–1238.

Rook GAW, Zumla A (1997) Gulf War syndrome: is it due to a systematic shift in cytokine balance towards a Th2 profile? Lancet, 349, 1831–1833.

Rubonis AV, Bickman L. (1991) Psychological impairment in the wake of disaster: the disaster-psychopathology relationship. Psychol Bull, 109:384–399.

Schuster MA, Stein BD, Jaycox LH, Collins RL, Marshall GN, Elliott MN, Zhou AJ, Kanousse DE, Morrison JL, Berry SH (2001) A national survey of stress reactions after the September 11, 2001, terrorist attacks. N Engl J Med, 345(20):1507–1512.

Sharpe M, Peveller R, Mayou R (1992) The psychological treatment of patients with functional somatic symptoms: a practical guide. Journal of Psychosomatic Research, 36, 515–529.

Skodol AE, Schwartz S, Doherenwnd BP, Levav I, Shrout PE, Reiff M (1996) PTSD symptoms and comorbid mental disorders in Israeli war veterans. British J Psychiatry, 169: 717–725.

Sloan P (1988) Post-traumatic stress in survivors of an airplane crash-landing: a clinical and exploratory research intervention. Journal of Traumatic Stress, 1, 211–229.

Southwick SM, Morgan A, Nagy LM, Bremner D, Nicolaou AL, Johnson DR (1993) Trauma-related symptoms in veterans of operation desert storm: a preliminary report. American Journal of Psychiatry, 150, 1524–1528.

Southwick SM, Morgan A, Darnell A, Bremner D, Nicolaou AL, Nagy LM (1995) Trauma-related symptoms in veterans of operation desert storm: a 2-year follow up. American Journal of Psychiatry, 152, 1150–1155.

Speckens AEM, VanHemert AM, Spinhoven P, Hawton KE, Bolk JH, Rooijmans HGM (1995) Cognitive behavioural therapy for medically unexplained physical symptoms: a randomised controlled trial. BMJ, 311, 1328–1332.

Speckens AEM, VanHemert AM, Bolk JH, Rooijmans HGM, Hengeveld MW (1996) Unexplained physical symptoms: outcome, utilization of medical care and associates factors. Psychological Medicine, 26, 745–752.

Straus SE (1999) Bridging the gulf in war syndromes. [commentary]. Lancet, 353, 162–63.

Summerfield D (1995) In Kleber RJ, Figley CR, Gersons BPR (Eds) Beyond Trauma: cultural and societal dynamics (pp. 17–30). New York: Plenum Press.

Unwin C, Blatchley N, Coker W, Ferry S, Hotopf M, Hull L (1999) Health of UK servicemen who served in Persian Gulf War. Lancet, 353, 169–178.

Verbrugge LM, Ascione FJ (1987) Exploring the iceberg. Common symptoms and how people care for them. Medical Care, 25, 59–69.

Vries M de, Soetekouw PMMB, Bleijenberg G, VanderMeer JWM (1998) The post-Cambodia complaints study, phase I: A study to nature, extent and cause (in Dutch). Nijmegen: St Radboud.

Tennen H, Affleck G (1990) Blaming others for threatening events. Psychol Bull, 108:209–232.

The Iowa Persian Gulf Study Group. (1997). Self-reported illness and health status among Gulf War veterans. JAMA, 277, 238–245.

Turnquist DC, Harvey JH, Anderson BL (1988) Attributions and adjustment to life-threatening illness. Br J Clin Psychol, 27:55–65.

Velden K van der. (1999) General Practice at work. Thesis. Erasmus University, Rotterdam.

Wegman DH, Woods NF, Bailar JC (1997) Invited commentary: how would we know a Gulf War Syndrome if we saw one? American Journal of Epidemiology, 146, 704–710.

Weiner B (1995) Spontaneous causal thinking. Psychol Bull, 97:74–84.

Wessely S, Nimnuan C, Sharpe M (1999) Functional somatic syndromes: one or many? Lancet, 354, 936–939.

Wessely S (2002) Preliminary notes on Nato-Russia advanced research workshop on social and psychological consequences of chemical, biological and radiological terrorism. Nato Scientific and Environmental Affairs Division (internet site).

Weyerman AG, Norris FH, Hyer LE (1996) Examining comorbidity and posttraumatic stress disorder in a Vietnam veteran population using the MMPI-2. Journal of Traumatic Stress, 9, 353–360.

Wilkinson CB (1983) Aftermath of a disaster: the collapse of Hyatt Regency Hotel skywalks. American Journal Psychiatry, 140, 1134–1139.

Winje D (1996) Long-term outcome of trauma in adults: the psychological impact of a fatal bus accident. Journal of Consulting and Clinical Psychology, 1996, 1037–1043.

Wong PTP, Weiner B (1981) When people ask 'why' questions, and the heuristics of attributional research. J of Personality and Social Psychol, 40:650–663.

Wyke S, Hunt K, Ford G (1998) Gender differences in consulting a general practitioner for common symptoms of minor illness. Social Science Medicine, 46, 901–906.

Yzermans CJ, Zee J van der, Oosterhek M, Spreeuwenberg P, Kerssens J, Donker G, Schadé E. (1999) Gezondheidsklachten en de vliegramp Bijlmermeer. Een inventariserend onderzoek. Amsterdam, Academic Medical Center/Utrecht, NIVEL.

Yzermans CJ, Donker GA, Becker HE, Oosterhek M, Schadé E (2003) Psychological symptoms six years after a plane crash. Submitted for publication.

Yzermans CJ, Gersons BPR (2002) The chaotic aftermath of an airplane crash in Amsterdam: a second disaster. In: Havenaar JM, Cwikel JG, Bromet EJ (eds) Toxic Turmoil; psychological and societal consequences of ecological disasters. New York: Kluwer Academic/Plenum publishers, 85–99.

Impact of medicines on Public Health: EURO-MED-STAT

Pietro Folino-Gallo · Tom Walley · Kees DeJoncheere · Robert vander Stichele
on behalf of the EURO-MED-STAT Project

Impact of medicines on public health: background of the EURO-MED-STAT Project

Several thousand medicinal products are presently licensed and marketed in the European Union countries. The overall use of active ingredients is in the order of tons per day and the expenditure more than € 90 billions per year (€ 56 billions of which are paid by national health care systems).

This wide utilisation of medicines has an important impact on public health and exerts its influence by four different ways:

Medicines cause intended therapeutic effects: i.e. improving or preventing diseases and relieving symptoms.

Medicines may cause medication errors and other medicine-related problems: patients taking a medicine for no medically valid indication, patients receiving a wrong medicine or the right medicine in the wrong way, patients failing to receive the medicine they need, patients experiencing adverse drug reactions.

Medicines pose an economic burden and impose an opportunity cost: pharmaceutical expenditure accounts for a large proportion of health care spending and it is rising faster than any other area of health care.

The use of pharmaceuticals has an ecotoxicological impact by releasing in the environment, via the wastewater, pharmacologically active substances (including endocrine disrupters and carcinogens) able to pollute drinking water, rivers, seas and soil.

Some official documents only consider the impact of medicines on health as their intended therapeutic effect, or in regard to the need to approve more medicines of high quality in a shorter time. But we will see that licensing new medicines is only one side, and perhaps not the most important, of the impact of medicines on public health.

Therapeutic effects of medicines

By their intended therapeutic effects, medicines are able to prevent or treat diseases and relieve symptoms. This is the reason why physicians prescribe and patients use medicines. The potential advantages of medicines are extensively promoted/advertised by pharmaceutical companies and as a result there is plentiful, sometime misleading, information about the clinical indications for medicines [1].

Some therapeutic classes represent important progress and have dramatically improved the therapeutic approach to several diseases.

Streptokinase and other fibrinolytic agents have substantially improved prognosis and survival rate of patients with acute myocardial infarction.

Antiulcer agents have changed a severe disease (with fatal complications), requiring gastric surgical resection, into a disease requiring only the assumption of few pills per day for a short time period with a substantial improvement of prognosis and quality of life of the patients. Avoiding surgical intervention of gastric resection, and all its complications, has meant a substantial gain for individual patients and public health and a substantial reduction in costs for hospitalisation.

Angiotensin converting enzyme inhibitors (ACE-Is) represent a milestone in the treatment of patients with congestive cardiac failure because they are able to improve symptoms and prolong survival of these patients. They are also able to slow the progression of renal failure in diabetic patients with microalbuminuria.

Antibiotics, together with a substantial improvement of sanitation, have helped displace infectious diseases as the major cause of death in many countries.

Thus medicines represent very useful tools for improving individual and public health, but these important advantages have also a down side: the possibility that treated patients have a not optimal outcome. Up to 40% of treated patients experience some medicine-related problem, which sometime may be life threatening. Use of medicines may cause medication errors and adverse drug reactions.

Medication errors and adverse drug reactions

Sporadic reports of medication errors were published before the 1990s. Steel et al. [2] reported in 1981 that more than half of therapeutic accidents in a teaching hospital were related to the utilisation of medicines. Ten years later an analysis of cardiac arrests [3] proved that medicines were the most important cause of iatrogenic cardiac arrest and that 64% of them were preventable. But with the publication in 1991 of the Harvard Medical Practice Study I and II [4, 5] medication errors became a scientific research topic. The Harvard Medical Practice Study is one of the most comprehensive studies of medical errors: a sample of 31 000 records was drawn from a population of more than 2.5 million patients in 51 hospitals in New York State. The first major result from the Harvard Medical Practice Study was that 3.7% of the hospitalised patients (1/27) experienced iatrogenic adverse events: death was the outcome in 14% of these patients. The second important result was that medicine related problems were the most common cause of adverse events (19%), more common than surgical infections (14%) or technical complications (13%). Both the Harvard studies showed that most of the medicine related problems were linked to errors and were preventable.

Similar results were performed few years later by The Quality in Australian Health Care Study (QAHCS) [6] which analysed 14 000 records from 28 hospitals in 2 Australian states. The percentage of adverse events was higher in the Australian study (16%) than in the Harvard study, partially because the Australian researchers were able to identify errors which occurred during the hospitalisation but were not diagnosed until later; however real differences could not be excluded.

Extrapolating the results from their study to the Australian population, the authors concluded that 470 000 hospitalisations and 3.3 million bed days were related to adverse events, with an estimated 18 000 deaths and 17 000 patients suffering permanent damage. The medicines, which were the most common cause of adverse events in the Australian study, were cardiovascular, antibiotics and antineoplastics.

A problem of particular relevance, but often under evaluated, is that of medication errors and adverse effects in children. The American Academy of Paediatrics [7] analysing more than 90 000 lawsuits for malpractice estimated that medication errors are the most frequent and the most expensive reason for lawsuits.

An evaluation of medicines used in a paediatric department in Belgium showed that 12% of the medicines were used inappropriately. An analysis enlarged to other Belgium hospitals obtained a percentage of errors in utilisation of medicines ranging from 12 to 21%.

The European Commission has estimated that over 50% of the medicines used in children have never actually been studied for paediatric use. This important lack of information about the appropriate use (indications and dosages) in children may result in an increased risk of medication problems. On the basis that children are 20% (about 75 million people) of the total EU population, the European Commission has proposed specific regulatory actions in this field, aimed to encourage studies so as to improve the quality of therapeutic care in children [8].

The scientific literature on medication errors has progressively enlarged and in 1998 Lazarou et al. [9] published a meta-analysis. They concluded that in 1994 more than two million patients (2 216 000) in US experienced a severe reaction to medicines, with a fatal outcome in more than 100 000 patients. There were wide methodological differences in the studies included in Lazarou's meta-analysis, and so the results must be interpreted cautiously. Nevertheless it appears clear that medication related problems are a relevant public health problem and they could represent between the fourth and sixth cause of death in the US.

In 1999 the Institute of Medicines (IOM) published its report "*To Err is Human*" [10] which estimated that up to 98,000 hospital deaths per year were due to medical errors. But the IOM report did not include figures from ambulatory patient care settings.

Medication problems are not limited to hospitals, and also happen in general practice. It has been estimated that 40% of the patients using a medicine have a negative outcome. It is generally thought that because hospital consumption is a small portion (between 5–15%) of the total medicine consumption, medication problems should be frequent also in general practice. The present trend to move away from in-patient treatment to out-patient treatment may lead to an increase in medication-error deaths in the community. In the US from 1983 to 1993, bed days decreased by 21% and the number of visits in out-patients clinics increased by 75%. In parallel, in the same period, medication-error deaths in hospitalised patients increased by 237%, while deaths in outpatients increased by 848% [11].

Comparatively little is known about medication errors outside hospital. Johnson et al. [12, 13] performed one of the most complete studies. They calculated that medication related problems accounted for 116 million extra visits to doctors per year, 76 million additional prescriptions, 17 million emergency department visits, 8 million admissions to hospital, 3 million admissions to long term care facilities and 199 000 additional deaths with a total cost higher than $ 76.6 billion.

Despite a growing scientific literature about the epidemiology of medication problems, there is still uncertainty about its frequency. A recent report of the UK Audit Commission [13] estimated that there were more than 1200 medicine-related deaths in the UK in the year 2000 (Fig. 1). These figures are, probably, a wide underestimation of the real entity of the problem.

The systems approach

Both the Harvard and Australian studies are relevant because they proved that medication errors happen and are frequent, even in tertiary care and teaching hospitals, and they can be subjected to systematic study. This has made possible a more modern approach, so that

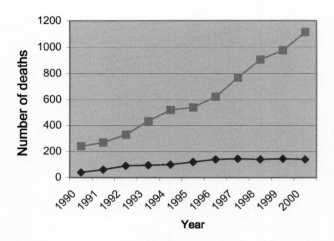

—■— Adverse effects of medicine in therapeutic area

—◆— Medication errors

Fig. 1. Number of deaths in England and Wales from medication errors and the adverse effects of medicines 1990 to 2000. Source: reference n. 14

medication errors are not seen as a rare, human and individual event (due to a "bad apple"), but rather the fault of the "system" where it happens. If the system is not safe, the error is more probable ("errors waiting to happen") and it will be more difficult to intercept and neutralise it. For this reason, systems analysis has two major objectives:
▶ the first one is to analyse the errors to understand their causes and create a setting where the individual error becomes less likely
▶ the second one is, if an error has happened, to intercept it and avoid or limit damage.

A strong multidisciplinary collaboration between specialists in public health, clinical pharmacology and management seems indispensable to clarify these issues, by using consistent definitions and methods.

Economic burden of medicines

The European Union is the largest pharmaceutical world market, ahead of Japan and the US. The total EU expenditure has been estimated to be more than € 90 billions (2/3 paid by national health systems).

This large expenditure on pharmaceuticals poses an economic burden and imposes an opportunity cost: pharmaceutical expenditure accounts for a large proportion of health care spending and it is rising faster than any other area of health care. We need to be sure that it constitutes good value. Here the wide variation between different countries identified by OECD may give cause for concern (Fig. 2).

Pharmaceutical expenditure as percentage of the health expenditure ranges from 11–12 percent in the Netherlands and Germany to 20–21 percent in Spain and France. This suggests wide differences in the national systems. We have also an idea of how great the pres-

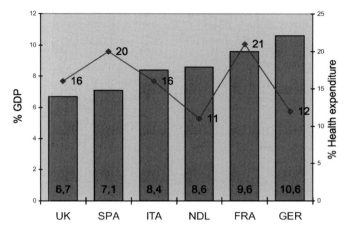

Fig. 2. Health expenditure as % of GDP (bars) and pharmaceutical expenditure as % of health expenditure (line) UK = United Kingdom; SPA = Spain; ITA = Italy; NDL = The Netherlands; FRA = France; GER = Germany. Source: OECD Health Data 2000

sure of pharmaceutical expenditure is on some national systems, especially France and Spain, and the potential advantages to these countries by curbing the pressure on their health systems.

The comparison of utilisation and expenditure data of antiplatelet agents in England give an estimation of the pressure a single medicine can exert on national systems. According to the data from the NHS Prescribing Pricing Authority, the number of items of antiplatelet agents prescribed has doubled in England between September 1996 and September 2001. In the same period the cost of these drugs increased 6.5 fold, from less than £ 2 million to £ 13 million. In September 2001, about 90% of the prescribed items were for aspirin and only a small amount of prescriptions for other agents (clopidogrel, dypiridamole, ticlopidine). But in the same period, the expenditure for aspirin was less than £ 4 million (1/3 of the total expenditure for anti platelet agents) while the expenditure for clopidogrel alone was more than £ 6 million.

These data raise two relevant questions that can be generalised to other medicines and therapeutic groups:

▶ Does clopidogrel (or other new medicines at higher cost) have an added value sufficient to justify its expenditure?
▶ What can we learn from international comparison of expenditure and utilisation of these medicines in other countries?

These are general questions which the EURO-MED-STAT project aims to answer.

A further factor increasing expenditure for medicines is the medicalisation of what in the past were considered non-medical problems. There are many examples of this, for instance, obesity. The Western world is suffering from an epidemic of obesity, with all its attendant morbidity and mortality. In the past, obesity would have been considered a matter for the individual to address rather than for prescribing but now the pharmaceutical industry offers new products to treat this condition. This in part redefines the condition as something worthy of medical attention even in the mildest cases. This is a difficult example because there is clearly morbidity involved here. So the situation is much easier for therapies such as minoxidil to improve hair growth, or botulinus toxin for cosmetic uses.

Many third party payers have restricted access to such medicines in their system. In parallel with this there is increasing medicalisation of risk. The best example of this is cardiovascular risk where we know that treatment with statins will lower a patient's risk of cardiovascular disease by approximately 30%. In practice we are often rushing to embrace such means to address cardiovascular risk rather than aggressively addressing smoking and other lifestyle changes first. This is also true of osteoporosis. Such preventive therapies are the major growth area in the pharmaceutical market in developed countries.

Environmental impact of medicines

Presence of medicines in the environment

Medicines are excreted, unchanged or as metabolites, by humans and enter the environment via the wastewater, often after treatment in sewage treatment works.

The first studies about eco-toxicological impact of medicines were performed in the 1970's, but in recent years residues of medicines for humans and animals have increasingly been researched in the environment. Until year 2000 more than 80 medicines, from a wide array of therapeutic classes (hormones, antibiotics, antineoplastics, non-steroidal anti-inflammatory agents, lipid lowering agents, cardiovascular medicines and others) had been detected in the environment (soil and water, including drinking water) [14] and reported largely in the non-medical scientific literature (Table 1). Similarly to pesticides, the concentration of medicines in the environment ranges from the detection limit in nanograms to micrograms per litre.

Table 1. Sample of medicines found in the environment

Therapeutic class	Surface water	Drinking water
Cardiovascular		
Atenolol	✓	
Furosemide	✓	
Lipid lowering		
Bezafibrate	✓	
Clofibric acid		✓
Antineoplastics		
Cyclophosphamide	✓	
Neurologicals		
Diazepam	✓	✓
Antibiotics		
Erythromycin	✓	
Lincomycin	✓	
Oleandomycin	✓	
Spiramycin	✓	
NSAIDs		
Ibuprofen	✓	
Antiulcer		
Ranitidine	✓	
Antiasthma		
Salbutamol	✓	
Tylosin	✓	✓

Source: reference n 20

The number of medicines investigated is so far only a fraction of the total number of licensed medicines. This is partly because the present procedure for licensing of medicines requires pre-clinical and clinical trials to assure their efficacy and safety, and ecotoxicological data is not required for approval. Thus the environmental impact of most medicines is largely unknown.

Risks of the medicine residues in the environment

Medicines are specifically designed to be highly active and most of the medicines detected in the environment have carcinogenic or endocrine-disrupter properties. It is thus reasonable to assume that other animals in the environment will be influenced by exposure to medicines and that chronic exposure of humans to sub therapeutic concentrations of medicines could represent a risk, which has never been assessed. Two examples can clarify the problem.

Clofibric acid is an antilipid agent whose use, during the 1980s was banned or severely restricted because of an increased mortality in users and a potential carcinogenic effect [15]. Fifteen years after these restrictions Buser et al. [16] examined the presence of clofibric acid in the North Sea. They sampled the water in four different points: two points in the open sea and two points in proximity of the coastline near the Elbe estuary.

During repeated samples, from June 1996 to April 1997, clofibric acid was detectable in all the four sample points. The presence of clofibric acid in the North Sea fifteen years after the severe restriction in its use was surprising. But the apparent absence of a concentration gradient from the coast to the open sea was more surprising. Both the restriction in therapeutic use and the absence of gradient suggest that there is a long-term contamination and a long persistence of clofibric acid in the environment.

Clofibric acid was also present, at comparable concentration, in repeated samples, in four lakes in Switzerland, where the medicine was never produced or manufactured, strongly confirming the hypothesis that medicine excreted by treated patients was, via wastewater, the main source of contamination.

The second example refers to diethylstilbestrol [17], a synthesised stilbene with biological properties similar to those of natural estrogens. Unlike estrogens, diethylstilbestrol was inexpensive to manufacture and it was prescribed widely for about 20 years, with an estimated 10 million Americans exposed to the medicine. In 1971 in US and in 1978 in Europe its use during pregnancy was banned because of the association with the development of cervicovaginal adenocarcinoma more than 15 years after in utero exposure. Presently, diethylstilbestrol is still used as antineoplastic agent and it is thus excreted in the environment but there is a lack of data about utilisation of this medicine in human and its presence and effects in the environment.

One more point of interest is how the utilisation of a single product is able to produce a strong environmental impact. In Germany, the use of a very common disinfectant (Mercurochrome) has been estimated to be responsible for the release into the environment of 150 kg of mercury per year. Taking in account that this agent has been largely used for many years, we can estimate that, at a European level, this single product is responsible for a total release in the environment of some tons of mercury.

The last point about ecotoxicological impact is the presence of some medicines into the drinking water. Several reports from Europe and US [15, 19–20] have described the presence of therapeutic medicines in the tap water. Analgesics and antirheumatic agents, diazepam, statins and other lipid lowering agents, antibiotics, antineoplastic agents and contrast media, have all been identified in drinking water, at concentrations ranging from nanograms to micrograms per litre.

For this reason several bodies at national level (Austria, Germany, The Netherlands and Sweden) have now started to fund projects on the impact of medicines pollution on human beings. Other public Institutions would be justified in paying extra attention to the risk posed to the environment by medicine residues and any efforts at pollution prevention, especially its minimisation, could have important consequences for improved patient health and pharmaceutical spending.

The EURO-MED-STAT protocol

An international collaboration of academics and government agencies was formed to undertake the EURO-MED-STAT project (appendix 1).

APPENDIX 1: **List of participants to the EURO-MED-STAT project**

Ingrid Rosian, Sabine Vogler
Austrian Institute of Health – Vienna

Robert vander Stichele
Heymans Instituut – University of Gent

Lasse Larsen, Bettina Ødegaard
Danish Medicines Agency Brønshøj

Jaana Martikainen
Finnish Social Insurances
Helsinki

Eric van Ganse, Guihlem Pietri
Unit of Pharmacoepidemiology
University of Lyon

Ulrich Schwabe
Ruprecht-Karls-Universität
Heidelberg

Athena Linos, Elena Riza
School of Medicine
University of Athens

Michael Barry, Lesley Tilson
National Centre for Pharmacoeconomics
Dublin

Pietro Folino (co-ordinator), G. Stirparo
National Research Council of Italy
Rome

Alessandra Righi
ISTAT-National Institute for Statistics – Rome

Mario Bruzzone, Emma Puca
Ministry of Health – Rome

Nello Martini, Antonio Addis
Ministry of Health – Rome

Jean Marie Hermans, Petra Jansen
Ministry of Health, Welfare and Sport
The Hague

Marit Ronning, Irene Litleskare
WHO Collaborating Centre for Drug Statistic Methodology –
Oslo

Antonia Faria Vaz, Francisco Batel Marques
INFARMED – National Institute of Pharmacy –
Lisbon

Alfonso Carvajal, Maria Sainz
Institute of Pharmacoepidemiology –
University of Valladolid

Karolina Antonov, Anders Carlsten
Apoteket – Corporation of Swedish Pharmacies –
Stockolm

Tom Walley
Prescribing Research Centre
University of Liverpool

Kees DeJoncheere
Regional Adviser for Pharmaceuticals and Technology
WHO – Regional Office for Europe

The European Commission DG-Health and Consumer Protection, within the Health Monitoring Programme, funds the project. Its aims are to develop a set of indicators, to be integrated into the EU Public Health Information Network (EUPHIN), for monitoring price, expenditure and utilisation of medicinal products in the EU member states.

The monitoring of price, utilisation and spending in a standardised manner could then be a requirement for each EU member state, allowing better comparison between countries and allowing each country to benchmark its performance against others. The project was broken into four tasks.

TASK 1: undertaking an inventory of data sources and a survey of available data in each EU Member State to address medicine utilisation in the community and in hospital, medicine expenditure and medicine prices.

TASK 2: to assess the reliability of the data and its comparability between countries: the data is to be collected by defined daily dose (DDD) and medicines classified by ATC code. Key questions on utilisation are whether the data covers all of the country or only regions, whether both community and hospital data are available, what the sources of such data were (wholesalers, pharmacies, prescribers), whether the data covers only reimbursed medicines or all the products, and Prescribed Only Medicines and/or OTC products; and an assessment of the quality of the data, its reliability and availability. Key questions on price and expenditure data are: kind of price (ex-factory, wholesaler, pharmacy, state reimbursed); community price and hospital price; and private spending versus public spending.

TASK 3: developing Standard Operating Procedures (SOPs) for data management (collection, validation and comparison). Standard Operating Procedures are essentially needed to overcome the difficulties arising from the national discrepancies in health systems, in the classification of medicinal products, and in recording utilisation and expenditure. The ATC/DDD methodology (WHO) [21] will be used for organising raw data and for structuring the analyses by therapeutic classes. The European Standard for Medicinal product identification (ENV 12610) [22] by the European Committee for Standardization (CEN) will be used as a standard for describing medicinal products and their packages. A set of utilisation, cost and expenditure indicators derived from the available validated data will then be selected for data comparison. A key point will be to establish the aims of each indicator and its intended audience. Each indicator will therefore be clearly defined (objective, definition, description, rationale and data collection). The SOPs will also state the level of access and confidentiality of data.

TASK 4: pooling and comparing the validated data with special reference to cardiovascular medicines. The validated data will be pooled and reported according to the established indicators. Cardiovascular products will serve as a test case for the process of pooling, comparing and reporting the validated data. They have been selected both because of their public health importance in treating very common diseases and because other EU public health projects are devoted to produce indicators on cardiovascular morbidity and mortality [23–26].

Perspectives

To date, several reports have analysed and tried to compare the European pharmaceutical systems. Wide discrepancies have been described. A systematic comparison of the number of licensed medicines in the European member states [27] showed wide differences between countries (the number of licensed packs in Germany is seven fold greater than in Sweden, the number of medicines mutually available in all the countries is very low, medicines withdrawn from a country are still available and even widely used in others). Wide differences have been described in consumption of antibiotics by Cars et al. (Fig. 3) and their paper [28], published in 2001 although with data referring to 1997, is a reference study because of the wide differences (e.g. French consumption 4 fold more than Dutch consumption) and the lack of more updated data.

Some comparative data from the EURO-Medicines database [27] referred to the consumption of antibiotics in 1999 and including a number of countries from Central and Eastern Europe (Fig. 4), showed that both total consumption and pattern of use differ widely between countries, and that each country has a specific and different pattern of usage.

From all these reasons (wide utilisation, medication-related problems, economic burden, environmental impact and wide variations in usage), a standardised means of monitoring medicine utilisation and expenditure internationally appears to offer several advantages. This monitoring is not simple to achieve because of the wide differences in national pharmaceutical policies in licensing, pricing, and reimbursing.

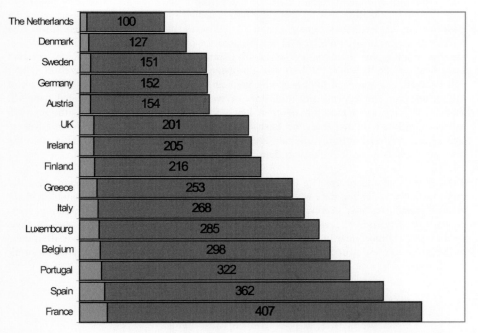

Fig. 3. Differences in the consumption of antibiotics for systemic use (J01) in the European Union countries in the year 1997. In blue consumption in DDD/1000 inh/day. In red index numbers. Source: reference n. 28

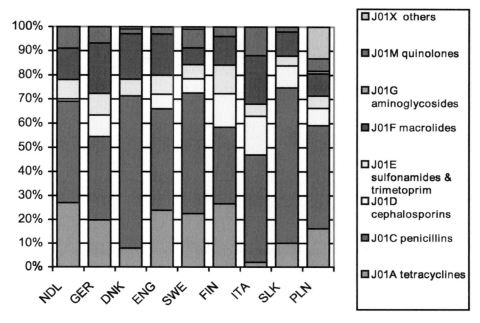

Fig. 4. Pattern of use (% of the total) of the different antibiotic classes in 11 European countries in the year 1999. NDL = The Netherlands; Ger = Germany; DNK = Denmark; ENG = England; SWE = Sweden; FIN = Finland; ITA = Italy; SLK = Slovakia; PLN = Poland; Source: EURO-Medicines database

The aim of the EURO-MED-STAT project is to analyse these differences and to propose specific indicators able to monitor and analyse them and move toward an improved level of harmonisation between the European Union member states, essential to assure an equal high standard of care to all European citizens.

Acknowledgements: EURO-MED-STAT is funded by the European Commission, D-G Health and Consumer Protection, within the Health Monitoring Programme.

References

1. Gottlieb S, Congress criticises drug industry for misleading advertising BMJ 2002; 325: 1379
2. Steel K, Gertman PM, Crescenzi C et al. Iatrogenic illness on a general medical service at a university hospital. New Engl J Med 1981; 304:638–642
3. Bedell SE, Deitz DC, Leeman D, DelBanco TL. Incidence and characteristics of preventable iatrogenic cardiac arrests. JAMA 1991; 265:2815–2820
4. Brennan TA, Leape LL, Laird NM, Hebert L, Localio R, Lawthers AG, Newhouse JP, Weiler PC, Hiatt HH. Incidence of adverse events and negligence in hospitalized patients. Results of The Harvard Medical Practice Study I. New Engl J Med 1991; 324:370–376
5. Leape LL, Brennan TA, Laird N, Lawthers AG, Localio AR, Barnes Ba et al. The nature of adverse events in hospitalized patients. Results of The Harvard Medical Practice Study II. New Engl J Med 1991; 324:377–384

6. Wilson McLR, Runciman WB, Gibberd RB, Harrison BT, Newby L, Hamilton JD. The quality in Australian Health Care Study. Med J Aust 1995; 163:458–471
7. American Academy of Pediatrics. Committee on Drugs and Committee on Hospital Care Prevention of Medication Errors in the Pediatric Inpatient Setting. Pediatrics 1998; 102:428–430
8. European Commission, Enterprise Directorate-General: Better medicines for children. Proposed regulatory actions on paediatric medicinal products. Consultation document Brussels February 28th 2002
9. Lazarou J, Pomeranz BH, Corey PN. Incidence of adverse drug reactions in hospitalized patients. JAMA 1998; 279:1200–1205
10. Kohn LT, Corrigan JM, Donaldson MS, eds: To err is human: building a safe health system. Washington DC; National Academic Press; 1999
11. Phillips DP, Christenfeld N, Glynn LN. Increase in US medication-error deaths between 1983 and 1993. Lancet 1998; 351:643–644
12. Johnson JA, Bootman JL. Drug related morbidity and mortality. A cost-of-illness model. Arch Intern Med 1995; 155:1949–1956
13. Johnson JA, Bootman JL. Drug related morbidity and mortality and the economic impact of pharmaceutical care Am J Health Syst Pharm 1997; 54:554–558
14. UK Audit Commission A spoonful of sugar London December 2001
15. Health Council of the Netherlands. Environmental risks of medicines. The Hague: Health Council of the Netherlands 2001 (in Dutch)
16. United Nations Department for Policy Coordination and Sustainable Development. Consolidated list of products whose consumption and/or sale have been banned, withdrawn, severely restricted or not approved by governments. Sixth issue. New York 1997 United Nations Publications
17. Buser HR, Muller MD, Theobald N Occurrence of the pharmaceutical drug clofibric acid and the herbicide mecoprop in various Swiss lakes and in the North sea Environ Sci Technol 1998; 32:188–192
18. Giusti RM, Iwamoto K, Hatch EE Diethylstilbestrol revisited: A review of the long term health effects. Ann Intern Med 1995; 122:778–788
19. Daughton CG. Environmental stewardship and drugs as pollutants Lancet 2002; 360:1035–1036
20. Zuccato E, Calamari D, Natangelo M, Fanelli R Presence of therapeutic drugs in the environment Lancet 2000; 355:1789–1790
21. WHO Collaborating Centre for Drug Statistics Methodology. ATC index with DDDs Oslo 2002
22. European Committee for Standardization. European prestandard ENV 12610 Medical informatics-Medicinal product identification. Brussels 1997
23. N Hammar: Monitoring of acute myocardial infarction and coronary heart disease Eur J Public Health 2002; 12:17–18
24. Salomaa V. Monitoring of stroke and other cerebrovascular diseases Eur J Public Health 2002; 12:18
25. S Sans: Monitoring of cardiovascular risk factors Eur J Public Health 2002; 12:18
26. S Giampaoli: Recommendations from the EUROCISS project Eur J Public Health 2002; 12:18
27. Folino-Gallo P, WalleyT, Frolich JC, Carvajal A, Edwards RI. Availability of medicines in the European Union. Results from the EURO-Medicines project. Eur J Clin Pharmacol 2001; 57:441–446
28. Cars, Mölstad S, Melander A. Variation in antibiotic use in the European Union. Lancet 2001; 357: 1851–1853

Health risks of psychosocial stress at work: evidence and implications for occupational health services

Johannes Siegrist

Introduction

The importance of work for health goes beyond traditional occupational diseases. Given the far reaching changes in the nature of work in advanced societies, health-adverse psychosocial work environments are becoming more prevalent. These psychosocial work environments are characterized by work pressure, frequent interruptions, information overload, and a low level of task control or autonomy. Irregular working hours, shift work and exposure to noise may aggravate adversity, as is the case with threats of job instability and redundancy, forced mobility and the prospects of involuntary retirement. As will be discussed, these psychosocial work factors affect people's health and well-being, and this needs to be considered under the purview of occupational health.

Why is work so important for human well-being? How does work contribute to the burden of stress and its adverse effects on health? In all advanced societies work and occupation in adult life are accorded primacy for the following reasons. First, having a job is often a prerequisite for continuous income and, thus, for independence from traditional support systems (family, community welfare etc.). Moreover, level of income determines a wide range of life's opportunities. Secondly, training for a job and achieving an appropriate occupational status are important parts of socialization. It is through education, job training, and status acquisition that personal growth and developments are realized, a core social identity outside the family is acquired, and goal-directed activity in human life is shaped. Furthermore, occupation defines an important criterion of social stratification. Finally, occupational settings produce the most pervasive and continuous demands during one's lifetime. They take up the largest amount of active time in midlife, thus providing a source of recurrent negative and positive cognitions, emotions and related behaviours.

Because adverse psychosocial work environments cannot be identified by direct physical or chemical measurements, theoretical models are needed to analyze them. A theoretical model is best understood as a heuristic device that selectively reduces complex reality to meaningful components. Two such theoretical models have received special attention in recent years: the demand-control and the effort-reward imbalance models.

The demand-control model is based on the premise that strain occurs when there is high psychological work demand in combination with a low degree of task control (Karasek and Theorell 1990). Low control at work is defined in terms of low level of decision latitude (authority over decisions) and a low level of skill utilization. While high demand/low control jobs are assumed to produce strain in those exposed ('job strain') this two-dimensional model offers a 'salutogenic' in addition to a 'pathogenic' perspective: jobs defined by high demands and a high level of decision latitude and skill utilization ('active jobs') promote personal growth and feelings of mastery or self-efficacy. These concepts are rooted in research on stress physiology and health psychology (Skinner 1996, Spector

1998, Steptoe and Appels 1989). More recently, the two-dimensional demand-control model was modified to include a third dimension, social support at work. The instrumental, cognitive and emotional change at work was shown to buffer strain reactions (House 1981, Johnson and Hall 1988). Accordingly, highest level of strain – and strongest effects on health – are expected in jobs defined by high demands, low control, and low social support (Karasek and Theorell 1990).

Demand-control theory offers a sociological conceptualization of work stress that is restricted to the situational aspects of the psychosocial work environment that does not take aspects of individual coping into account. In terms of policy implications, this has the advantage of pointing to the structural levels where change may be initiated (see below).

A second, more recently developed model – effort-reward imbalance – views work stress within a distributive justice framework, that is as a form of social exchange rooted in the notions of reciprocity and fairness (Siegrist 1996, see also Cosmides and Tooby 1992). This model assumes that effort at work is spent for the rewards of money, esteem, and career opportunities including job security. The model of effort-reward imbalance claims that lack of reciprocity between costs and gains (i.e. high 'cost'/low 'gain' conditions) elicits sustained strain reactions. For instance, having a demanding, but unstable job or spending continuously high effort without being offered any prospects for promotion cause high cost/low gain conditions. The emphasis on occupational rewards (including job security) reflects changes in the global economy and labour market with the growing importance of fragmented careers, job instability, under-employment, redundancy, forced occupational mobility, and their resultant financial consequences.

According to this model, strain reactions from high cost/low gain conditions are most intense and long-lasting in the following circumstances: a) lack of alternatives in the labour market that prevent people from giving up even unfavourable jobs, as the anticipated costs of disengagement (e.g. the risk of being laid-off) outweigh costs of accepting inadequate benefits; b) unfair job arrangements that may be accepted for a certain period of time for the strategic purposes of improving their chances for career promotion at a later stage; c) a specific personal pattern of coping with demands and eliciting rewards characterized by overcommitment may prevent people from accurately assessing cost-gain relations. 'Overcommitment' defines a set of attitudes, behaviours, and emotions reflecting excessive striving in combination with a strong desire for approval and esteem (Siegrist 1996). At the psychological level, experience of effort-reward imbalance is often paralleled by feelings of impaired self-esteem whereas experiencing a balance is assumed to promote 'salutogenic' feelings of satisfaction, enhanced self-worth and success.

While specific individual coping characteristics (overcommitment) are included in this model it nevertheless offers a clear distinction of the extrinsic and intrinsic components both at the conceptual and at the operational levels.

Psychosocial stress at work and health: selected empirical evidence

Over the past 15 years a substantial body of evidence has been obtained that documents the explanatory power of the two work stress models with regard to a variety of diseases and conditions of ill health in different occupational groups. Many studies testing the demand-control model have been summarized in several recent reviews (Schnall et al. 2000, Karasek et al. 1998, Hemingway and Marmot 1999, Stansfeld and Marmot 2002). Although several investigations showed no association between demand-control and health, the majority showed a positive association for the model or its components. In general, a relative risk of disease ranging from around 1.5 to 3.0 was observed in employees exposed to job

Table 1. Studies of effort-reward imbalance and cardiovascular risk (overview) (modified from J. Siegrist: Effort-reward imbalance at work and health. In. D. Ganster, P. Perrowe (eds.) Historical and Current Perspectives on Stress and Health, Vol. 2 (pp. 262–291), Elsevier, New York, 2002

First author (year)	Type of study	Cardiovascular outcome*	High effort/low reward (ERI) and/or over-commitment (OC)	Odds ratio (OR)
Siegrist 1990	prospective	acute MI, SCD, subclinical CHD	ERI + OC	ranging from 3.4–4.5
Bosma 1998	prospective	newly reported CHD	ERI + OC †	2.2
Kuper 2002	prospective	CHD	ERI + OC †	1.3
Peter 1998	cross-sectional	prevalence of hypertension	ERI only	♂ 1.6
		prevalence of high LDL cholesterol	OC only	♀ 1.3
Peter 2002	case-control	acute MI versus healthy control (men)	ERI only	1.7
Siegrist 1997	cross-sectional	prevalence of high LDL cholesterol	ERI only	3.5
Joksimovic 1999	follow-up	coronary restenosis following CHD	OC only	2.8

Abbreviations: CHD = coronary heart disease; LDL = low density lipoprotein cholesterol; MI = myocardial infarction; SCD = sudden cardiac death; † proxy measure of effort-reward imbalance at work

strain, and the magnitude of the population-attributable risk of job strain for prevalent diseases such as coronary heart diseases was found to be 10–15% (Schnall et al. 2000).

In the recent past, there has been a rapid growth of evidence demonstrating a similar contribution of the effort-reward imbalance model (Marmot et al. 2002, Schnall et al. 2000, Siegrist 2002). This evidence with regard to cardiovascular and other disease is presented here in greater detail because research conducted in association with the Northrhine-Westphalian Public Health Research Network made a significant contribution to its development (see Acknowledgement). This network provided opportunities of developing and conducting comparative research based on this theoretical model, especially with Scandinavian and British research teams (see below). In addition, a small scale study of associations of effort-reward imbalance with musculoskeletal pain and with depressive symptoms was conducted in a sample of 316 male and female employees of a public transport enterprise within Northrhine-Westphalia. To our knowledge, this was the first time that the explanatory role of this model with regard to musculoskeletal pain was explored (Joksimovic et al. 2002, Larisch et al. 2002).

The review first summarizes available evidence for the model with regard to cardiovascular risk and disease, mainly coronary heart disease (CHD) (see Table 1), and then provides an overview of study results for other health indicators (see Table 2).

In relation to CHD and its major risk factors, two prospective observational studies, a follow-up study and three cross-sectional or case-control studies have reported findings with partial or full confirmation of the model's basic hypotheses (see Table 1). A German study of blue-collar workers, covering some 2000 person-years (Siegrist et al. 1990), and the Whitehall II study of British civil servants based on an original sample of 10 308 men and women followed over a mean 5.3 years (Bosma et al. 1998) are prospective investigations. Although a Swedish cohort study of some 5720 healthy employed men and women is also prospective, baseline data only are currently available (Peter et al. 1998). Two further

Table 2. Studies of effort-reward imbalance and other health outcomes (overview) (modified from J. Siegrist: Effort-reward imbalance at work and health. In. D. Ganster, P. Perrowe (eds.) Historical and Current Perspectives on Stress and Health, Vol. 2 (pp. 262–291), Elsevier, New York, 2002

First author (year)	Type of study	Health outcome	High effort/low reward (ERI) and/or over-commitment (OC)	Odds ratio (OR)		
Stansfeld 1998	prospective	functioning: physical (I), men-tal (II), social (III)	ERI + OC †	I ♂1.4 ♀2.0	II 1.7 2.3	III 1.6 1.8
Stansfeld 1999	prospective	psychiatric disorder	ERI + OC †	♂2.5 ♀1.6		
Stansfeld 2000	prospective	alcohol dependence (men)	ERI + OC †	1.9		
Kuper 2002	prospective	physical functioning, mental functioning (SF36)	ERI + OC † ERI + OC †	1.4 2.2		
Tsutsumi 2001	cross-sectional	depression	ERI OC	3.7 3.1		
Pikhart 2001	cross-sectional	self-rated health	ERI	2.6		
Rugulies 2000	cross-sectional	back pain psychosomatic symptoms, self-rated health	ERI	ranging from 1.9–3.6		
Killmer 1999	cross-sectional	burn-out: exhaustion (I), de-personalization (II)	ERI OC	3.6 1.8	2.0 2.3	
Joksimovic 2002	cross-sectional	musculoskeletal pain	ERI OC	ranging from 1.9–4.3		
Larisch 2002	cross-sectional	depression	ERI OC	5.9 5.9		

†: proxy measure of effort-reward imbalance at work

studies are of a cross-sectional nature, one representing a large case-control study of 951 male and female CHD patients and 1147 healthy controls (Peter et al. 2002), and one analyzing associations of psychosocial work stress with cardiovascular risk factors in a group of 179 male middle-managers (Siegrist et al. 1997). A follow-up study of 106 coronary patients who underwent coronary angioplasty was conducted to explore the role of effort-reward imbalance in predicting coronary restenosis following coronary angioplasty (Joksimovic et al. 1999).

With regard to incident CHD during a mean 5-year observation period, effort-reward imbalance assessed at baseline was associated with a relative risk of 2.2 in the Whitehall II study and of approximately 4.0 in the German blue-collar study. This excess risk could not be explained by established biomedical or behavioural risk factors, as these variables were taken into account in multivariate statistical analysis (see Table 1).

It should be noted that the original questionnaire measuring effort-reward imbalance was not available at baseline screening of the Whitehall cohort. Therefore, proxy measures have been constructed to measure the model. Interestingly, the findings derived from the 5-year observation period have recently been replicated for a period of 11 years of the same cohort where effort-reward imbalance at work still predicted incident CHD in a significant way (Kuper et al. 2002).

Adjusting for major cardiovascular risk factors in multivariate statistical models, such as hypertension, hyperlipidemia or elevated fibrinogen, might, in fact, result in 'overadjustment' as these risk factors are partly influenced by stress-induced sustained activation of the autonomic nervous system as well. Indeed, several cross-sectional investigations have documented associations of effort-reward imbalance and the prevalence of hypertension, hyperlipidemia or a co-manifestation of these two cardiovascular risk factors (Peter et al. 1998; Marmot et al. 2002).

Additional evidence not reported here is available from a Finnish prospective study that did not provide an explicit measure of the model, but documented a significantly elevated risk hazard of cardiovascular mortality (RH: 2.3) among men whose work was defined by a combination of high demands with low income, a finding that the authors interpreted in the framework of the effort-reward imbalance model (Lynch et al. 1997a). In the same study it was also found that progression of carotid atherosclerosis, as established by ultrasound technique, was most advanced in the subgroup of workers exposed to high demands and low economic rewards (Lynch et al. 1997b).

Overall, evidence strongly supports the theory that high cost/low gain conditions at work are associated with an increased risk of cardiovascular disease. Results further illustrate that a combination of information on perceived structural conditions and on personal coping characteristics has more explanatory power than an approach that is restricted to only one of these two model components.

Additional health outcomes were explored in the Whitehall II study and other investigations (see Table 2). Mild to moderate psychiatric disorders, subjective health functioning, and alcohol dependence were all significantly associated with effort-reward imbalance in the Whitehall II study (Stansfeld et al. 1998, 1999, 2000, Kuper et al. 2002).

Another investigation was conducted in 190 male and female employees of a small Japanese plant during a time of economic hardship. After adjustment for age, gender, occupational status and job type effort-reward imbalance was associated with a 3.7 increased risk of depression. Similarly, the odds ratio of overcommitment was 3.1 (Tsutsumi et al. 2001). In a study conducted in four post-communist countries in Central and Eastern Europe with a total of 3941 working subjects, the age-sex adjusted odds ratio of effort-reward imbalance for poor self-rated health was 2.6 (Pikhart et al. 2001).

In the United States, a study of 258 room cleaners in four large hotels reported increased risks of low back pain, upper back pain, severe bodily pain, psychosomatic symptoms and poor self-rated health when exposed to effort-reward imbalance at work (Rugulies & Krause 2000). Similarly, in a group of 316 male and female employees of a public transport enterprise in Germany, scoring high on overcommitment was associated with musculoskeletal pain in the neck, in the hip and in lower extremities (Joksimovic et al. 2002).

Emotional exhaustion and burnout were two health indicators determined to be associated with effort-reward imbalance in a study of 202 nurses in a German university hospital. Moreover, feeling burn out was more frequent in nurses with a high level of overcommitment (Bakker et al. 2000; Killmer 1999). Two additional large-scale studies reinforced the notion that overcommitment affected health outcomes. One was a representative cross-section survey of 1636 employed Dutch men and women (Jonge et al. 2000) and the other was the above mentioned Whitehall II study (Kuper et al. 2002).

In summary, both the extrinsic and the intrinsic components of the effort-reward imbalance model are now considered significant risk factors for the development of stress-related diseases and ill-health, in particular CHD, depression, some forms of addiction and poor self-rated health. Current evidence indicates that adverse effects on health are prevalent among men and women in midlife and early old life, and that these effects are not restricted to modern Western societies.

Implications for occupational health services

What are the policy implications of this new information? First, it is possible to identify dimensions of work-related stress in a wide range of occupations using standardized, well-tested questionnaires. These questionnaires measuring the effort-reward imbalance model as well as the demand-control model are now available in a number of languages for use in international studies. Thus, we can obtain further scientific evidence demonstrating associations between adverse psychosocial work environments and health indicators in working populations. Secondly, it is possible to use these measures to evaluate the amount of work-related stress in specific businesses or occupational groups. Information can then be fed back to those concerned, for instance to serve as a basis of monitoring activities or stress prevention programs. A third possible application concerns legal procedures and compensation claims regarding the afflictions of work life on health. However, the quantitative evidence on the proportion of a health risk that is attributable to work-related stress is confined to the level of populations, not individuals. Thus, the 'etiological fraction' that is attributable to adverse work conditions can hardly be transferred to the individual case, for instance in the context of justification of a compensation claim (Rockhill et al. 1998).

Probably the most significant policy implication concerns the design and implementation of work site stress prevention and health promotion programs. Both approaches, the effort-reward imbalance and the demand-control model, offer specific suggestions in this respect. Whereas propositions derived from the demand-control model are related to measures of job redesign, job enlargement, job enrichment, skill training and enhanced participation (Karasek and Theorell 1990, Karasek 1992), the focus of the effort-reward imbalance model is on adequate terms of exchange between efforts and rewards. Examples of such measures include the development of compensatory wage systems, the provision of models of gain sharing and the strengthening of non-monetary gratifications. Moreover, ways of improving promotional opportunities and job security need to be explored. Supplementary measures are interpersonal training and social skills development, in particular leadership behaviour and stress management techniques with the aim of reducing excessive ways of being committed to work and of strengthening successful coping processes at the individual and group level (Aust et al. 1997, Puls et al. 2002).

These developments have consequences for both occupational health and physicians. Because these new challenges require interdisciplinary teamwork including expertise from behavioural and social sciences, the role for occupational health continues to expand. Moreover, primary intervention measures need to be developed and implemented at specific worksites and in close collaboration with employers and employees. The nature of this collaboration is 'bottom-up' rather than 'top-down', as evidenced by the establishment of discussion groups. This may create some resistance as it weakens the traditional expert role of physicians. On the other hand, developing an intervention is a creative process where new ideas and interpretations are generated. A generic model of work stress, such as demand control or effort-reward imbalance, provides no more than a frame of reference that needs to be elaborated by a 'local theory' (Theorell 1998). A local theory takes into account the context and climate of the work setting and the characteristics of people involved in order to meet the specific needs and expectations.

This new knowledge also affects the core tasks of occupational physicians. For instance, combining work stress information with biomedical information (e.g. by using ambulatory monitoring techniques) may help in detecting high-risk individuals (e.g. identification of 'occult' hypertension; see Schnall et al. 2000). This would enable more tailored individual or group specific interventions. In addition, there are far-reaching implications of this information on secondary prevention, such as physician's decision-making processes on return to work (e.g. after cardiac events) or diagnostic decisions on work ability or early retirement (Gaudemaris 2000).

In conclusion, significant progress has been achieved in the scientific study of associations between an adverse psychosocial work environment and health. While further tasks remain to be solved by researchers the main challenge now consists in applying this knowledge to worksite health promotion measures. Occupational health services should play a decisive role in this process.

Summary

This contribution provides a selective overview of recent progress in the study of psychosocial stress at work and its impact on the workers' health. Epidemiological investigations based on two theoretical models of work stress – the demand-control model and the effort-reward imbalance model – have generated new evidence on elevated risks of coronary heart disease, cardiovascular risk factors, depression, musculoskeletal pain, alcohol dependence, burn out, and poor self-rated health with exposure to an adverse psychosocial work environment. Research results with regard to the effort-reward imbalance model are reviewed in more detail than the demand-control model, given the author's and his co-worker's longstanding involvement in this research development (partly in association with the Northrhine-Westphalian Public Health Research Network).

In general, findings from prospective and cross-sectional investigations demonstrate significantly elevated odds ratios ranging from approximately 1.3 to 3.5. Evidence is more consistent for men than for women, but is found in a variety of blue- and white-collar occupations in different countries.

Implications of this research for occupational health services are discussed, with particular reference to the development and implementation of new primary prevention approaches including more comprehensive assessment and counselling for high risk individuals and groups.

In conclusion, significant progress has been achieved in an important field of occupational public health research. While further research questions need to be answered, the main challenge now consists of applying this knowledge to worksite health promotion.

Acknowledgement

I acknowledge the support of research reviewed here by grants from the German Research Foundation (DFG) and the Federal Ministry of Research and Technology (Northrhine-Westphalian Public Health Research Network). Moreover, the European Science Foundation's Program on 'Social Variations in Health Expectancy in Europe' provided excellent opportunities for conducting comparative investigations. A more extensive version of this contribution is given in J. Siegrist: Effort-reward imbalance at work and health. In D. Ganster, P. Perrowe (Eds.) Historical and current perspectives on stress and health, volume 2, pp 261–291. Elsevier, New York 2002.

References

Aust B, Peter R, Siegrist J (1997) Stress management in bus drivers: a pilot study based on the model of effort-reward imbalance. Int J Stress Management 4:297–305
Bakker AB, Killmer C, Siegrist J, Schaufeli WB (2000) Effort-reward imbalance and burnout among nurses. J Adv Nursing 31:884–891

Bosma H, Peter R, Siegrist J, Marmot M (1998) Two alternative job stress models and the risk of coronary heart disease. Am J Public Health 88:68–74

Cosmides L, Tooby J (1992) Cognitive adaptations for social exchange. In: Barkow JH, Cosmides L, Tooby (eds) The Adapted Mind: Evolutionary Psychology and the Generation of Culture. Oxford University Press, New York, pp 163–228

Gaudemaris R de (2002) Clinical issues: return to work and public safety. In: Schnall PL, Belkic K, Landsbergis P, Baker D (eds) The Workplace and Cardiovascular Disease. Occupational Medicine, Vol. 15. Hanley & Belfus, Philadelphia, pp 223–230

Hemingway H, Marmot M (1999) Psychosocial factors in the aetiology and prognosis of coronary heart disease: systematic review of prospective cohort studies. BMJ 318:1460–1467

House J (1981) Work, Stress and Social Support. Addison-Wesley, Reading MA

Johnson JV, Hall E (1988) Job strain, work place, social support, and cardiovascular disease. Am J Public Health 78:1336–1342

Joksimovic L, Siegrist J, Meyer-Hammer M, Peter R, Franke B, Klimek W, Heintzen M, Strauer BE (1999) Overcommitment predicts restenosis after cronary angioplasty in cardiac patients. Int J Behav Med 6:356–369

Joksimovic L, Starke D, Knesebeck O von dem, Siegrist J (2002) Perceived work stress, overcommitment and self-reported musculoskeletal pain: a cross-sectional investigation. Int J Behav Med 9:122–138

Jonge J de, Bosma H, Peter R, Siegrist J (2000) Job strain, effort-reward imbalance and employee well-being: a large-scale cross-sectional study. Soc Sci Med 50:1317–1327

Karasek R A, Theorell T (1990) Healthy Work. Stress, Productivity, and the Reconstruction of Working Life. Basic Books, New York

Karasek R, Brisson C, Kawakami N, Houtman I, Bongers P, Amick B (1998) The job content questionnaire (JCQ): an instrument for internationally comparative assessments of psychosocial job characteristics. J Occup Health Psychol 4:322–355

Karasek R (1992) Stress prevention through work reorganization: a summary of 19 international case studies. Conditions of Work Digest 11:23–41

Killmer C (1999) Burnout bei Krankenschwestern. LIT-Verlag, Münster

Kuper H, Singh-Manoux A, Siegrist J, Marmot M (2002) When reciprocity fails: effort-reward imbalance in relation to CHD and health functioning within the Whitehall II study. Occupation and Environmental Medicine (in press)

Larisch M, Joksimovic L, Knesebeck Ovd, Starke, D, Siegrist J (2002) Berufliche Gratifikationskrisen und depressive Symptome. Psychother Psych Med, 52:1–7

Lynch J, Krause N, Kaplan GA, Tuomilehto J, Salonen JT (1997) Work place conditions, socioeconomic status, and the risk of mortality and acute myocardial infarction: the Kuopio ischemic heart disease risk factor study. Am J Public Health 87:617–622

Lynch J, Krause N, Kaplan GA, Salonen R, Salonen JP (1997) Work place demands, economic reward, and progression of carotid atherosclerosis. Circulation 96:302–307

Peter R, Alfredson L, Hammar N, Siegrist J, Theorell T, Westerholm P (1998) High effort, low reward, and cardiovascular risk factors in employed Swedish men and women: baseline results from the WOLF Study. J Epidemiol Community Health 52:540–547

Peter R, Siegrist J, Hallqvist J, Reuterwall C, Theorell T, SHEEP Study Group (2002) Psychosocial work environment and myocardial infarction: improving risk estimation by combining two alternative job stress models in the SHEEP study. J Epidemiol Community Health 56:294–300

Pikhart H, Bobak M, Siegrist J, Pajak A, Rywik S, Kyshegyi J, Gostautas A, Skodova Z, Marmot M (2001) Psychosocial work characteristics and self-rated health in four post-communist countries. J Epidemiol Community Health 55:624–630

Puls W, Inhester ML, Wienold H (2002) Stress management trainings as a component of workplace prevention of substance use disorders. Sucht 48:271–283

Rockhill B, Newman B, Weinberg C (1998) Use and misuse of population attributable fractions. Am J Public Health 88:15–19

Rugulies R, Krause N (2000) The impact of job stress on musculoskeletal disorders, psychosomatic symptoms and general health in hotel room cleaners. Int J Behavioral Med 7:16

Schnall PL, Belkic K, Landsbergis P, Baker D (2000) The workplace and cardiovascular disease. Occupat Med. State of the Art Reviews 15:1–374

Siegrist J, Peter R, Junge A, Cremer P, Seidel D (1990) Low status control, high effort at work and ischemic heart disease: prospective evidence from blue-collar men. Soc Sci Med 31:1129–1136

Siegrist J (1996) Adverse health effects of high effort – low reward conditions at work. J Occup Health Psychol 1:27–43

Siegrist J, Peter R, Cremer P, Seidel D (1997) Chronic work stress is associated with atherogenic lipids and elevated fibrinogen in middle-aged men. J Intern Med 242:149–156

Siegrist J (2002) Effort-reward imbalance at work and health. In: Ganster D, Perrowe P (eds) Historical and Current Perspectives on Stress and Health, Vol. 2. Elsevier, New York, pp 262–291

Skinner EA (1996) A guide to constructs of control. J Personality and Social Psychol 71:549–570

Spector PE (1998) A control theory of job stress process. In: Cooper CE (ed) Theories of Organizational Stress. Oxford University Press, Oxford, pp 153–169

Stansfeld S, Fuhrer R, Shipley MJ, Marmot MG (1999) Work characteristics predict psychiatric disorder: prospective results from the Whitehall II study. Occup Environm Med 56:302–307

Stansfeld S, Bosma H, Hemingway H, Marmot M (1998) Psychosocial work characteristics and social support as predictors of SF-36 functioning: the Whitehall II Study. Psychosom Med 60:247–255

Stansfeld S, Head J, Marmot M (2000) Work-related factors and ill health: The Whitehall II Study. HSE Books, London

Stansfeld S, Marmot M (eds) (2002) Stress and the heart. Psychosocial pathways to coronary heart disease. BMJ Books, London

Steptoe A, Appels A (eds) (1989) Stress, Personal Control and Health. Wiley, Chichester

Tsutsumi A, Kayaba K, Theorell T, Siegrist J (2001) Association between job stress and depression among Japanese employees threatened by job loss in comparison between two complementary job stress models. Scand J Work Environ Health 27:146–153

Accreditation and professionalisation in (public) health related education – consequences of Bologna

Jürgen v. Troschke · Daniela Mauthe · Georg Reschauer · Karl Kälble

The change of job outlines and qualification requests in (public) health related education

The German Health and social system is located in a fundamental process of change and modernisation that also concerns the health professions and their qualification. Reorganisation and change concern the historical grown structures and regulation systems of social security, their standards and values and the institutional and professional organisation. This process is connected with social, especially demographic and economic changes that are characterized by increasing life expectancy, aging and decreasing birth rates, singularisation of life forms, differentiation of social relations, ethnical plurality and interculturality, chronicle impairments, expansion of helping systems. There is a growing influence of international interconnections, globalisation and migration on the further development.

The image of health professions is no longer characterized by physicians and nursing staff. With the increasing meaning of the health care sector as service branch the structures of professions became more and more complex and now walk ahead with new challenges. The creation of new professions and disciplines as well as the professionalisation of tasks are accompanied by the higher qualification or the turning of health professions into graduate professions.

In the context of institutionalisation of Public Health in Germany there are – along with the postgraduate programs in Public Health at universities – numerous and various health related personnel training and further education developed and offered in comparison to 1999. In 2001 there where 42% more health related course of studies with a total number of 280 (Kälble 2002).

It is obvious that students as well as potential employers require quality assurance (by accreditation and evaluation) and transparency.

The new graduation system in Germany

One new development in the German Education System in the introduction of Bachelor and Master's Degree courses similar to those in the Anglo-Saxon System. With the amended Framework Law of Higher Education (Hochschulrahmengesetz – HRG) passed in 20 August 1998 and the applied decisions from the Standing Conference of the Ministers of Education and Cultural Affairs of the federal states in Germany (Kultusministerkonferenz – KMK) on the 3 December 1998 and on the 5 March 1999 the basic conditions were created for German higher education institutions to introduce – on a test-period basis – degree programs leading to Bachelor and Master (BA/MA) degrees – parallel to the existing long one-tier programs. Initiated was this process by the multiple lamented deficits of the higher education system (e.g. expensive education, long periods of training as well as Germany's descending international competitiveness in the field of higher education).

The aim connected with the introduction of the new graduation system is to enlarge and elaborate the creative scope of the higher education institutions, to shorten the standard period of study, to improve the international compatibility of German university degrees, to enhance the student mobility and to increase the quotas of foreign applicants for a place at university. As a result it is aimed to enhance the country's international attractiveness.

The most important structural objectives concerning the BA/MA programs can be summarized like this: the standard period of study for Bachelor degree programs is at least three and not more than four years, for Master degree programs the standard period of study is at least one and not more than two years. Consecutive study programs should not exceed five years. BA/MA degree programs have to be modularized and have to include a credit system. Bachelor degree and Master degree are qualifying for a profession. The BA represents a first degree qualifying for a profession, the MA is a further degree qualifying for a profession. BA/MA programs can be offered at universities as well as at universities of applied sciences that means the qualification is cross-institutional regulated. The conferred degrees by universities and universities of applied sciences should not be differentiated by supplements characterizing the type of higher education institution (e.g. FH). Nevertheless the performance profile characterizing the type of higher education institution should be expressed. The "Diploma Supplement" gives further details about the studies forming the basis of the degree. The description of the degree has to emphasize the distinction of the training opportunities in "more application-" or "more theory-oriented".

In accordance with the higher education compass (Hochschulkompass) – the internet service of the Association of Universities and other Higher Education Institutions in Germany (Hochschulrektorenkonferenz – HRK) to inform about German higher education institutions and their degree programs – until February 2003 about 749 Bachelor courses and 869 Master courses (altogether = 1.618; these are 15% of all offered degree programs) will be offered by higher education institutions in Germany.

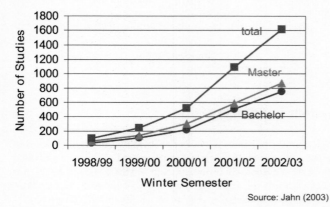

Source: Jahn (2003)

Fig. 1. Quantitative Development of Bachelor and Mester degree programmes at German higher education institutions

The two-tier degree structure in the European context

The introduction of Bachelor and Master degree programs in Germany is related to the process of standardization in the European higher education system and the so called Bologna Process. With the further development of European integration an increasing necessity for the similarity of education systems can be realized.

The Sorbonne-Declaration

In May 1998 the Ministers in charge of higher education of France, Germany, Italy and United Kingdom signed in Paris at the Sorbonne University the so-called Sorbonne-Declaration on the "Harmonisation of the architecture of the European Higher Education System". Other European countries joined the Declaration. One of the most important objectives of the European Ministers of Education is the construction of a European Higher Education Area (EHEA) by 2010 to promote the co-operation of higher education institutions within Europe.

The Sorbonne-Declaration aims
- to support student and teacher mobility within Europe and the integration in the European labour market,
- to introduce the interchangeability and flexibility in higher education systems, especially by encouraging co-operation between institutions,
- to facilitate continuing education and the recognition of study periods in Europe,
- to improve the readability of higher education qualifications in Europe through a common degree level system for undergraduates (Bachelor degree) and graduates (Master and doctoral degree).

The Bologna Process – towards the European higher education area

On 19 June 1999, 29 European Ministers in charge of higher education signed in Bologna the Declaration on establishing the European Area of higher education by 2010 and promoting the European System of higher education world-wide. The Ministers affirmed in the Bologna Declaration their intention to:
- adopt a system of easily readable and comparable degrees (also through the implementation of the Diploma Supplement);
- adopt a system essentially based on two main cycles (undergraduate and graduate);
- establish a system of credits (such as ECTS);
- promote mobility by overcoming obstacles;
- for students, access to study and training opportunities and to related services;
- for teachers, researchers and administrative staff, recognition and valorisation of periods spent in a European context researching, teaching and training, without prejudicing their statutory rights;
- promote European co-operation in quality assurance;
- promote the necessary European dimensions in higher education.

In the context of the Bologna follow-up conference taking place on 19 May 2001 in Prague, the Ministers in charge of higher education of 33 European signatory countries arranged following steps to support, supervise and adapt the process of establishing a European

Area of higher education and to assess the progress achieved and to set directions and priorities for the coming years.

In the Prague Communiqué the Ministers

► reaffirmed their commitment to the objectives of the Bologna Declaration;
► appreciated the active involvement of the European University Association (EUA) and the National Unions of Students in Europe (ESIB);
► took note of the constructive assistance of the European Commission;
► made comments on the further process with regard to the different objectives of the Bologna Declaration;
► emphasised as important elements of the European higher education area:
► lifelong learning;
► involvement of students;
► enhancing the attractiveness and competitiveness of the European higher education area to other parts of the world (including the aspect of transnational education).

On Ministers decision the next follow-up meeting for the Bologna process should take place in September 2003 in Berlin.

The so called Bologna Process is an ambitious programme for the reform of higher education with the aim not only to enhance the international competitiveness of the universities and their graduates but also to gradually adapt the education offered by the universities to the changing needs of the information society in the 21st century (the transformation of our industrial society into a knowledge- and information-based-society).

The accreditation process in Germany

The introduction of the new degrees is changing German higher education more rapidly and profoundly than any other reform measure during the last decades. As defined in the Bologna Declaration, the study structure of the European Higher Education Area should essentially be characterised by two cycles – undergraduated and graduated. The introduction of new degree structures and programs goes in many countries hand in hand with the implementation of new quality assurance mechanisms, often in the form of accreditation.

Accreditation is a central instrument to support the necessary processes of changes in European higher education systems. Accreditation serves to assure quality when implementing new (ex ante steering) degree programs and also to monitor existing ones (ex post steering). Accreditation, i. e. certification of a degree program, will take place after review of the standards for content and specialisation, the vocational relevance of the degree to be awarded and the coherence and consistency of the general conception of the degree program. It will be awarded for a limited period of time within the frame of a transparent, formal and external peer review. After this time the degree programme has to be reviewed. The process of a peer review is steered by agencies which are also reviewed through regular external evaluation. The instrument of accreditation of certificate degree programs is relatively new in Europe but is increasingly gaining acceptance in the countries involved in the Bologna process.

To ensure quality in higher education teaching and study and to provide reliable orientation and enhance transparency for students, employers and higher education institutions alike, the German Accreditation Council (Akkreditierungsrat) was established in 1999 following a resolution of the Standing Conference of the Ministers of Education and Cultural Affairs of the federal states in Germany (Kultusministerkonferenz – KMK) adopted on 3 December 1998.

It is an independent institution that

▶ co-ordinates and monitors the accreditation procedure for all Bachelor and Master study programs at universities and universities of applied sciences

▶ accredits accreditation agencies, whose activities it also co-ordinates. Germany was thus the first country in western Europe to have an official national accreditation institution

▶ works as a central documentation office to guarantee transparency with respect to compatibility and equivalency of study courses.

The Accreditation Council is made up of 17 members, who are representatives of the federal states, higher education institutions, students and professional practice (on behalf of both employer and employee organisations).

In Germany, the Standing Conference of Ministers of Education has decided in spring 2002 to apply the accreditation procedure to all existing and future study programs, not just the newly created Bachelor and Master programs.

The German accreditation agencies

At the moment, however, only new Bachelor and Master programs are accredited. The procedure is carried out on a voluntary basis on the one hand by regional accreditation agencies such as the "Institute of Accreditation, Certification and Quality Assurance" (Akkreditierungs-, Certifizierungs- und Qualitätssicherungs-Institut – ACQUIN), the "Agency for Quality Assurance through Accreditation of Study Courses" (Agentur für Qualitätssicherung durch Akkreditierung von Studiengängen – AQAS), the "Central Evaluation and Accreditation Agency of Hannover" (Zentrale Evaluations- und Akkreditierungsagentur Hannover – ZEvA). On the other hand profession specific accreditation agencies are involved in the accreditation process, as the "Accreditation Agency for Study Programs in Special Education, Care, Health and Social Work" (Akkreditierungsagentur für Studiengänge im Bereich Heilpädagogik, Pflege, Gesundheit und Soziale Arbeit – AHPGS), the "Accreditation Agency for Study Programs in Engineering and Informatics" (Akkreditie-

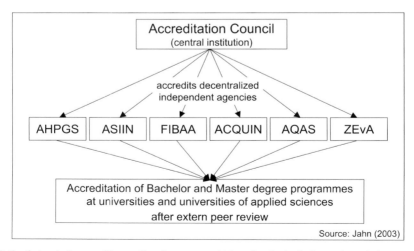

Fig. 2. Accreditation System in Germany (Co-operation of government, higher education institutions and practice)

rungsagentur für Studiengänge der Ingenieurwissenschaften und der Informatik – ASIIN) and the "Foundation for International Business Administration Accreditation" (FIBAA).

The basic examination schedules specific to each region (Länder) determine whether or not new study programs are introduced. The present tendency is towards accrediting not just Bachelor/Master programs but all the programs offered at tertiary level.

The Accreditation Agency for Study Programmes in Special Education, Care, Health and Social Work (AHPGS)

The dynamics of the previous sketched development revealed an urgent need of co-ordination and quality assurance. In this context the German Coordinating Agency for Public Health (DKGW) is involved in the foundation of an accreditation agency for study programs in the fields of (public) health and social work.

Therefore the DKGW benefits from various experiences, pronounced resources and manifold preparatory work relating to this topic. In 1995 representatives of the DKGW went on an educational trip to Public Health centers in the United States to support the international relations. In this context the representatives visited the Council on Education for Public Health (CEPH) in Washington. Co-operation and support of the establishment of accreditation procedures in Germany were reconciled with the Executive Director P. Evans. In the context of the European Symposia – organized and realized by the DKGW – the discussion of quality standards in teaching public health played an important role. The subject of the 2nd European Symposium in 1996 in Graz/Austria was "International co-ordination of the institutionalisation of Public Health". The subject of the 3rd European Symposium in February 2000 in Zürich/Switzerland was "Harmonisation of Public Health Education Programmes in Europe". Inter alia P. Evans (Council on Public Health Education – CEPH) from Washington gave lectures on the accreditation system in the United States and J. Bury (Association of Schools of Public Health in the European Region ASPHER) reported about the European experience in the accreditation of Public Health education programs.

In the context of a research project for the Federal Ministry of Education and Research (BMBF) in 1997/98 the DKGW made a total inquiry about all health related study programs offered at German higher education institutions and published the results as a Guide for the studies (DKGW publication series, volume 9). The great demand for this publication is an indicator for the urgent need of first year students as well as potential employers for transparency and quality assurance.

In March 2002 K. Kälble – staff member of the DKGW – received a DFG scholarship for "Change and professionalisation of the Health Professions in Germany. An analysis from the perspective of the sociology of occupations and the sociology of professions.

In this context the DKGW developed into an information office for questions about education and advanced training in Public Health. Numerous publications recommended the DKGW as central national information point.

In the Committee Training and Education of the German Association of Public Health (Deutsche Gesellschaft für Public Health – DGPH) the representatives of universitary postgraduate programs in Public Health and the DKGW elaborated standards for the basic course of universitary postgraduate programs in Public Health.

In October 1999 the DKGW organized and realized for the DGPH and other scientific societies a great international Public Health Congress in Freiburg "Public Health – Development and Potential" with more than 1 400 participants. The congress offered with various events the possibility to discuss and work on questions of professionalisation in health professions.

In order to guarantee a quality management and to promote the professionalisation in health related professions, the DKGW was engaged in the foundation of the Accreditation Agency for Study Programs in Special Education, Care, Health and Social Work (AHPGS). Initial members of the AHPGS are the dean conference nursing science (33 universities/ universities of applied sciences), the assemblies of the departments social work (73 universities/universities of applied sciences) and remedial education (8 universities/universities of applied sciences) as well as the DKGW. On 17 December 2001 the AHPGS itself gets the accreditation from the national Accreditation Council.

The AHPGS promotes the quality and transparency of German university/university of applied sciences study courses for health and social professionals. The AHPGS focuses with its work to guarantee uniform and international comparable quality standards in the new Bachelor and Master degrees through accreditation procedures. Therefore a continual information exchange with other national and international accreditation agencies as well as university representatives, practitioners, organisations and associations will be realized.

Because of the good preconditions not only the standards and criteria for the accreditation of Bachelor and Master degrees of the national accreditation board could be secured, also the further development of graduate profession and of professionalisation in health related professions could positively influenced. Therefore workshops and conferences should be held in co-operation with the involved partners.

References

Accreditation Council (1999) Accrediting Accreditation Agencies and Accrediting Degree Programmes leading to Bakkalaureus/Bachelor's and Magister/Master's Degrees – Basic Standards and Criteria – amended on 30 November 1999 and last revised on 17 December 1999. – www.accreditation_council.de/criteria.htm (14. 3. 2003)

Accreditation Council (2000) Key Points for an Akkreditierungsrat (Accreditation Council) System to Monitor the Accreditation Agencies – adopted on 17 August 2000. – www.accreditation_council.de/monitoring.htm (14.03.2003)

Accreditation Council (2001) Frame of Reference for Bachelor's/Bakkalaureus and Master's/Magister Degree Courses – adopted on 20 June 2001. – www.accreditation_council.de/frame_of_reference.htm (14. 3. 2003)

Center of Accreditation and Quality Assurance of the Swiss Universities (Organ für Akkreditierung und Qualitätssicherung der Schweizerischen Hochschulen – OAQ) Accreditation and evaluation in Europe. – www.oaq.ch (14. 3. 2003)

Hochschulrahmengesetz (HRG) Bekanntmachung der Neufassung des Hochschulrahmengesetzes vom 19. Januar 1999. In: Ministerium für Wissenschaft, Forschung und Kunst Baden-Württemberg (Hrsg) (2002) Hochschulrecht Baden-Württemberg. Stuttgart, S 239–255

Jahn H (2003) Entwicklung im deutschen Hochschulwesen im Kontext des Bologna-Prozesses. Lecture at the Conference of the committees of AHPGS, 21./22.2.2003 in Windenreute

Kälble K, Troschke Jv (1997) Aus- und Weiterbildung in den Gesundheitswissenschaften/Public Health. Schriftenreihe der Deutschen Koordinierungsstelle für Gesundheitswissenschaften an der Abteilung für Medizinische Soziologie der Universität Freiburg, Bd 8. Deutsche Koordinierungsstelle für Gesundheitswissenschaften, Freiburg

Kälble K, Troschke Jv (1998) Studienführer Gesundheitswissenschaften. Schriftenreihe der Deutschen Koordinierungsstelle für Gesundheitswissenschaften an der Abteilung für Medizinische Soziologie der Universität Freiburg, Bd 9. Deutsche Koordinierungsstelle für Gesundheitswissenschaften, Freiburg

Kälble K (1999) Gesundheitsbezogene Studiengänge an Universitäten und Fachschulen. In: Bundesvereinigung für Gesundheit (Hrsg) Gesundheit: Strukturen und Handlungsfelder. Luchterhand Verlag, Neuwied (Grundwerk/Loseblattwerk)

Kälble K, Troschke Jv (2001) Gesundheitswissenschaftliche Aus- und Weiterbildung in Deutschland: Entwicklung, Entwicklungsstand, die europäische Perspektive und die Herausforderung durch das neue Graduierungssystem. Zeithichschrift für Gesundheitswissenschaften, 4. Beiheft: Public Health – Entwicklungen und Potentiale: 39–53

Kälble K, Reschauer G (2002) Wandel der Berufsbilder und Qualifikationsanforderungen in den Gesundheitsberufen. Public Health FORUM 34:2–4

Kälble K (2001) Bachelor und Master für gesundheitsbezogene Berufe – neue Entwicklungen und Akkreditierung. Prävention 3:67–73

Klüsche W, Sieger M, Störmer N, Troschke Jv (2001) Die Akkreditierungsagentur für Studiengänge im Bereich Heilpädagogik, Pflege, Gesundheit und Soziale Arbeit (AHPGS). Prävention 3:74–76

Reschauer G, Wildner, M (2002) Public-Health-Ausbildung in Deutschland. Public Health FORUM 36:6–7

Tauch, Ch.; Rauhvargers, A. (2002): Survey on Master Degrees and Joint Degrees in Europe. – www.bologna-berlin2003.de/pdf/Survey_Master_Joint_degrees.pdf (14. 3. 2003)

Troschke Jv (1999) Aus-, Fort- und Weiterbildung in den Gesundheitswissenchaften. In: Polak G (Hrsg) Das Handbuch Public Health – Theorie und Praxis: Die wichtigsten Public Health Ausbildungsstätten. Springer Verlag, Wien, S 205–216

Subject Index

A

abstract characteristics   24, 27
abuse of alcohol   92
access to services   275
acute day hospital treatment   153, 164, 170
adolescent   63, 158–159, 283, 285, 288–289
advice   51–52, 69, 91, 132, 293, 299, 302–303
age-related challenges   84
allergies   57, 63
antidiabetic drug   213
– therapy   204
antigenic set   135
antihypertensive medications   204
– therapy   204
anxiety disorder   146
archiving   259–260, 262, 264, 266
arterial hypertension   203
asthma   63, 110–112, 114, 117, 327
atherosclerotic process   220
attributive validity   132

B

balanced information   276
behavioural disorder   30, 145
benefit packages   83
bio terrorism   5, 7
blood glucose   205
building   321

C

cancer   3–6, 37, 64, 66, 68, 92, 146, 227–231,
    233–238, 240–242, 247, 287, 309, 316, 332
cardiac illnesses   220
– rehabilitation   219–225
– – programs   223–224
– – service   219
cardiovascular diseases   64, 205, 212, 220–221,
    225
cardiovascular events   203
case-control studies   227, 357
children   42, 48, 60–61, 68, 71, 76, 81–82, 86, 93,
    100, 104, 110–117, 137, 141, 247, 260, 275–277,
    279, 281–285, 287–292, 318, 344–345, 354
– immunizations   68
chronic diseases   48, 63–64, 69, 83, 86–87, 132,
    133

citizen-oriented health care system   132–133
clinical decision-making   248–249
– guidelines   215
– responsibilities   204
– trials in children   114
co-ordination   132, 253, 290, 370
communal hygiene   68
communication   45, 108–109, 114, 117, 131–133,
    169, 178, 260, 284, 290, 296, 306, 308, 337
community intervention   5
community-psychiatry approach   154
comorbidities   205, 210, 221
complete abstract number   30
consumer's profiting   293
– role   132
controls   65, 93, 100, 139, 210–211, 229, 242, 358
coronary heart disease   203
cost-benefit studies   142
cost-containment policies   83
counselling   99–100, 103–106, 109, 183, 212,
    215, 220, 222–223, 361
country-specific public health information   11
cross-border cooperation   53
curative care   69, 133
– interventions   3

D

data analysis   123–124, 126, 260–262, 294
– archiving   262, 264
– production   260–261
data-based quality circle   104–105
day assessment   205
deinstitutionalization   148, 153, 170, 187, 201
dementia   64, 148, 206
demographic picture   81
dental public health   245
diabetes mellitus   203
disabilities   5, 156–157, 166–167, 203, 275,
    319
disasters   5–7, 77, 317–321, 325, 336–341
discrete choice   295
discrimination   145–146, 149
disease management programs   83, 207
– mapping   233–234
dissemination   52–53, 165, 184, 259–260, 262,
    264, 270

distance   73, 150, 295–297, 300–306, 308–311
distribution of services   67
doctor-patient-interaction   132–133
documentation   70, 104–106, 156, 183–184, 205,
    262, 264–265, 266, 369
DRG   69, 297–298, 315–316
drug utilization   99–100, 103, 105–110, 115, 117

E
eco-toxicological impact   348
economic growth rates   82
– outcomes   219
– transformation   92
efficiency   45, 69, 76, 83–85, 110, 189, 215, 297,
    308
elderly   47, 54, 63, 66–68, 82, 100–101, 117, 140,
    142, 146–147, 204, 210, 220, 222–223, 260,
    275
emancipation   131
empowerment   131, 133, 177
environmental changes   90
– control   3
EUPHA-presidency   15
European Day Hospital Evaluation   168
European Journal of Public Health   33–34
evidence-based guidelines   8, 52
– dentistry   245
– health information   276, 285
– treatment   101
exchange of information   9–10, 137
expert judgment   65

F
fee-for-service agreements   67
female diseases   119
financial equilibrium   293
financing structure   82
first-line combination therapy   204
formal area   123, 125

G
gender   25, 97, 119–127, 132, 196, 203, 208, 210,
    231, 281, 286, 294–296, 304, 329–330, 359
– bias   119–123, 125
– insensitivity   121
– research   119–120
general practitioners   48, 102, 111, 116, 137,
    141–142, 216, 293–294, 296, 316, 337
globalisation   5, 7–8, 365
guidance documents   215

H
health care costs   4–5, 7, 156, 167, 189
– providers   207
– system   8, 43, 53, 56–58, 63–64, 67, 69, 71,
    73, 75, 77, 82, 84–86, 103, 106, 109, 145–149,
    190, 204, 215–216, 245, 281, 343
– utilisation   67
health determinants   25, 54, 60, 62, 65
– education   4–5, 7, 18, 114, 150
– – programs   65, 115

– facilities   65, 293
– impact   73–74, 77
– inequalities   27, 66
– insurance   3, 37, 64, 67, 71, 82–83, 85–87,
    102, 248
– outcomes   103, 358–359
– policy   3–4, 30–31, 45, 47, 51–53, 56–57, 59–
    60, 69, 74–76, 78, 90–91, 94, 106–108, 113,
    133, 146, 153, 155, 168, 173, 224, 275
– priorities   65–66, 70
– promotion   4, 7, 18, 22, 25–26, 30, 43, 45,
    57, 65, 67, 69, 76, 92–93, 132–133, 260, 284–
    285, 287–288, 360
– related behaviours   285–287
– research   3, 31, 47, 51–52, 55–56, 119, 127
– sciences   89–92, 94, 119, 127
– services   3–8, 15, 22, 25, 27, 29, 44, 53–57,
    69, 74, 76–77, 83, 90–91, 93, 96, 149, 153, 173,
    179, 192, 260, 276, 282–284, 288, 294, 309,
    361
– – financing   66
– status   5–6, 44–45, 71, 107, 207, 230, 233,
    278, 281, 283, 291, 341
– targets   76
healthcare professionals   137, 139, 222
healthier society   73
healthy cities   5
– regions   5
– schools   5
high blood pressure   204
high-risk populations   8
HIV infection   6
home-based rehabilitation   219, 223
hospitalisation, costs for   344
hospital network's structure   296
hospital setting   154–155, 166–168
hypercholesterolemia   203
hypertension   3, 101, 203–205, 207, 209–217,
    220, 222–223, 357, 359–360

I
immigrants   4, 81–82, 86
implementation of policies   36, 288
improvement   41, 51, 66, 90, 102, 109, 111–112,
    125, 133, 146, 153, 163, 166–167, 173, 215,
    221, 272, 284, 304, 306, 312, 344
in-patient treatment   168, 171, 345
income   355
inequality   91
influenza   135–143, 140–142
information systems   12, 31, 54, 69, 275–276,
    291
innovative ideas   11
interaction   29, 52, 57, 62–63, 100, 105, 107,
    110, 131, 176, 216, 306, 311, 325, 334, 339
intersectoral research   52
intervention possibilities   282

J
job instability   355–356

L
lack of information 345
life expectancy 5, 42, 59, 63–64, 71, 89–90, 92–
    93, 95–97, 146, 365
life-long prolongation 223
lifestyle factors 57, 60, 227, 229–231, 240
– habits 222
local health facilities 293

M
measurement of utility 294
medical assessment 220
– guidelines 246
medicalisation 4, 347–348
medication errors 343–346
medicine intake 166
medicine-related problem 343–344
mental disorder 145–148, 150–151, 154, 156–
    157, 163, 170, 187, 190, 200, 207, 340
– health 48, 66, 145, 148, 150, 153, 165–168,
    173–177, 179–180, 183, 185–187, 189–192,
    194–196, 198–199, 279, 339
– health care 146, 148–149, 153–154, 167, 173,
    176–177, 181, 184–187, 189–191, 198
– – system 145, 148–149, 170, 190–191, 195
– health education 150
– health services 153–155, 164, 166–168, 173,
    175–176, 178–180, 182–183, 186–187, 192–
    194, 196, 199–200, 337
– hospitals 145, 147–149, 190
methodological area 123, 125
microalbuminuria 205
migration 6, 37, 77, 173, 179–180, 293, 297,
    300, 302, 304, 306, 308–309, 311–312, 365
morbidity 31, 47, 66, 82–83, 99–100, 106–107,
    112–113, 116, 133, 136–138, 176, 233, 283,
    347, 351, 354
mortality 3–4, 31, 42, 63–64, 66, 89–97, 99–101,
    116, 133, 136, 140–142, 146–148, 219–220,
    224, 227–231, 233–242, 310, 316, 347, 349,
    351, 354, 359, 362
motivation 48, 132, 222
multicenter trials 204
multifactorial nature 219
multimorbidities 215
mutations 135
myocardial infarction 219–220, 224–225, 343,
    354, 357, 362

N
national surveillance network 137, 139
natural experiment 42, 90, 92
networks 44, 57, 62, 66–67, 99, 132, 309
new public health 7, 11, 43, 45, 52
newly formed viruses 135
non-communicable diseases 3, 90, 93
nutrition 5, 31, 48, 71, 260

O
obesity 48, 63, 210–211, 222, 292, 347
occupational diseases 355

– health 355, 360
– health services 355, 360–361
– injuries 64
open source 259
osteoarthritis 64
out-patient treatment 345
outcome measures 153, 168, 187, 200
overmedicalization 121
overweight 63, 210

P
participation 9, 18–19, 24, 28, 44, 113, 122, 133,
    178, 206, 213, 323, 360
patient empowerment 131
– migration 293–294, 296, 299, 306, 309, 311
– trusts 309
patient-centred care 131–133
– medicine 131–132
– model 131
perinatal outcomes 71
pharmaceutical expenditure 343, 346–347
pharmacological treatment 215
Poisson distribution 234
policy- and decision-makers 52
policy-makers 9–10, 12, 336
political differences 35
– support 6
pollution 90
post-marketing surveillance and drug utilisation
    studies 114
post-traumatic stress disorder 175, 319
pre-study doctor's questionnaire 206
prenatal care 68
prescription-related morbidity 100–101
prescriptions 67, 111–113, 115–117, 293, 345,
    347
prevalence 4, 25, 27, 47, 111–113, 147, 203–205,
    208, 210–213, 215–216, 222, 233, 248, 319,
    324, 357, 359
– of obesity 203
prevention 3, 5–8, 31, 37, 41–42, 44–45, 57, 60–
    63, 66–67, 70, 73, 76–77, 83, 86–87, 93, 99–
    100, 139, 149–150, 216, 224, 227, 242, 251–
    252, 260, 350, 360, 362
preventive health services 63
– pharmacotherapy 223
– programmes 3–4, 6, 73
primary care sector 204
– prevention 4, 150, 361
proactive platform 9–10
problem based learning 251
professional guidelines 6
promotion 17, 25, 30, 43–45, 54, 70, 74, 76,
    102, 282, 285, 356
prospective surveys of off-label use and unli-
    censed use of drugs 114
provider-centred health care system 133
psychological effects 220, 337–338
– stress 322, 324
psychosocial well-being 221, 249
public health education 204

- impact   154, 168, 173
- outcomes   69
- perspective   3, 103, 133, 292
- policy   5, 8, 42, 56, 65–66, 70, 105, 119, 153
- priorities   66
- professionals   9–10, 220
- research   4, 6–8, 22, 37, 52, 62, 103, 119–120, 122–123, 126, 284, 361
- sciences   119
- services   6–7, 44
- system   5, 64, 224
- targets   65
- training   7, 12, 74
public justification   91
Public Use   266

Q
quality assessment of research   27
- assurance   8, 84, 103, 105–106, 123, 132, 163–164, 184, 201, 248, 260, 365, 367–368, 370
- management   245, 248, 371
- of care   48, 56, 131, 132, 153, 159, 345
- of life   43–44, 47, 64, 66, 103–104, 153–154, 156–157, 166, 175–177, 181, 190, 192, 194–196, 199, 207, 219, 225, 249, 253, 281–285, 291–292, 344

R
range of disciplines   37
RCTs   154–155, 163, 166, 180, 246, 250–252
redeployment   66
reductionism   131
redundancy   355–356
regional health councils   66
rehabilitation   44–45, 76, 83, 85, 132, 170, 219–225, 253, 255
- programs   200, 221–223
- service   70, 220, 222, 224
rehospitalisation   221
reputation   155, 167, 295–297, 300–304, 306, 308, 310–311
respiratory diseases   136, 140–142
responsibilities   49, 65, 105, 113
revascularization procedures   220
risk equalisation   83
- factors   3–4, 7, 25, 64–65, 120, 150, 203, 207, 220–224, 228–230, 233, 236, 238, 240–241, 339, 354, 357–359, 361–362

S
safety   43, 57, 61, 64–65, 68, 71, 99–100, 102, 106, 110, 113, 115, 164, 168, 177, 285, 349, 362
- standards   65
schizophrenia   146, 148, 150, 173, 177–179, 187, 190–192, 194–198, 200–201
scientific practice   259
Scientific Use Files   261

scope for collaboration   36
secondary analysis   260, 262–263
- prevention   59, 76, 220–225, 248, 360
self-healing   131
self-help groups   132, 149
service utilization   207
shared database   269–270, 272
shared decision-making   131
skills-building workshops   10
social aid programs   68
- inequality   149
- problems   44, 131, 327
- rehabilitation   164
- security   44, 66–67, 90, 94–95, 365
- status   94–95, 219
societal responsibility   8
socio-ecological concept   94
socio-economic inequalities   5
- status   222–223, 229–230, 233, 240–241
solid judgement method   28
solidarity   8, 69, 81–83, 86
source   106, 121, 191, 230, 259, 261, 349, 355
standardised screening instrument   282
subjective health perception   282
substance misuse   159
substantial area   123, 125
- reduction   344
supervised programs   219
systematic reviews   65, 106, 109, 246, 253–254

T
therapeutic accidents   344
- treatments   142
traffic-related injuries   64
transparency   260, 263, 365, 368–371
traumatic event   318–320, 324, 334–335
treatment standards   153

U
under-employment   356
unequivocal evidence   203
urine glucose   205
utilisation   66, 106, 110–111, 115, 174, 283–284, 343–345, 347, 349, 351–352

V
virological tests   137

W
waiting times   6, 261, 295–296, 300–304, 306, 308, 310–312
well-established methodologies   154
WHO   3, 4–5, 10–11, 13, 35, 37, 47–48, 52, 59, 63, 70, 79, 89, 96, 111, 136–137, 140, 145–147, 150–151, 167, 190–191, 204, 217, 219, 221, 225, 230–231, 241, 243, 281, 350–351, 354
work stress   356, 358, 360–363
worksite health promotion   361

Printing: Saladruck Berlin
Binding: Stürtz AG, Würzburg